*Workbook for*

# Textbook of Basic Nursing

**TENTH EDITION**

**CAROLINE BUNKER ROSDAHL, RN-C, BSN, MA**
Staff Nurse
Hennepin County Medical Center
Minneapolis, Minnesota

Vice President Emeritus
Nursing and Health Careers
Anoka-Hennepin Technical College
Anoka, Minnesota

Board of Directors
University of Minnesota School of Nursing Alumni Association and Nursing Foundation
Minneapolis, Minnesota

**MARY T. KOWALSKI, RN, BA, BSN, MSN**
Professor / Director / Instructor, Retired
Vocational Nursing and Health Careers
Cerro Coso Community College
Ridgecrest, California

Wolters Kluwer | Lippincott Williams & Wilkins
Health
Philadelphia • Baltimore • New York • London
Buenos Aires • Hong Kong • Sydney • Tokyo

*Acquisitions Editor:* Elizabeth Nieginski
*Product Manager:* Annette Ferran
*Editorial Assistant:* Zachary Shapiro
*Design Coordinator:* Joan Wendt
*Illustration Coordinator:* Brett MacNaughton
*Manufacturing Coordinator:* Karin Duffield
*Prepress Vendor:* Aptara, Inc.

10th Edition



9 8 7 6 5 4 3 2
Printed in China

ISBN-13: 978-1-60547-773-2
ISBN-10: 1-60547-773-7

Care has been taken to confirm the accuracy of the information presented and to describe generally accepted practices. However, the authors, editors, and publisher are not responsible for errors or omissions or for any consequences from application of the information in this book and make no warranty, expressed or implied, with respect to the currency, completeness, or accuracy of the contents of the publication. Application of this information in a particular situation remains the professional responsibility of the practitioner; the clinical treatments described and recommended may not be considered absolute and universal recommendations.

The authors, editors, and publisher have exerted every effort to ensure that drug selection and dosage set forth in this text are in accordance with the current recommendations and practice at the time of publication. However, in view of ongoing research, changes in government regulations, and the constant flow of information relating to drug therapy and drug reactions, the reader is urged to check the package insert for each drug for any change in indications and dosage and for added warnings and precautions. This is particularly important when the recommended agent is a new or infrequently employed drug.

Some drugs and medical devices presented in this publication have Food and Drug Administration (FDA) clearance for limited use in restricted research settings. It is the responsibility of the health care provider to ascertain the FDA status of each drug or device planned for use in his or her clinical practice.

No endorsement of specific actions of LPN/LVNs in violation of state statutes or Board of Nursing rules was intended or implied in this book. Each nurse must assume the responsibility to practice within the rules and guidelines of the state and of the healthcare area within which he or she is employed.

LWW.COM

# Contents

Answers to the activities and questions in the Workbook are available as Instructor Resources on thePoint

CHAPTER 1

# The Origins of Nursing

## SECTION I: TESTING WHAT YOU KNOW

**Activity A** *Match the Roman Matrons in Column A with their contributions in Column B.*

**Column A**

____ 1. Phoebe

____ 2. Saint Paula

____ 3. Fabiola

____ 4. Saint Helena

**Column B**

a. Established first gerontological facility

b. First deaconess and visiting nurse

c. Established inns and hospitals for pilgrims

d. Namesake of the first free hospital in Rome in 390 AD

**Activity B** *Match the nurses in Column A with their contributions in Column B.*

**Column A**

____ 1. Melinda Ann Richards

____ 2. Isabel Hampton Robb

____ 3. Lillian Wald

____ 4. Florence Nightingale

**Column B**

a. Founded the school of nursing at Johns Hopkins University

b. Continued to care for the sick when nursing was considered menial

c. Organized school of nursing at Massachusetts General Hospital

d. Founded American public health nursing

**Activity C** *Mark each statement as either "T" (True) or "F" (False). Correct any false statements.*

1. T F Lillian Wald and Mary Brewster founded the first Visiting Nurse Service.
2. T F The Nightingale lamp is a common component of the nursing pin.
3. T F An insignia is a distinguishing badge of authority or honor.
4. T F Hippocrates is the acknowledged "Father of Medicine."
5. T F Nursing curricula should focus mainly on theoretical knowledge.

**Activity D** *Fill in the blanks.*

1. A physician repeats the ____________ oath when graduating from a school of medicine.
2. Nightingale was born in ____________ in 1820 to wealthy English parents.
3. The ____________ and the Staff of Aesculapius are the modern symbols of medicine.
4. The word *nurse* is derived from the Latin word which means "to ____________."

**Activity E** *Consider the following figure.*

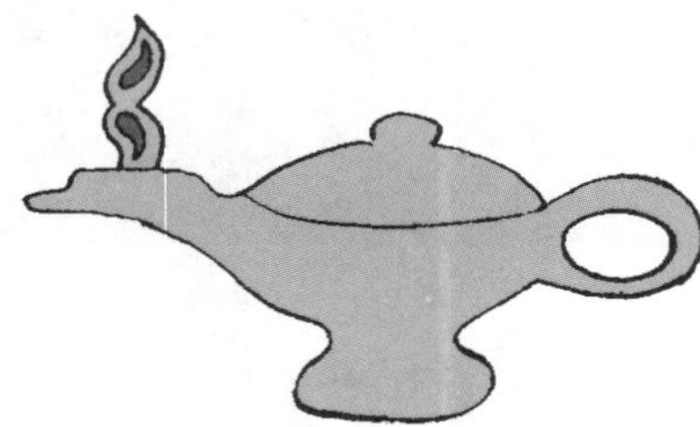

1. Explain the significance of the "Nightingale lamp."

______________________________

______________________________

2. List the various names of the "Nightingale lamp."

______________________________

______________________________

**Activity F** ***Names of some of the pioneer nursing schools are given below in random order. Write the correct sequence in which they were established in the boxes provided.***

1. Thompson Practical Nursing School in Brattleboro
2. Young Women's Christian Association (YWCA)
3. Household Nursing Association School of Attendant Nursing
4. American Red Cross

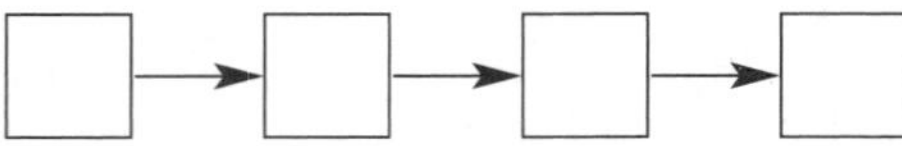

**Activity G** ***Briefly answer the following questions.***

1. Which three nursing programs were established on the basis of the Nightingale plan?

______________________________

______________________________

2. Which period is known as the "dark ages of nursing"?

______________________________

______________________________

3. Which factors create a need for more healthcare in the public sector?

______________________________

______________________________

4. Which qualities are required to become a nurse?

______________________________

______________________________

5. What is the importance of nursing uniforms?

______________________________

______________________________

6. Which religious symbols are represented on nursing pins?

______________________________

______________________________

7. What was the impact of World War I on nursing?

______________________________

______________________________

## SECTION II: APPLYING WHAT YOU KNOW

**Activity H** ***Answer the following questions, which involve Nightingale's principles.***

Nightingale opened the first nursing school outside a hospital in 1860. Some principles of the Nightingale School for Nurses are still taught today.

1. A social worker wants to pursue a nursing course. Her friend is a registered nurse in the hospital.
   a. The social worker inquires about the principles taught by the Nightingale Nursing School. What should the nurse's answer include?
   b. The social worker is also interested in knowing some of the Nightingale School's innovations in the field of nursing. What should the nurse's response include?

2. A nurse is taking care of a 60-year-old client who is paralyzed. When discussing the growth of home care in the 20th century with the nurse, the client's relative asks about other factors that are expected to continue in the 21st century. What should the nurse's response include?

## SECTION III: GETTING READY FOR NCLEX

**Activity I** *Answer the following questions.*

1. What attributes should a nurse possess for a successful career? (Select all that apply.)
   - **a.** Personal conviction
   - **b.** Aggressive personality
   - **c.** Flexibility
   - **d.** Sense of spirituality
   - **e.** Good education
2. When Florence Nightingale entered the battlefield near Scutari, Turkey, she and the nurses had few supplies and little outside support. Which of the following interventions did Nightingale insist on, which immediately reduced the mortality rate?
   - **a.** Seeking more funds and support
   - **b.** Establishing sanitary conditions
   - **c.** Procuring more medications
   - **d.** Continuing the nurses' education
3. Individuals who influenced nursing during the medieval and ancient periods are given below in random order. Write the correct sequence.
   - **a.** Pastor Theodor Fliedner
   - **b.** Hippocrates
   - **c.** Fabiola
   - **d.** Phoebe
4. A female candidate for nursing wishes to enroll in courses offered to women by the Young Women's Christian Association (YWCA). Which of the following courses would she be able to pursue in the YWCA?
   - **a.** A 3-month program to train women in simple nursing care
   - **b.** Home nursing education to teach lay women
   - **c.** A vocational school-based nursing program
   - **d.** An associate's degree nursing program
5. A nurse is practicing at a healthcare center. Why would he or she require additional education and skills while working in this environment?
   - **a.** To earn more money
   - **b.** To specialize in a particular field
   - **c.** To provide primary healthcare
   - **d.** To improve accuracy of assessment
6. Which of the following changes did the Greeks bring about in the field of nursing?
   - **a.** Hospitals or hostels were set up to care for the sick.
   - **b.** Hospitals were set up for people with incurable diseases.
   - **c.** Hospitals were set up for pregnant women.
   - **d.** Therapy was administered by priests.
7. A nurse is caring for a client with a chronic disease at the client's home. Why should the nurse put greater emphasis on teaching the client and family?
   - **a.** Family members may need to operate sophisticated equipment.
   - **b.** Family members may need to provide primary healthcare.
   - **c.** Family members may need to understand higher levels of skill.
   - **d.** Hospital stays may need to be reduced.
8. Which has been the most influential among the latest nursing trends? (Select all that apply.)
   - **a.** Changes in nursing education
   - **b.** Limitations on payment for healthcare
   - **c.** Longer duration of hospital stay
   - **d.** Lifestyle factors and greater life expectancy
   - **e.** Better working conditions

9. Nursing during wartime has long been important. During which war did the first emergency training of nurses occur?
   a. Crimean War
   b. American Civil War
   c. World War I
   d. World War II

10. Some principles of the Nightingale school of nurses are still taught today. What key principles are as increasingly important today, as in Nightingale's time, in a healthcare system in which clients' conditions are more medically complex and clients move quickly from one healthcare system to another? (Select all that apply.)
    a. Prevention is better than a cure
    b. Working as a member of a team
    c. Teaching is a part of nursing
    d. Nurses must always follow the physician's orders
    e. Nursing is a science profession only

CHAPTER 2

# Beginning Your Nursing Career

## SECTION I: TESTING WHAT YOU KNOW

**Activity A** ***Match the nursing roles in Column A with their corresponding activities in Column B.***

| Column A | Column B |
|---|---|
| ____ 1. Advocate | a. Documents client care and client response |
| ____ 2. Teacher | b. Helps clients understand their rights and responsibilities |
| ____ 3. Care provider | c. Assists clients in preventing illness and injury before they occur |
| ____ 4. Communicator | d. Helps clients achieve maximum level of wellness |

**Activity B** ***Match the organizations in Column A with the eligible members in Column B.***

| Column A | Column B |
|---|---|
| ____ 1. National organizations | a. LPN |
| ____ 2. American Nurses Association (ANA) | b. RN/LPN |
| ____ 3. National Federation of Licensed Practical Nurses (NFLPN) | c. Student affiliates |
| ____ 4. National League for Nursing (NLN) | d. RN |

**Activity C** ***Mark each statement as either "T" (True) or "F" (False). Correct any false statements.***

1. T F To achieve licensure as a medical doctor, the graduate must take a licensure exam before practicing.
2. T F The RN nurse is responsible for diagnosing and treating clients.
3. T F RNs recite the Practical Nurse's Pledge at graduation.
4. T F A theoretical framework provides a reason and a purpose for nursing actions.
5. T F An RN can assist in surgery.
6. T F An advanced practice nurse provides bedside care and reports reactions to medications or treatments to the RN.
7. T F In a permissive licensure, the nurse may practice nursing without a license, but the use of the registered nurse or licensed practical nurse title is forbidden.

**Activity D** ***Fill in the blanks.***

1. The ____________ assistant is trained academically and clinically to practice medicine under the supervision of a doctor of medicine or osteopathy.

2. A clinical nurse specialist certificate is available in __________ areas of nursing.
3. The American Nurses Credentialing Center (ANCC) of the American Nurses Association grants advanced certificates in a total of __________ fields.
4. Generalist nursing certificates are available in __________ specialties.
5. The LPN/LVN works under the direct or indirect supervision of a physician or an __________.

**Activity E** ***Names of the various national organizations that were established to provide educational programs and professional publications for nurses are given below in random order. Write the correct sequence in which they were established in the boxes provided.***

1. Health Occupations Students of America (HOSA)
2. National League for Nursing (NLN)
3. National Federation of Licensed Practical Nurses (NFLPN)
4. National Association for Practical Nurse Education and Service (NAPNES)

☐ → ☐ → ☐ → ☐

**Activity F** ***Briefly answer the following questions.***

1. What is the role of a nurse as a student?

__________________________________________

__________________________________________

2. List some of the provisions made by state organizations for nursing.

__________________________________________

__________________________________________

3. What are the key program areas listed as crucial to nursing by the International Council for Nursing (ICN)?

__________________________________________

__________________________________________

4. What is the purpose of the National Federation of Licensed Practical Nurses (NFLPN)?

__________________________________________

__________________________________________

5. What is the role of the National League for Nursing (NLN)?

__________________________________________

__________________________________________

6. What are the features of an approved nursing school?

__________________________________________

__________________________________________

## SECTION II: APPLYING WHAT YOU KNOW

**Activity G** ***Answer the following questions based on a nurse's career.***

The ability of a nurse to act independently depends on his or her professional background, motivation, and work environment. Programs offered by various nursing organizations allow an LPN to become an RN.

1. What are some of the nursing programs an LPN can pursue to obtain an RN license?
2. An RN is interested in specialization and wants to know which fields are certified by the American Nurses Credentialing Center (ANCC) of the American Nurses Association. List some of these fields.
3. A nurse wants to know about the licensing law that is practiced in different states.
   a. Is it important for the nurse to seek licensure? Give reasons for your response.
   b. What are the two different types of licensure that can be pursued by the nurse?
4. A student asks the nursing instructor whether it is important for nurses to be familiar with nursing theories. What should the instructor's response be? Give reasons for your response.

## SECTION III: GETTING READY FOR NCLEX

**Activity H** *Answer the following questions.*

1. An LPN/LVN is newly appointed in a hospital. Which of the following functions would this nurse be involved in?
   a. Directing other nurses who work in the same hospital
   b. Reporting a client's condition to the RN
   c. Assisting in surgery
   d. Teaching practical nursing students
2. A licensed practical nurse caring for a client understands that the planning phase of the nursing process involves which of the following steps?
   a. Observing, recording, and reporting significant changes
   b. Carrying out prescribed therapeutic regimens and protocols
   c. Reporting information gained from assessment/data collection
   d. Applying nursing knowledge and skills to promote and maintain health
3. An advanced practice nurse is interested in achieving an ANCC certificate. To do this, which of the following courses should the nurse specialize in?
   a. Adult nursing
   b. Diagnostic testing
   c. Psychiatric nursing
   d. Community health nursing
4. The National Association for Practical Nurse Education and Service (NAPNES) has listed some of the standards of nursing practice of the LPN/LVN, including which of the following? (Select all that apply.)
   a. Using appropriate knowledge, skills, and abilities
   b. Using principles of nursing to meet clients' needs
   c. Executing principles of crisis intervention to maintain safety
   d. Holding a current license to practice nursing in accordance with the state's law
   e. Taking responsible actions in case of unprofessional conduct by a healthcare provider
5. A nurse in a maternity ward has been assigned the responsibility of teaching clients the precautions and practices to be followed for healthy living. Which activity is the nurse expected to perform to achieve this task?
   a. Conduct prenatal classes during pregnancy
   b. Conduct team meetings
   c. Document client care and client response
   d. Motivate clients to achieve goals
6. An RN is conducting classes for nursing students. A student asks the RN about the importance of projecting a professional image. What should the RN's response include? (Select all that apply.)
   a. "It helps the nurse represent his or her school."
   b. "It helps maintain the safety of the client."
   c. "It helps protect the rights of the nurse."
   d. "It helps the nurse follow work ethics."
   e. "It enhances the nurse's skills in front of the client."
7. An LPN has recently moved to a new state and is seeking employment. What are the laws that the LPN needs to be aware of?
   a. The nurse must hold a license to practice nursing.
   b. The nurse must be familiar with legal responsibilities.
   c. The nurse must follow rules set by an RN.
   d. The nurse must obtain confirmation of completion of a course.
8. Which of the following activities is a nurse involved in during the implementation phase? (Select all that apply.)
   a. Applying nursing knowledge and skills to promote and maintain health
   b. Assisting the client and family with activities of daily living
   c. Identifying health goals in the nursing plan
   d. Reordering the priorities in the care plan
   e. Following the rules prescribed by the RN

**9.** There are several types of nursing education that lead to licensure as a practical/vocational nurse. Which practical/vocational nursing schools are eligible to take licensure examination? (Select all that apply.)

**a.** County

**b.** State

**c.** Commonwealth

**d.** Territory

**e.** Province

**10.** Many nursing programs base their curricula on nursing theories. These theoretical frameworks provide reasons and purposes for nursing actions. What is Florence Nightingale's theory of nursing called?

**a.** Natural healing

**b.** Independent functioning

**c.** Self-care

**d.** Adaptation

CHAPTER 3

# The Healthcare Delivery System

## SECTION I: TESTING WHAT YOU KNOW

**Activity A** *Match the organizations in Column A with their roles in Column B.*

**Column A**

____ 1. Joint Commission

____ 2. Continuous quality improvement (CQI)

____ 3. Health maintenance organization (HMO)

____ 4. Social Security Disability Insurance (SSDI)

**Column B**

a. Monitors quality of ongoing care

b. Caters to employees who are unable to work

c. Assigns recognition to hospitals

d. Offers health services

**Activity B** *Match the health insurance or payment systems in Column A with their appropriate characteristics in Column B.*

**Column A**

____ 1. Private insurance

____ 2. Group insurance

____ 3. Health maintenance organization (HMO)

____ 4. Medicaid

**Column B**

a. Fixed monthly charge

b. No monthly premium

c. Cost is high

d. Premium is low

**Activity C** *Mark each statement as either "T" (True) or "F" (False). Correct any false statements.*

1. T F Because healthcare recipients are involved in the management of their own health, they are often referred to as clients instead of patients.

2. T F The principles of excellent nursing care are universal.

3. T F Home health nursing and hospice care have greatly enhanced the quality of healthcare available in the home.

4. T F The Joint Commission establishes appropriate quality and care standards.

5. T F Imagery is often used in tuberculosis therapy.

6. T F Relaxation therapy includes the use of very fine needles inserted into specific energy points underneath the skin to balance the body's flow of energy.

7. T F Prospective payment is a reimbursement system in which a predetermined amount is allocated for treating individuals with specific diagnoses.

8. T F Health maintenance organizations (HMOs) offer insurance for a fixed yearly charge.

**Activity D** *Fill in the blanks.*

1. The skilled nursing facility (SNF) provides ____________ hour nursing care under the supervision of a registered nurse.
2. ____________ is a type of insurance program for employees who have become unable to work.
3. Generally, Medicaid is for people over the age of ____________, those who are blind or disabled, or members of families receiving Aid to Families With Dependent Children.
4. The fee or premium paid in advance to the HMO is called the ____________ fee.
5. The ____________ system of prospective payment is based on medical diagnoses.
6. ____________, a healing method originating from Chinese medicine, is based on Chi, which is believed to be the energy of life.

**Activity E** *Consider the following figure.*

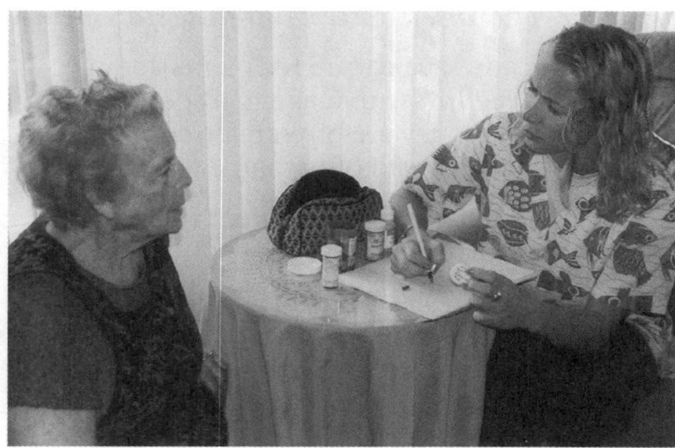

1. Explain the benefits of teaching clients about the medication and treatment program.

______________________________________________

______________________________________________

2. Explain the advantages of teaching older adults about the medication and treatment program.

______________________________________________

______________________________________________

**Activity F** *Briefly answer the following questions.*

1. What are some of the changes in healthcare that have been identified for this century?

______________________________________________

______________________________________________

2. What are the features of managed care for clients?

______________________________________________

______________________________________________

3. What are the results of financial constraints and influence of managed care plans on client care?

______________________________________________

______________________________________________

4. What are the areas of specialization of an intensive care unit (ICU)?

______________________________________________

______________________________________________

5. What are the advantages of telehealth care?

______________________________________________

______________________________________________

6. What are some of the main responsibilities of the members of a healthcare team?

______________________________________________

______________________________________________

## SECTION II: APPLYING WHAT YOU KNOW

**Activity G** *Answer the following questions concerning the nurse's role in helping clients understand the healthcare system.*

Nurses involved in acute and extended care facilities are expected to help clients with programs associated with the healthcare services and assist with any queries regarding the services provided.

1. A client has been admitted into a specialized care clinic that is too far from his home for his wife to be able to travel every day. The client's wife asks if anyone can help her handle the situation.
   a. How can the nurse help this client?
   b. What are some of the possible client representative services that are available to the client?
2. A nursing student has been asked to list some of the healthcare trends in this century. What trends should the student's list include?
3. A newly recruited nurse in an emergency ward asks the RN what services are available to clients in various healthcare systems. Which services should the nurse mention for the following healthcare systems?
   a. An acute care facility
   b. Managed care system
4. A nurse is updating a client about the Medicare program. What information should the nurse provide to the client? Answer in detail.

## SECTION III: GETTING READY FOR NCLEX

**Activity H** *Answer the following questions.*

1. Which type of nurse supervises the care of clients in a skilled nursing facility (SNF)?
   a. Registered nurse (RN)
   b. Licensed practicing nurse (LPN)
   c. Licensed vocational nurse (LVN)
   d. Nursing assistant (NA)
2. A nurse is providing respite care for a client. Which of the following services will the nurse provide? (Select all that apply.)
   a. Part-time supervision of clients with chronic medical conditions
   b. Relief for the primary caregivers of the client
   c. Part-time supervision of clients with mental illness
   d. Accessing clients via telephone or computer link
   e. Finding housing for the client's family
3. Which of the following benefits are obtained as a result of using a telehealth service? (Select all that apply.)
   a. Decreased unscheduled visits to the physician
   b. Supervised intensive care
   c. Minimized risk of acute problems
   d. Increased medication compliance
   e. Reduced hospital expenses
4. A nurse is caring for employees at an automobile spare parts factory. Which of the following interventions are most applicable for this nurse?
   a. Screening of common disorders
   b. Supervising the administration of immunizations
   c. Preventing accidents
   d. Checking the quality of medications
5. A client's family requires the help of a representative in obtaining required services. Which of the following services is the representative required to perform?
   a. Ensuring the quality of nurses providing care
   b. Helping the client's family find housing
   c. Providing health counseling
   d. Providing help during hospital admission
6. Which of the following is a feature of Medicare?
   a. Allows payment through monthly premiums
   b. Provides free or subsidized treatment
   c. Provides special service plans for the homeless
   d. Requires advance payment of capitation fee
7. Which of the following is a feature of chiropractic therapy?
   a. Manipulation of the spinal column and joints
   b. Rehabilitation techniques after injury
   c. Treatment using herbs and aromas
   d. Insertion of needles underneath the skin

8. A client is opting for treatment using Therapeutic Touch. Which of the following actions will be performed by a Therapeutic Touch practitioner?
   a. Teaching the client to think deeply
   b. Instructing the client to recall events
   c. Teaching the client about the energy field
   d. Instructing the client on management of disorders

9. A nurse is teaching a group of corporate executives about the available incentive programs that encourage employees to practice healthy habits. Which of the following health practices should the nurse discuss?
   a. Employee works more productively
   b. Employee undergoes regular physical examinations
   c. Employee uses telehealth to access the physician
   d. Employee uses the community health service

10. Nurses work in a variety of healthcare facilities. Which of the following types of healthcare facilities include community services? (Select all that apply.)
    a. Hospitals
    b. Extended care facilities
    c. Walk in care
    d. Home healthcare
    e. Care in schools and facilities

CHAPTER 4

# Legal and Ethical Aspects of Nursing

## SECTION I: TESTING WHAT YOU KNOW

**Activity A** *Match the organizations in Column A with their functions in Column B.*

| Column A | Column B |
|---|---|
| ____ **1.** State Board of Nursing | **a.** Conducts the NCLEX-RN and NCLEX-PN-exams |
| ____ **2.** United Network of Organ Sharing (UNOS) | **b.** Initiates, regulates, and enforces the provisions of the Nurse Practice Act |
| ____ **3.** National Council of State Boards of Nursing (NCSBN) | **c.** Ensures fairness in the receipt of donated organs |

**Activity B** *Match the legal terms in Column A with their definitions in Column B.*

| Column A | Column B |
|---|---|
| ____ **1.** Battery | **a.** Improper, injurious, or faulty treatment of a client that results in illness or injury |
| ____ **2.** Tort | **b.** Harm done to a client as a result of neglecting duties, procedures, or ordinary precautions |
| ____ **3.** Negligence | **c.** Injury that occurred because of another person's intentional or unintentional actions or failure to act |
| ____ **4.** Malpractice | **d.** Physical contact with another person without that person's consent |

**Activity C** *Mark each statement as either "T" (True) or "F" (False). Correct any false statements.*

**1.** T F Slander refers to a written statement or photograph that is false or damaging.

**2.** T F Nurses should give endorsements to the sale and promotion of commercial products or services.

**3.** T F Nurses should assist the clients in preparing legal wills.

**4.** T F In brain death, there is cessation of heartbeat without external stimuli.

**5.** T F Nurses may accept gifts from clients in return for the care that they provide.

**6.** T F Brain death is also known as clinical death.

**7.** T F The Good Samaritan Act protects a nurse from liability if the nurse gives emergency care in a reasonable and prudent manner within the limits of first aid.

**8.** T F Every client has a right to know the identity of nurses.

**Activity D** *Fill in the blanks.*

1. ____________ refers to moral principles and values that guide human behaviors.
2. ____________ consent means that tests, treatments, and medications have been explained to the client, as well as outcomes, possible complications, and alternative procedures.
3. Examples of nursing crimes of ____________ are participation in an illegal abortion, euthanasia, or mercy killing.
4. The Nurse ____________ Act defines and regulates the practice of nursing in the United States.
5. The ____________ is responsible for the NCLEX examinations.
6. ____________ of care is a legal term that implies that a healthcare professional has prematurely stopped caring for a client.
7. The right to ____________ means that a client has the right to expect that his or her property will be left alone.

**Activity E** *Consider the following figure.*

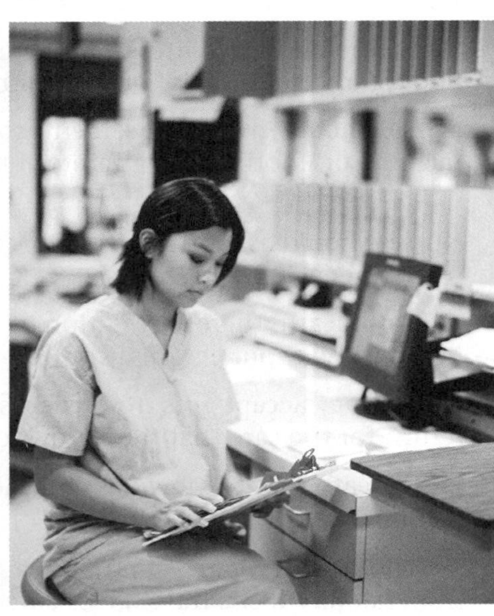

1. The nurse is updating a client's medical records on the computer. What care should the nurse take when doing so?

______________________________________________

______________________________________________

2. What is the importance of confidentiality in the relationship between the nurse and the client?

______________________________________________

______________________________________________

3. What can a nurse be held liable for if a client's confidentiality is breached?

______________________________________________

______________________________________________

4. What should a nurse do if held liable for breaching a client's confidentiality?

______________________________________________

______________________________________________

**Activity F** *Important events in the history of nursing and medicine are given below in random order. Write the correct sequence in which the events occurred in the boxes provided.*

1. The passing of the Patient Self-Determination Act (PSDA) by the federal government.
2. Adoption of A Patient's Bill of Rights by the American Hospital Association (AHA).
3. Recommendation of the Uniform Determination of Death Act to the states for enactment.
4. Implementation of the NCLEX examination in a computerized form called computerized adaptive testing (CAT).

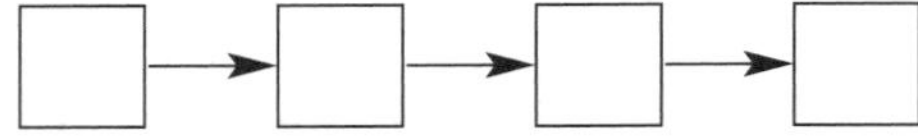

**Activity G** *Briefly answer the following questions.*

1. How does the Good Samaritan Act help nurses?

______________________________________________

______________________________________________

2. What is a living will?

______________________________________________

______________________________________________

3. What are the various criteria for clinical death?

______________________________________________

______________________________________________

4. Explain the purpose and the components of the Nurse Practice Act.

______________________________

______________________________

5. Enumerate various responsibilities of healthcare clients.

______________________________

______________________________

6. What is the purpose of the NCLEX examinations?

______________________________

______________________________

7. What are some of the logical precautions that nurses should take while on duty?

______________________________

______________________________

## SECTION II: APPLYING WHAT YOU KNOW

**Activity H** *Answer the following questions, which involve the nurse's role in management of situations that require ethical conduct.*

Before caring for clients, the nurse is responsible for becoming familiar with the ethical standards of the healthcare profession and the laws that are carefully designed to protect both the nurse and the clients.

1. A 12-year-old client visits the healthcare facility for optical tests and correction of hypermetropia.
   a. Which precautions should the nurse follow while assessing the client?
   b. What should the nurse consider about the client's rights in this case?
2. An 18-year-old female client with a dislocated shoulder complains to the hospital staff that the assigned nurse used abusive language and that the assessment was conducted in a very forceful manner.
   a. What offense can this nurse be held liable for?
   b. How should the nurse have behaved with the client?
3. A woman visits a local healthcare center and wishes to undergo sterilization. What are the legal issues that the nurse should make the client aware of?
4. A client admitted to the hospital in the last stages of lung cancer has prepared a living will stating that artificial methods of sustaining life must not to be used in his case.
   a. When will the client's living will go into effect?
   b. If this client goes into a coma, should the nurse provide artificial nutrition and hydration to maintain this client's health?

## SECTION III: GETTING READY FOR NCLEX

**Activity I** *Answer the following questions.*

1. A nurse photographs a cancer client without his knowledge or prior permission and sends the photographs to a healthcare magazine. What does this action on the part of the nurse amount to?
   a. Slander
   b. Malpractice
   c. Libel
   d. Assault
2. Which of the following clients admitted to a healthcare center should the nurse identify as belonging to a "vulnerable" category? (Select all that apply.)
   a. A 65-year-old diabetic
   b. A 17-year-old girl with gastroenteritis
   c. A 79-year-old man with goiter
   d. A 39-year-old woman in labor
   e. A 15-year-old mentally ill boy with tetanus
3. A nurse in the pediatric care unit of a hospital discovers that the scale for weighing babies is giving errors in its readings. What should the nurse do?
   a. Temporarily weigh the babies on an adults' scale
   b. Take two weight readings and take the average of the readings
   c. Buy a new weighing scale
   d. Report the errors in the weighing scale to the concerned authorities

4. Which of the following are the rights of a hospitalized client regarding nursing care? (Select all that apply.)
   a. To know the identity of nurses, including the student nurses
   b. To know the financial implications of treatment choices and available payment methods
   c. To have all communications and records pertaining to the client's health care treated as confidential
   d. To obtain free or subsidized treatment from the healthcare center
   e. To get special care compared with other clients

5. A nurse who has been newly recruited to a healthcare facility is expected to give competent and efficient care to the clients. For what kinds of offense could a nurse be held liable? (Select all that apply.)
   a. Failing to report defective or malfunctioning equipment
   b. Giving emergency first aid treatment to clients irrespective of any inconvenience caused
   c. Failing to meet established standards of safe care for clients
   d. Endorsing commercial products and services
   e. Failing to prevent injury to clients, other employees, and visitors

6. What symptoms present in a client would determine brain death?
   a. Partial unresponsiveness to external stimuli
   b. Fixed or dilated pupils
   c. Minimal presence of cephalic reflexes
   d. Hypothermia of the body

7. Which of the following bodies has legislative power to initiate, regulate, and enforce the provisions of the Nurse Practice Act?
   a. National Council of State Boards of Nursing (NCSBN)
   b. United Network of Organ Sharing (UNOS)
   c. State Board of Nursing
   d. Pharmacy Board

8. A nurse was practicing as an LPN without a license. What does this offense amount to?
   a. Felony
   b. Malpractice
   c. Libel
   d. Falsification

9. The daughter of a client who is being sustained on a life support system mentions to the nurse that the client has written a living will. What does the living will allow the client to do?
   a. Bequeath his wealth and property to persons of his choice
   b. Donate organs for transplantation
   c. Seek compensation from the hospital for his immediate relatives in case of his demise
   d. Demand that no artificial life-sustaining methods be used in his case

10. A nurse administers the wrong medication to a client, and the client is harmed as a result of this medication. For what type of offense might the nurse be liable?
    a. Felony
    b. Malpractice
    c. Assault
    d. Falsification

CHAPTER 5

# Basic Human Needs

## SECTION I: TESTING WHAT YOU KNOW

**Activity A** ***Match the needs of the clients in Column A with the appropriate nursing interventions in Column B.***

| Column A | Column B |
|---|---|
| ____ 1. Water and fluids | a. Show love, affection, and belonging |
| ____ 2. Inability to take in food and nutrients | b. Provide reading or video materials |
| ____ 3. Social needs | c. Provide tube feedings |
| ____ 4. Spiritual needs | d. Weigh the client regularly |

**Activity B** ***Match the needs in Column A with their appropriate level in Maslow's hierarchy of needs in Column B.***

| Column A | Column B |
|---|---|
| ____ 1. Freedom from threats | a. Physiologic |
| ____ 2. Opportunities for innovation and creativity | b. Self-esteem |
| ____ 3. Water, food, and sleep | c. Self-actualization |
| ____ 4. Recognition of strength and choice | d. Security and safety |

**Activity C** ***Mark each statement as either "T" (True) or "F" (False). Correct any false statements.***

1. T F Primary needs must be met to give quality to life.
2. T F Elimination of waste products is one of the survival needs.
3. T F Goose flesh is a mechanism that assists in temporary regulation of body temperature.
4. T F In Maslow's hierarchy of needs, a need at any given level of the hierarchy is more urgent to a person if the needs above it are satisfied.
5. T F Self-actualization is related to a person's perception of self.
6. T F Illness or injury can cause a person to regress to a lower level of functioning.
7. T F Relationships with others, including family and community, can always be addressed before the basic physiologic needs are met.
8. T F Maintaining warmth for a newborn is a second-level need.

**Activity D** ***Fill in the blanks.***

1. Human needs are thought of in progressive levels, known as a ____________.
2. Any form of ____________ is needed to maintain optimum health.

3. The normal oral temperature in Celsius is ____________.

4. ____________ self-esteem directly relates to disorders such as chemical dependency.

5. The term ____________ implies a fully functioning person.

**Activity E** *Consider the following figure.*

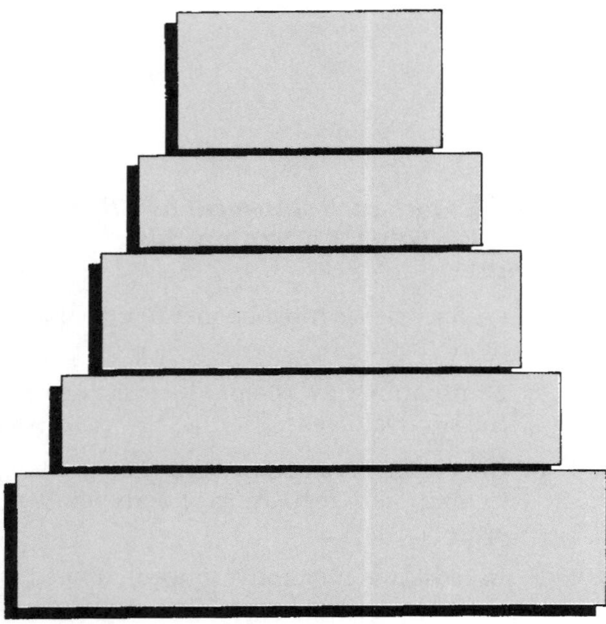

1. Maslow described a theory of human needs in which simple, basic needs are identified in relation to more complex, higher-level needs. Fill in Maslow's hierarchy of needs, placing each type of need in the appropriate position in the given figure.

**Activity F** ***The needs Maslow described in his theory of human needs are given below in random order. Write the correct sequence in which these needs must be fulfilled, in order from most basic to most complex, in the boxes provided.***

1. Security and safety
2. Self-actualization
3. Love
4. Physiologic
5. Self-esteem

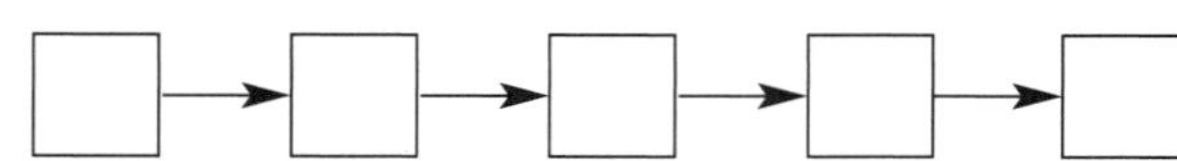

**Activity G** ***Briefly answer the following questions.***

1. What does Maslow's theory of human needs state?

____________________________________________

____________________________________________

2. What are the basic physiologic needs?

____________________________________________

____________________________________________

3. List some of the factors that can threaten the body's need for temperature regulation.

____________________________________________

____________________________________________

4. What is the core temperature survival range for the human body in Celsius and Fahrenheit degrees?

____________________________________________

____________________________________________

5. What are the characteristics of a self-actualized person?

____________________________________________

____________________________________________

## SECTION II: APPLYING WHAT YOU KNOW

**Activity H** ***Answer the following questions, which involve the nurse's role in management of basic human needs.***

In order to help clients prevent risks or threats to their basic human needs, the nurse should be familiar with the basic human needs and identify each client's specific needs.

1. A client is asthmatic and has breathing problems. What are the basic nursing interventions for this client?

2. A teenaged client has been rescued from a fire and is to undergo surgery for severe burns on his hands. The client has been traumatized by the accident and is mentally unprepared for the surgery. How should the nurse encourage the client?
3. A client has a fever and feels nauseated when eating. She has been diagnosed with malnutrition. What should the nurse do to ensure that the client's need for food and nutrients is fulfilled?
4. A client has constipation and is facing problems with elimination of waste products. What are the nursing interventions for these problems?
5. There was a train derailment, and several clients were admitted to the hospital and underwent surgery for fractured bones and other injuries. The clients are recovering after the surgery but have not yet started to move around and walk independently. What are the nursing interventions that may ensure quick recovery of these clients?
6. A client was involved in an accident that has impaired her vision. The client is a tailor by profession, and her condition has affected her hopes and self-esteem. How can the nurse help this client regain self-esteem?

## SECTION III: GETTING READY FOR NCLEX

**Activity I** *Answer the following questions.*

1. After heart surgery, a client has severe weakness. What nursing intervention ensures that the client's nutritional status is maintained?
   a. Maintaining calorie counts
   b. Evaluating oxygenation status
   c. Teaching the client range of motion exercises
   d. Providing the client warm milk
2. Which of the following needs should the nurse identify as a second-level needs for clients in a general ward according to Maslow's hierarchy of needs?
   a. Self-esteem
   b. Security and safety
   c. Social needs
   d. Spiritual needs
3. A client has been admitted into care in an unconscious state with hypothermia. Which of the following symptoms should the nurse identify as the body's mechanism to regulate the body temperature? (Select all that apply.)
   a. Shivering
   b. Goose flesh
   c. Cough
   d. Perspiration
   e. Drowsiness
4. A client who works as a carpenter sustained serious injuries to his hands in an accident and is now spending many sleepless nights worried about how his injury will affect his future. What should the nurse do?
   a. Consult the physician to provide medication to the client to promote sleep
   b. Assist the client to regain positive self-esteem by encouraging independence
   c. Provide the client safe, comfortable, and quiet surroundings to promote sleep
   d. Work together with physical therapists to assist the client with rehabilitation
5. A nurse is trying to identify which of her clients has achieved self-actualization. What characteristics should the nurse observe the client for? (Select all that apply.)
   a. The client is comfortable enough to plan ahead and be creative.
   b. The client feels that his or her contributions are appreciated by family, friends, and employers.
   c. The client is able to cope with life's situations, deal with failure, and be free of anxiety.
   d. The client is self-confident, and thinks well of himself or herself, and is well thought of by others.
   e. The client has a sense of humor, is self-controlled, and deals with stress in productive ways.

6. A nurse is assigned to care for clients who have been rendered homeless due to a natural disaster. Which of the following should the nurse identify as the primary need of the clients?
   a. Security and safety
   b. Societal needs
   c. Self-esteem needs
   d. Family and community needs

7. The nurse is caring for a client who was exposed to extreme heat during an accident in a factory. What nursing intervention is important to ensure that the client meets the need for temperature regulation?
   a. Give the client a cold water bath
   b. Closely monitor the client's temperature
   c. Give the client warm milk
   d. Keep the client covered at all times

8. The nurse is caring for a group of older adults. Which of the following are nursing interventions for these clients' basic physiologic needs?
   a. Assisting clients to attend places of worship
   b. Providing regular entertainment
   c. Assisting with hygiene and elimination
   d. Performing a safety check in the home environment

9. The nurse is legally bound to report any suspected abuse in clients. A client reports spousal battering. Which of the following is the primary basic need that the nurse knows is threatened by abuse?
   a. Safety and security
   b. Love
   c. Self-esteem
   d. Self-actualization

10. A client has experienced a stroke. Which of the following human needs is addressed first?
   a. Nutrients
   b. Shelter
   c. Love
   d. Safety and security

CHAPTER 6

# Health and Wellness

## SECTION I: TESTING WHAT YOU KNOW

**Activity A** *Match the key terms in Column A with their definitions in Column B.*

**Column A**

____ 1. Homeostasis

____ 2. Disease

____ 3. Morbidity

____ 4. Mortality

____ 5. Defense mechanisms

____ 6. Domestic violence

**Column B**

a. Internal stress reducers, even though they may not be truthful or effective ways of adapting to a stressful situation

b. Refers to the number of people with an illness or disorder relative to a specific population

c. Balance of all of the components of the human organism

d. The fastest-growing public health problem in the United States today

e. Change in the structure or function of body tissues, biological systems, or the human mind

f. Refers to the chances of death associated with a particular illness or disorder

**Activity B** *Match the illnesses and diseases in Column A with their appropriate implications in Column B.*

**Column A**

____ 1. Acute illness

____ 2. Chronic illness

____ 3. Organic disease

____ 4. Functional disease

**Column B**

a. Occurrence of detectable structural change in one or more organs that also alters usual function

b. Interferes with the continuum for a short period of time

c. A disorder in which a structural cause cannot be identified

d. Results in long-term health impairment

**Activity C** *Mark each statement as either "T" (True) or "F" (False). Correct any false statements.*

1. T F Genetic makeup contains risk factors that we can control.

2. T F In a systemic infection, the area of invasion is limited to one area or organ.

3. T F High-level wellness is called optimum health.

4. T F Baby-boomers are the large number of people born after World War II.

5. T F The number one cause of death in adolescents in America is motor vehicle accident injury.

6. T F A deficiency of several vitamins, or general malnutrition, is more common in the United States than deficiency of a single vitamin.

**Activity D** *Fill in the blanks.*

1. Chemicals that cause cancer are described as ____________.
2. Pregnant women who smoke increase the chances of ____________ or premature births.
3. ____________ is a mental or physical tension exerted upon an individual's homeostasis.
4. ____________ drinking is defined as having five or more alcoholic drinks in 1 day at least once per month.
5. The prostate-specific antigen (PSA) test is used as a screening tool and to determine the effectiveness of treatment after prostate ____________ is diagnosed.
6. The growth exhibited by abnormal tissue or tumors is termed ____________.
7. Malignant cells tend to spread to other parts of the body by a process called ____________.

**Activity E** *Briefly answer the following questions.*

1. List some of the factors a nurse needs to be aware of regarding health and wellness.

______________________________________________

______________________________________________

2. How does the World Health Organization (WHO) define health?

______________________________________________

______________________________________________

3. What do primary and secondary healthcare services do?

______________________________________________

______________________________________________

4. What does Maslow's theory on the wellness–illness continuum state?

______________________________________________

______________________________________________

5. What are the benefits of quitting smoking with regard to the time passed after the last cigarette?

______________________________________________

______________________________________________

## SECTION II: APPLYING WHAT YOU KNOW

**Activity F** *Answer the following questions, which involve the nurse's role in health promotion.*

A nurse's role in managing health and wellness involves assisting clients with health promotion.

1. A 24-year-old client who wishes to maintain her health and reduce stress levels seeks information from the nurse.
   a. The client asks the nurse how much exercise is recommended, in general, for Americans. What should the nurse's reply be?
   b. Which two defense mechanisms should the nurse identify as internal stress reducers?
   c. What are some of the common eating disorders in young women in the United States that the nurse can identify and monitor for in this client?

## SECTION III: GETTING READY FOR NCLEX

**Activity G** *Answer the following questions.*

1. Which of the following should the nurse recognize as a general cause of infection?
   a. Alteration in the structure of a biological system
   b. Adverse reaction to a drug
   c. Invasion by harmful microorganisms
   d. Response to a disease
2. Which of the following are environmental issues affecting health that the nurse should be aware of? (Select all that apply.)
   a. Air pollutants
   b. Soil erosion
   c. Deforestation
   d. Toxic chemicals
   e. Radon poisoning

**3.** Which of the following is included in the 10 leading causes of morbidity and mortality in the United States?

**a.** Cirrhosis
**b.** Appendicitis
**c.** Cancer
**d.** AIDS

**4.** A nurse working in a healthcare center in the U.S. has observed that many clients have bad eating habits. What are some of the programs the nurse can implement to improve the diet of these clients? (Select all that apply.)

**a.** Educate clients about healthy choices for school lunches.
**b.** Encourage clients to buy food only from reputable stores.
**c.** Educate clients about the benefits of vegetarian food.
**d.** Facilitate worksite nutritional programs.
**e.** Encourage home-delivered meals for the elderly.

**5.** Which of the following is included in the 10 leading health indicators in the United States?

**a.** Tobacco use
**b.** Alcohol use
**c.** Malnutrition
**d.** Stress

**6.** Which of the following illnesses should the nurse identify as acute?

**a.** Arthritis
**b.** Cold
**c.** Asthma
**d.** Cancer

**7.** Which of the following categories of clients would require long-term care?

**a.** Clients with chronic illnesses
**b.** Clients with functional diseases
**c.** Elderly clients
**d.** Clients with organic diseases

**8.** A client has been advised to perform various physical activities. The nurse should inform the client that which of the following are benefits of physical activity? (Select all that apply.)

**a.** Maintains blood pressure
**b.** Improves flexibility
**c.** Increases levels of good cholesterol
**d.** Helps manage diabetes
**e.** Minimizes the risk of tuberculosis

**9.** A client working in a steel factory complains of being uncomfortable with the level of noise at work. What information should the nurse provide this client?

**a.** "Wear protective ear devices."
**b.** "Seek consultation for ear drops."
**c.** "Seek a change in career."
**d.** "This is normal; don't worry."

**10.** Which of the following factors has the greatest effect on bone density loss in postmenopausal women?

**a.** Lack of activity and exercise
**b.** Family history of osteoporosis
**c.** Poor eating habits
**d.** Loss of the estrogenic hormones

CHAPTER 7

# Community Health

## SECTION I: TESTING WHAT YOU KNOW

**Activity A** *Match the branches of the Department of Health and Human Services in Column A with the services they provide in Column B.*

| Column A | Column B |
|---|---|
| ____ 1. Agency for Healthcare Research and Quality (AHRQ) | a. Conducts research projects in 27 separate institutes on thousands of health-related subjects |
| ____ 2. Centers for Medicare and Medicaid Services (CMS) | b. Provides for the safety of foods and cosmetics and the safety and effectiveness of pharmaceuticals, biological products, and medical devices |
| ____ 3. Food and Drug Administration (FDA) | c. Administers Medicare and Medicaid programs and the Children's Health Insurance Program |
| ____ 4. National Institutes of Health (NIH) | d. Conducts research designed to improve quality of healthcare, including information on costs and client safety |

**Activity B** *Match the types of pollution in Column A with their adverse effects on human health in Column B.*

| Column A | Column B |
|---|---|
| ____ 1. Air pollution | a. Typhoid fever, dysentery, and infectious hepatitis |
| ____ 2. Water pollution | b. Loss of hearing and stress |
| ____ 3. Land pollution | c. Asthma and sinusitis |
| ____ 4. Noise pollution | d. Risk of cancer |

**Activity C** *Mark each statement as either "T" (True) or "F" (False). Correct any false statements.*

1. T F Health concerns are based on a community's demographics as well as a nation's overall health and economy.
2. T F The United Nations Children's Fund (UNICEF) helps children, especially those in developed countries.
3. T F Indian Health Service (IHS), a branch of the Department of Health and Human Services, provides health surveillance to monitor and prevent outbreaks of disease.
4. T F The mission of the Centers for Disease Control and Prevention (CDC) is to promote health and quality of life by preventing and controlling disease, injury, and disability.
5. T F The Food and Drug Administration (FDA) develops and tests products itself.

6. T F Healthcare workers come into contact daily with issues and concerns involving bloodborne pathogens.
7. T F The mission of the National Safety Council (NSC) is to educate and influence society to adopt safety, health, and environmental policies, practices, and procedures.

**Activity D** *Fill in the blanks.*

1. Communities are studied as a part of ___________ which is the study of populations.
2. The study of mutual relationships between living beings and their ___________ is known as bionomics.
3. ___________ is a chemical element that occurs in nature as a byproduct of the disintegration of radium.
4. Lead poisoning, which is known as ___________ continues to be a significant public health problem.
5. The ionizing waves of energy that penetrate objects are known as ___________.
6. ___________ populations are subgroups in a community with unique or special healthcare needs.

**Activity E** *Briefly answer the following questions.*

1. What are the focus areas of nursing research supported by the National Institute of Nursing Research (NINR)?

   ________________________________________

   ________________________________________

2. List the direct care services offered by the Visiting Nurses Association (VNA).

   ________________________________________

   ________________________________________

3. What are the services offered by the American Red Cross?

   ________________________________________

   ________________________________________

4. What are the advances in public health that have contributed to an increase in the life expectancy of the average American?

   ________________________________________

   ________________________________________

## SECTION II: APPLYING WHAT YOU KNOW

**Activity F** *Answer the following questions, which involve the nurse's role in community health.*

The nurse helps clients to understand the roles and functions of community health organizations and provides information to appropriate organizations regarding the nature of assistance required by the community.

1. What are the health-related functions of WHO and UNICEF?
2. What is the role of a nurse practitioner (advanced practice nurse) in a community health center?
3. What is the role of a nurse who is part of the healthcare team of Planned Parenthood of America?

## SECTION III: GETTING READY FOR NCLEX

**Activity G** *Answer the following questions.*

1. A nurse is required to monitor the health status of a community. Which of the following factors should the nurse consider to determine community health? (Select all that apply.)
   a. Birth rate
   b. Sex ratio
   c. Mortality rate
   d. Teen pregnancy
   e. Population density

2. Which of the following is the main function of the World Health Organization (WHO)?
   a. Helps children in developing countries
   b. Helps countries during natural disasters
   c. Provides health-related information to the public
   d. Provides a network of hospitals and health centers
3. Which of the following is the responsibility of the United States Public Health Service (USPHS)?
   a. Pollution control
   b. Insect control
   c. Air quality control
   d. Sanitation control
4. Which of the following offices of the Office of Public Health and Science (OPHS) provides health information to both consumers and healthcare professionals?
   a. Office of the Surgeon General
   b. Office of Emergency Preparedness
   c. National Health Information Center
   d. National Vaccine Program Office
5. Which of the following should the nurse identify as being regulated by the Food and Drug Administration (FDA)? (Select all that apply.)
   a. Complex medical devices
   b. Medications
   c. Radiation-emitting products
   d. Sources of air pollution
   e. Sources of water pollution
6. A client wants to know how the nurse would effectively dispose of biohazardous materials. What should the nurse's response include?
   a. Medical equipment companies provide recycling kits.
   b. Biohazardous materials are disposed of at dumping grounds.
   c. Medical equipment companies provide containers and bags.
   d. Biohazardous materials are incinerated in bins.
7. Which of the following is the standard set by the Occupational Safety and Health Administration (OSHA) for ensuring education and protection of healthcare workers?
   a. Standard to prevent musculoskeletal disorders
   b. Standard to control animal-borne diseases
   c. Standard to provide health education
   d. Standard to prevent alcohol and substance abuse
8. Which of the following is one of the roles of the American Public Health Association (APHA)?
   a. Provides services to needy children and families
   b. Provides health resources for medically underserved people
   c. Provides services to elderly people
   d. Provides better personal and environmental health
9. Which of the following is a role of an advanced practice nurse in a community health center?
   a. Maternal and prenatal care
   b. Psychological screenings
   c. Administration of medication
   d. Performing medical diagnoses
10. Which of the following is a focus area of nursing research supported by the National Institute of Nursing Research (NINR)?
   a. Safety and health protection in the workplace
   b. Occupational exposure to bloodborne pathogens
   c. Reduction of risks for disease and disability
   d. Prevention of occupational hazards

CHAPTER 8

# Transcultural Healthcare

## SECTION I: TESTING WHAT YOU KNOW

**Activity A** ***Match the terms in Column A with their definitions in Column B.***

**Column A**

____ **1.** Culture

____ **2.** Subcultures

____ **3.** Race

____ **4.** Ethnicity

**Column B**

**a.** Common heritage shared by a specific culture

**b.** Implies genetic characteristics associated with having ancestors from a specific part of the world

**c.** Accumulated learning for generational groups of individuals within structured or nonstructured societies

**d.** Groups within dominant cultures

**Activity B** ***Match the subcultures in Column A with their health belief in Column B.***

**Column A**

____ **1.** Anglo American

____ **2.** African American

____ **3.** Latino or Hispanic

____ **4.** Asian American

**Column B**

**a.** Illness and misfortune occur as punishment from God, referred to as castigo de Dios, or by an imbalance of "hot" or "cold" forces within the body.

**b.** Illness is caused by infectious microorganisms, organ degeneration, and unhealthy lifestyles.

**c.** Health is the result of a balance between yin and yang energy; illness results when equilibrium is disturbed.

**d.** Supernatural forces can cause disease and influence recovery.

**Activity C** ***Mark each statement as either "T" (True) or "F" (False). Correct any false statements.***

**1.** T F The technique for compressing the energy pathway points is called acumassage.

**2.** T F Acupuncture, acupressure, food, and herbs are used to restore balance.

**3.** T F Cultural and religious traditions are always followed by every member of a community.

**4.** T F The mix of ethnic groups in the United States continually changes.

**5.** T F Kosher laws govern dietary practices for Muslims.

6. T F Culture is influenced by environment, expectations of society, and national origin.

_______________

**Activity D** ***Fill in the blanks.***

1. __________ is the accumulated learning for generational groups of individuals within structured or nonstructured societies.
2. Racial mixing has blurred the __________ characteristics of individuals.
3. __________ is a belief based on preconceived notions about certain groups of people.
4. __________ sensitivity is the understanding and tolerance of all cultures and lifestyles.
5. Buddhists believe that hard work and right living enables people to attain __________.
6. __________ is the common heritage shared by a specific culture.
7. ________ are groups within dominant cultures.
8. The belief that supernatural forces dominate is called __________.
9. Transcultural communication is facilitated through the use of a professional __________.
10. Caring for clients while taking into consideration their religious and sociocultural backgrounds is called __________.

**Activity E** ***Consider the following figure.***

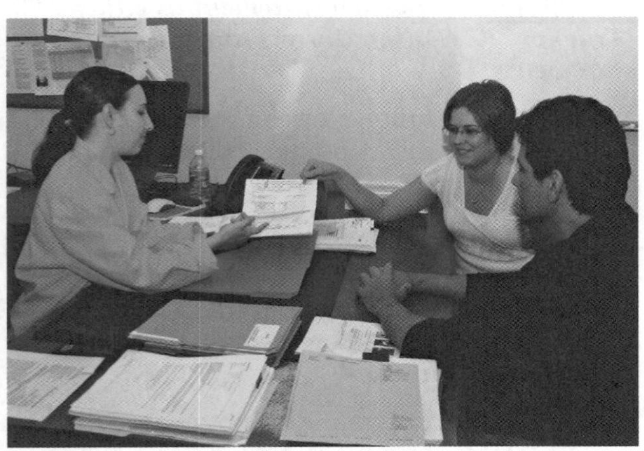

1. What are the qualities that an interpreter should possess?

**Activity F** ***Briefly answer the following questions.***

1. What does culture consist of?

_______________

2. What are the racial categories according to the federal government standards?

_______________

3. Which are the four subcultures identified by the Centers for Disease Control and Prevention (CDC)?

_______________

4. List the culturally influenced components that are common to many members of a cultural group.

_______________

5. List the people who perform rituals as part of the healing process in various ethnic and religious groups.

_______________

## SECTION II: APPLYING WHAT YOU KNOW

**Activity G** ***Answer the following questions, which involve the nurse's role in managing care for clients from diverse cultures.***

The nurse assists clients belonging to different cultures with health improvement.

1. What concepts identified by the American Nurses Association (ANA) for nursing care for clients from diverse cultures should the nurse be aware of?
2. A nurse is caring for clients belonging to various ethnic groups. What information should

the nurse have regarding ethnic groups' retaining their cultural heritage?

3. A nurse is caring for clients of various cultures. What are the critical factors involved in nursing care for diverse cultures?

## SECTION III: GETTING READY FOR NCLEX

**Activity H** *Answer the following questions.*

1. A nurse is assigned to work in a healthcare facility in an area with a culture with which she is unfamiliar. Which of the following assessments should the nurse perform as part of transcultural nursing? (Select all that apply.)
   a. The nurse's own cultural background
   b. Language and communication patterns of the client
   c. Living habits of the client
   d. Religious beliefs and practices of the client
   e. Intellectual level of the client
2. How does cultural sensitivity help a nurse provide better care?
   a. By understanding language and communication
   b. By understanding ethnic medicine
   c. By understanding and accepting others' behaviors
   d. By understanding religious beliefs and practices
3. Which of the following health belief systems is dominated by supernatural forces?
   a. Scientific/biomedical
   b. Magicoreligious
   c. Holistic medicine
   d. Hot–cold theories
4. An Asian couple visits the healthcare center with their 2-year-old child, who has a mild temperature. In relation to beliefs about personal space and touching, what approach should the nurse take when caring for this client?
   a. Kiss the child on the cheeks
   b. Touch the child on the arm
   c. Hug the child tightly
   d. Touch the child on the head
5. A nurse is appointed to care for a Muslim client. What beliefs or practices should the nurse be aware of when dealing with this client?
   a. Observe kosher dietary laws
   b. Prohibit pork and alcohol
   c. Decline tests on holy days
   d. Belief in faith healing
6. A Buddhist client with depression visits the healthcare center. Which of the following principles of Buddhism can the nurse use to help the client overcome depression?
   a. Live a natural life
   b. High appreciation of life
   c. Attain pain-free existence
   d. Emphasis on public health
7. A client wants to know the reason for the higher percentage of non-whites diagnosed with mental illness in the United States. Which of the following should the nurse's response include?
   a. Family conflicts
   b. Poverty
   c. Stressful lifestyle
   d. Genetic disorders
8. A nurse caring for a client recognizes the patient's need for spiritual support. Which of the following interventions should the nurse perform?
   a. Recite spiritual stories to the client
   b. Accompany the client to religious places
   c. Ask the client to contact a spiritual leader
   d. Ask the client to listen to spiritual discourses
9. In which of the following health beliefs are the physical and biomedical processes studied and manipulated to control life?
   a. Holistic
   b. Scientific
   c. Magicoreligious
   d. Yin-yang

**10.** A nurse is caring for a Muslim-Arab female client. Which of the following is the most expected reaction of the client when the nurse is conducting an assessment?

**a.** Looks the nurse directly in the eye
**b.** Exhibits no facial expressions
**c.** Does not object to touch
**d.** Makes eye-to-eye contact

CHAPTER 9

# The Family

## SECTION I: TESTING WHAT YOU KNOW

**Activity A** *Match the alternative family types in Column A with their definitions in Column B.*

**Column A**

____ 1. Cohabitation

____ 2. Gay or lesbian

____ 3. Communal

____ 4. Foster

**Column B**

a. Several people living together

b. Children living in temporary arrangements with paid caregivers

c. Unmarried individuals in a committed partnership living together

d. Intimate partners of the same sex living together

**Activity B** *Match the family types in Column A with their definitions in Column B.*

**Column A**

____ 1. Nuclear family

____ 2. Extended family

____ 3. Single-parent family

____ 4. Binuclear and reconstituted families

**Column B**

a. Consists of the nuclear family and other related people

b. Involves an adult head of the house with dependent children

c. After divorce, both parents continue to assume a high level of childrearing responsibilities

d. A two-generation unit consisting of a husband, a wife, and their immediate children

**Activity C** *Mark each statement as either "T" (True) or "F" (False). Correct any false statements.*

1. T F The response to major stressors can be depicted in two phases: adjustment and adaptation.

2. T F Child launching begins when the first child leaves home to live independently and ends when the last child leaves home.

3. T F Birth order does not play a large role in shaping the experiences of siblings.

4. T F A married couple that lives together with their children is a nuclear dyad.

5. T F Dual-worker families are nuclear families in which both parents work outside the home.

6. T F The likes and dislikes of an individual determine his or her recreational pursuits.

**Activity D** *Fill in the blanks.*

1. The ___________ function is significant for society because it is necessary for maintaining human life on earth.
2. Fixed retirement income is not sufficient for many people because of ___________.
3. ___________ is an essential family task that relates to Maslow's hierarchy of basic human needs in guiding children toward acceptable standards of elimination, food intake, sexual drive, respect for others and their possessions, and sense of spirituality.
4. A family's coping ability is significantly compromised during a ___________.
5. In the ___________ family, partners commute a long distance, usually on weekends, to be together.
6. An extended family that lives together in one house or in close proximity to one another is called a ___________ network.

**Activity E** *Consider the following figure.*

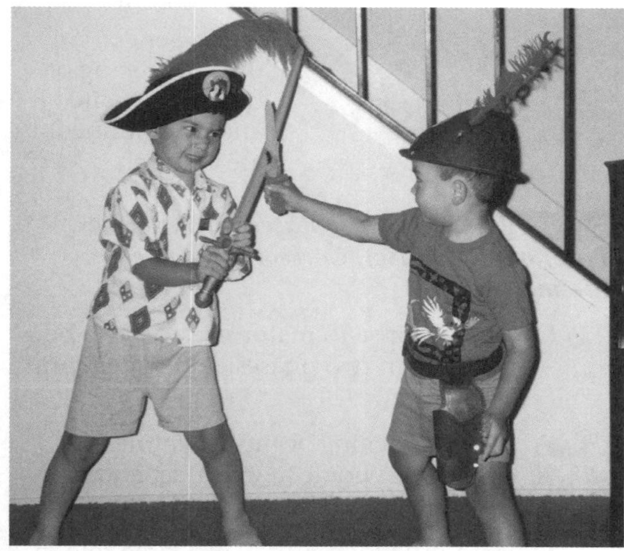

1. What is the role of siblings in the family?

___________

___________

**Activity F** *The stages of the family are given below in random order. Write the correct sequence of their occurrence in the boxes provided.*

1. Contracting family stage
2. Transitional stage
3. Expanding family stage

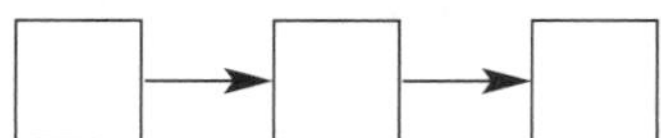

**Activity G** *Briefly answer the following questions.*

1. What factors have influenced modern society's perceptions of family?

___________

___________

2. What are the five basic family functions?

___________

___________

3. What health and social problems do families living in poverty face?

___________

___________

4. What are the five universal characteristics that families share?

___________

___________

## SECTION II: APPLYING WHAT YOU KNOW

**Activity H** *Answer the following questions, which involve the nurse's role in the management of stress.*

The nurse helps clients to overcome stress and pressure.

1. A nurse is caring for a client with stress. The client has been recently divorced and is caring for her school-age child.
   a. What are the responsibilities of the client in the given situation?

2. A nurse is caring for a client who has lost a foot due to a pressure ulcer.
   a. What issues related to the family should the nurse consider when caring for this client?
   b. How would the client's illness affect the family financially?

3. A nurse is conducting a seminar for young adults on addictions and their ill effects.
   a. What types of addictions should the nurse talk about?
   b. How is the family affected by addiction?

## SECTION III: GETTING READY FOR NCLEX

**Activity I** *Answer the following questions.*

1. Why is it important for a nurse to understand various family forms?
   a. To provide informed care
   b. To provide judgmental care
   c. To provide standardized care
   d. To provide friendly care

2. Which of the following belong to a single-adult household?
   a. A career-oriented young adult
   b. Unmarried individuals living together
   c. Couple who work in different shifts
   d. Couple with no children

3. The nurse is caring for a client who has given birth. The nurse understands that both parents are working and not very stable financially. Which of the following would be the most appropriate suggestion with regard to caring for the child?
   a. Work in different shifts
   b. Take the child to the workplace
   c. Stay at home to care for the baby
   d. Arrange for foster care

4. A client arrives at the healthcare facility accompanied by her male partner. The nurse understands that the two are unmarried individuals in a committed partnership. To what kind of family do they belong?
   a. Foster
   b. Communal
   c. Cohabitation
   d. Nuclear

5. A nurse is caring for a client in his 80s, who is assisted by his grandchildren. Which of the following should the nurse suggest to help the client cope with a decline in his physical faculties? (Select all that apply.)
   a. Reduce physical activity
   b. Provide adequate diet
   c. Ensure sufficient rest
   d. Have a good sense of humor
   e. Keep the client indoors

6. Although every family is unique, families share universal characteristics. Which of the following should the nurse recognize as the client's family's universal characteristics? (Select all that apply.)
   a. Is a large social system
   b. Performs certain basic functions
   c. Has structure
   d. Has its own cultural values and rules
   e. Moves through stages in its life cycle

7. A client's self-esteem has been negatively impacted by a recent divorce. What problems is the client at higher risk for developing later in life as a result of changes in self-esteem? (Select all that apply.)
   a. Chemical dependency
   b. Eating disorders
   c. Depression
   d. Schizophrenia

8. The nurse is documenting the family functions for a new mother with a 3-month-old infant. Which basic family function is significant for this mother and for society in maintaining human life on earth?
   a. Physical
   b. Emotional
   c. Economic
   d. Reproductive

9. A client tells the nurse about an intimate relationship that is leading to possible marriage. What stage of family should the nurse document on the chart?
   a. Establishment
   b. Contracting
   c. Transitional
   d. Expanding family

10. Individuals and families respond to both stressors in many ways, but the response to major stressors can be depicted in two phases. The nurse practitioner has documented in the chart that the client's family is in the adjustment phase. What occurs during the adjustment phase?
    a. May deny or ignore the stressor
    b. Realize that regaining stability will involve changes in the family structure
    c. Friends and community can provide assistance with the problem-solving process during the stressful period
    d. Rules, roles, boundaries, and patterns of behavior within the family are altered as needed in order to regain stability.

CHAPTER 10

# Infancy and Childhood

## SECTION I: TESTING WHAT YOU KNOW

**Activity A** *Match the age in Column A with the major levels of cognitive development during that age in Column B.*

| Column A | Column B |
|---|---|
| ____ **1.** 3 months | **a.** Develop preferred sleeping position, cry to signal needs |
| ____ **2.** 6 weeks | **b.** Laugh, squeal, look at objects for several seconds, reach for and grasp objects |
| ____ **3.** 2 to 3 months | **c.** Smile, babble, follow lights, react to sounds |
| ____ **4.** 8 weeks | **d.** Develop social smile, respond to pleasurable interactions such as looking at human faces |

**Activity B** *Mark each statement as either "T" (True) or "F" (False). Correct any false statements.*

**1.** T F Sucking milk provides comfort and relieves tension and anxiety in the infant.

**2.** T F The toddler phase consists of ages 1 to 12 months.

**3.** T F Solid foods provide babies with necessary iron and vitamins and the opportunity to learn to take food from a spoon, to chew, and to swallow.

**4.** T F Tantrums are more common when children are hungry, tired, frustrated, or feeling neglected.

**5.** T F After age 7 years, children can think abstractly.

**6.** T F A baby is called a newborn or neonate during the first 4 weeks after birth.

**Activity C** *Fill in the blanks.*

**1.** According to Piaget's theory of cognitive development, infants develop an understanding of object ____________, the knowledge that an object seen in a particular spot, but temporarily hidden from view under a blanket, continues to exist and will return to view when it is uncovered.

**2.** Babies experience ____________ anxiety when they distinguish between people they recognize and strangers, clinging to familiar persons and pulling away from strangers.

**3.** ____________ is the term given to handling and self-stimulation of the genital organs.

**4.** The change from feeding only breast milk or formula to incorporating a variety of solid foods is called ____________.

**5.** During ____________, a child's behavior may go backward to that of an earlier stage of development. This may also occur during illness.

**6.** The process of growth and development follows cephalocaudal and ____________ directions.

**Activity D** *Briefly answer the following questions.*

1. What are the characteristics of the process of growth and development?

___

___

2. What is parallel play in toddlers?

___

___

3. What is toddlerhood?

___

___

4. What causes bed-wetting, and what are some interventions for it?

___

___

## SECTION II: APPLYING WHAT YOU KNOW

**Activity E** *Answer the following questions, which involve these theories.*

When discussing the growth and development of an infant with a client, the nurse refers to various theories and phases of development.

1. A nurse is discussing Erikson's theory of psychological development with a client.
   a. What does Erikson's psychological theory state?
   b. What are the main points of Erikson's theory on which the nurse should focus?
2. A nurse is explaining cognitive development in children to a client, with the help of Piaget's theory of cognitive development.
   a. What does Piaget's theory of cognitive development state?
   b. What should the nurse explain about the four levels of cognitive development?

## SECTION III: GETTING READY FOR NCLEX

**Activity F** *Answer the following questions.*

1. Which of the following should the nurse identify as a common fear faced by preschoolers?
   a. Accidents
   b. Darkness
   c. Crowds
   d. Fire
2. What are the characteristics displayed by infants during the preoperational phase?
   a. Child internalizes actions
   b. Child investigates and explores the environment
   c. Child can think in the abstract
   d. Child learns to control body movement
3. What kind of play do older school-aged children indulge in?
   a. Cooperative play
   b. Interactive play
   c. Play with the entire class
   d. Structured games with defined roles
4. What should a nurse communicate to parents about how they can offer anticipatory guidance in their child's growth and development?
   a. Recognize the child's pace of learning abilities
   b. Recognize the child's responses to stimuli
   c. Recognize the child's genetic inclination
   d. Recognize the child's likes and dislikes
5. What is the most important psychosocial challenge experienced by an infant?
   a. Trust in primary caregivers
   b. Feeling of loneliness
   c. Forming food habits
   d. Adjustment to the external environment

6. A nurse is caring for an infant who has been diagnosed with nursing bottle mouth. The nurse knows that which of the following is the effect of nursing bottle mouth?
   a. Dry mouth
   b. Fungal infection
   c. Serious dental condition
   d. Mouth ulcers
7. What instructions should a nurse give to caregivers in order to handle toddler tantrums in public?
   a. Pacify the toddler
   b. Divert the attention of toddler
   c. Remove the child from public view
   d. Give in to the toddler's demands
8. What instruction should a nurse give to caregivers in order to handle a toddler's separation anxiety?
   a. Accept the emotional reactions of the toddler
   b. Deal with the toddler firmly
   c. Teach the toddler to control anxiety
   d. Spend time with the toddler
9. What advice should a nurse offer to a caregiver whose preschooler is experiencing sibling rivalry?
   a. Individualize attention
   b. Separate the siblings
   c. Discourage tattling
   d. Separate objects shared by preschoolers
10. The mother of an infant wants to know what to expect for this infant's normal growth and development until age 2. According to Piaget's theory of cognitive development, what should the nurse tell this mother?
   a. The infant will investigate and explore the environment and look at things from their own point of view.
   b. The infant will internalize actions and can perform them in the mind.
   c. The infant can think in the abstract.
   d. The infant can learn by touching, tasting, and feeling.

CHAPTER 11

# Adolescence

## SECTION I: TESTING WHAT YOU KNOW

**Activity A** ***Match the theory in Column A with its fundamental basis in Column B.***

| Column A | Column B |
|---|---|
| ____ 1. Erikson's theory | a. Cognitive development |
| ____ 2. Piaget's theory | b. Psychosocial development |

**Activity B** ***Match the stages of adolescence in Column A with their main characteristics in Column B.***

| Column A | Column B |
|---|---|
| ____ 1. Early adolescence | a. Desire for independence |
| ____ 2. Middle adolescence | b. Grapple with everyday issues |
| ____ 3. Late adolescence | c. Fluctuations in self-assurance |

**Activity C** ***Mark each statement as either "T" (True) or "F" (False). Correct any false statements.***

**1.** T F The developmental period between puberty and maturity is known as adolescence.

**2.** T F Piaget's theory describes the psychosocial development of adolescents.

**3.** T F Peer groups can influence adolescents in many ways.

**4.** T F Parents, teachers, and counselors can help adolescents form a healthy sexual attitude.

**5.** T F The birth control measures that are used to prevent pregnancy never fail.

**6.** T F Adolescents may take risks with their health and relationships to define their identity, to exert their independence, and to prove that they are maturing.

**7.** T F Homosexual activities at a temporary and experimental stage do not affect heterosexuality later.

**8.** T F During the preadolescence stage, boys often mature faster than girls.

**Activity D** ***Fill in the blanks.***

**1.** Adolescence spans the ages between ____________ years.

**2.** According to Piaget, the person from 12 to 15 years of age enters stage IV of cognitive development, known as ____________ operations.

**3.** ____________ is marked by eating minimal amounts of food.

**4.** The ____________ needs are prominent during the period of adolescence.

**5.** The early adolescence stage is also referred to as a/an ____________ stage.

**6.** By the age of ____________ years, girls normally experience menarche.

**Activity E** *Consider the following figure.*

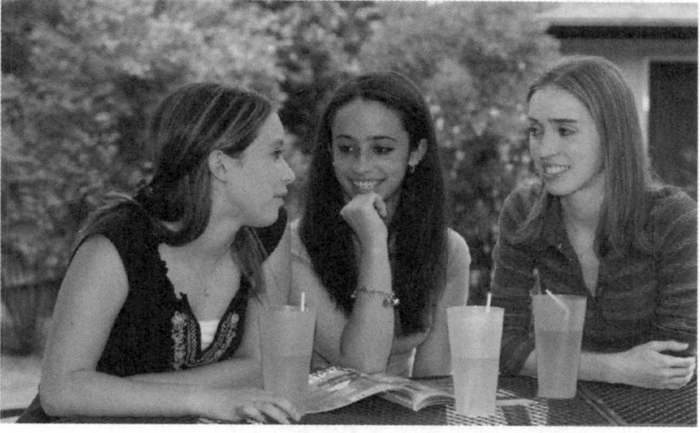

1. Explain the peer group.

______________________________

______________________________

2. Explain the importance of the peer group in adolescents' lives.

______________________________

______________________________

**Activity F** *Briefly answer the following questions.*

1. What is the importance of adults' respect toward adolescents?

______________________________

______________________________

2. Explain the role of family caregivers and other trusted adults in adolescents' sexual lives.

______________________________

______________________________

3. Why does adolescence prove to be challenging for families?

______________________________

______________________________

4. List some of the risk-taking behaviors observed in adolescents.

______________________________

______________________________

5. What pubertal changes are visible in girls during adolescence?

______________________________

______________________________

6. What are the problems likely to be faced by homosexual youths?

______________________________

______________________________

7. What are the characteristics that mark adolescence?

______________________________

______________________________

## SECTION II: APPLYING WHAT YOU KNOW

**Activity G** *Answer the following questions, which involve the nurse's role in management of such situations.*

A nurse's role in teaching involves assisting the client during pubertal changes that take place in the body, providing sex education, helping clients overcome peer pressure, and assisting them in developing good nutritional habits.

1. A nurse is taking care of a teenager who complains about involuntary discharge of semen while sleeping. The nurse observes that the client is confused and does not know about the pubertal changes that are taking place in his body. How should the nurse help the client?
2. During the nursing assessment of a minor injury, a girl reveals to the nurse that she is interested in having an intimate relationship with her boyfriend but does not know much about sex.
   a. How can the nurse help this client form a healthy sexual attitude?
   b. Why is it important to provide sex education to teenagers?
   c. Why do sexually active adolescents need counseling?

3. A man who is being assessed for high blood pressure reveals to the nurse that he is worried about his 18-year-old son, who has started using drugs and alcohol and does not listen to him.
   a. Why do adolescents take risks with their health and relationships?
   b. What should the nurse suggest to the client to help his son overcome peer pressure?
4. A client tells the nurse that her 16-year-old daughter does not eat proper food and seems to be fond of eating junk food only.
   a. How do eating disorders develop in teenaged girls?
   b. Why should adolescents be encouraged to develop good nutritional habits?

## SECTION III: GETTING READY FOR NCLEX

**Activity H** *Answer the following questions.*

1. A client reveals to the nurse that she was involved in homosexual activities during her adolescence and that now she is interested in a male friend but is afraid to have an intimate relationship with him because of her sexual history. What should the nurse explain to the client to allay her fears?
   a. Homosexual activities cause physical harm and the client needs to be assessed.
   b. Homosexual activities at an experimental level do not affect heterosexuality later.
   c. Sexual identity developed during adolescence is permanent.
   d. This is abnormal and a physician should be consulted immediately.
2. While taking care of a teenager in the early adolescence stage, what behavior of the client should the nurse anticipate?
   a. Childish way of appearing, thinking, and behaving
   b. Seclusion and moodiness
   c. True attitude of maturity
   d. Introspection and fluctuations in self-assurance
3. The mother of a teenager is worried because her son does not listen to her and makes his own decisions in almost all matters. What advice should the nurse give the client?
   a. "Making independent decisions is a natural task of adolescence."
   b. "Do not interfere in your son's life; he is growing up."
   c. "It is very risky to allow your son to make his own decisions."
   d. "Force your son to listen to you and follow your decisions."
4. A nurse is assessing a group of clients between 15 and 16 years of age to prepare a survey report on development of adolescents during middle adolescence. What relevant characteristics should the nurse include in her checklist? (Select all that apply.)
   a. Show increased interest in opposite sex
   b. Develop better relationships with parents
   c. Form ideas about the future
   d. Take more responsibility for self-care and personal cleanliness
   e. Spend more time alone
5. The father of a 14-year-old girl is worried because his daughter is very inactive and has no interest in school activities that could help her make educational and career choices in the future. What should the nurse suggest to the client to solve the problem?
   a. Skill development is part of cognitive growth that is observed in clients 12 to 15 years of age; she still has time and will develop slowly.
   b. Adult encouragement and guidance are needed for skill development.
   c. Force her to take part in various school activities.
   d. Skills developed during the teen years do not affect educational and career choices made by adolescents in the future.
6. A teenaged client, while being assessed for fever, reveals to the nurse his confusion regarding sexuality. How can a nurse help sexually active adolescents form healthy sexual attitudes?
   a. By providing sex education
   b. By preventing them from getting involved in intimate relationships at this age
   c. By convincing them to have intimate relationships only after they get married
   d. By educating them about sexually transmitted diseases

**7.** A teenager visiting the primary care provider for an annual physical exam tells the nurse about college plans. What is the major developmental task the nurse knows occurs for teenagers?

**a.** Infrequent emotional turmoil

**b.** Slow physical growth from year to year

**c.** Formation of cultural image

**d.** Establishment of goals for the future

**8.** A teenager expresses a desire for independence from parents with the school nurse. In what stage is this considered a main behavior?

**a.** Early adolescence

**b.** Middle adolescence

**c.** Late adolescence

**d.** Early adulthood

**9.** Several risk-taking behaviors occur during adolescence. On what topics of risk-taking behaviors should parents be prepared to provide guidance and effective strategies? (Select all that apply.)

**a.** Noncompliance with a medical regimen

**b.** Sexual promiscuity

**c.** Use of illicit substances

**d.** School truancy

**e.** Taking a new job

**10.** A teenage girl is very concerned about her appearance and does not want to gain weight. The teenager frets continuously about her fear of becoming fat. She has been diagnosed with anorexia nervosa. What is a key characteristic of someone with anorexia nervosa?

**a.** Eats minimal food

**b.** Has pattern of binge eating on the weekends

**c.** Over use of laxatives

**d.** Eats three times a day immediately followed by induced vomiting

CHAPTER 12

# Early and Middle Adulthood

## SECTION I: TESTING WHAT YOU KNOW

**Activity A** ***Match the age range in Column A with the appropriate period transition in Column B.***

| Column A | Column B |
|---|---|
| ____ 1. 18–22 years | a. Career choice |
| ____ 2. 22–28 years | b. Self-identity |
| ____ 3. 28–33 years | c. Settling down |
| ____ 4. 33–39 years | d. Payoff years |
| ____ 5. 40–45 years | e. Change of career |
| ____ 6. 45–65 years | f. Getting into the adult world |

**Activity B** ***Mark each statement as either "T" (True) or "F" (False). Correct any false statements.***

1. T F The tasks of early adulthood center on relationships, career choices, and family establishment.
2. T F The individual's choices and circumstances are more influential than chronological age in determining patterns of development.
3. T F The developmental task of middle adulthood is intimacy versus isolation, as adults face midlife transitions.
4. T F Individuals choose to establish relationships with others or to remain detached from others in early adulthood.
5. T F The tasks of generativity occur during middle adulthood.

**Activity C** ***Fill in the blanks.***

1. The tasks of ____________ occur when middle adults decide to pass on learning and share skills with younger generations.
2. According to Erikson and other theorists, developmental challenges depend on individual characteristics, support from society, and ____________ influences.
3. For biologic reasons, women in their 30s must make specific decisions related to ____________.
4. Many adults consider a return to school during their ____________ years, enrolling in colleges and universities in their free time without work.

**Activity D** *Consider the following figure.*

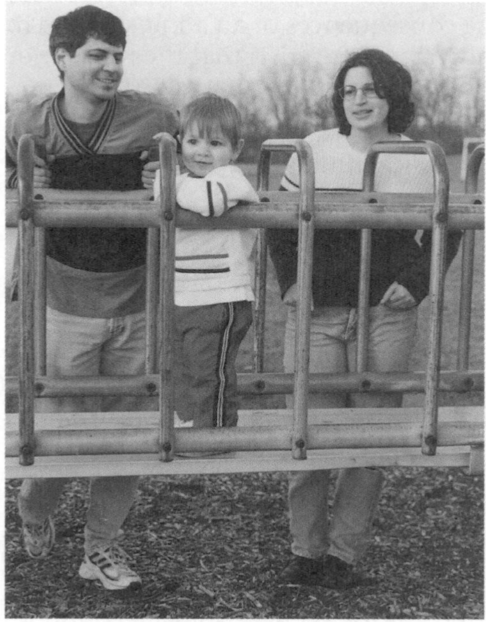

1. Give the significant aspect of the young adult period for starting and shaping a family.

______________________________________________

______________________________________________

**Activity E** ***The following section integrates concepts based on the theories of early adulthood. Stages of development in early adulthood are given below in random order. Write the correct sequence of stages in the boxes provided.***

1. Reappraising commitments
2. Establishing adult relationships
3. Starting a family
4. Choosing a career

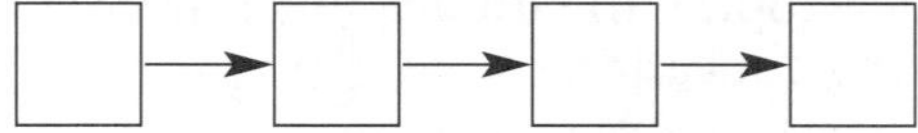

**Activity F** ***Briefly answer the following questions.***

1. What are the various methods that can help older adults plan for retirement?

______________________________________________

______________________________________________

2. What is indicated by the term "sandwich generation"?

______________________________________________

______________________________________________

3. What are the challenges likely to be faced by a divorced adult?

______________________________________________

______________________________________________

4. What are the changes that take place in the lives of adults in their 30s?

______________________________________________

______________________________________________

5. Why do some couples in their 20s choose to postpone marriage?

______________________________________________

______________________________________________

## SECTION II: APPLYING WHAT YOU KNOW

**Activity G** ***Answer the following questions, which involve the nurse's role in management of early adulthood and women's issues.***

The nurse assists clients for guidance and helps clients build a strong family unit.

1. A nurse is addressing a meeting in which parents are being informed about the patterns of young adults leaving home. What information should the nurse include?
2. A teenaged client is discussing with the nurse her relationships with others. Which relationships should the nurse encourage?
3. A couple with young children asks the nurse about the factors that contribute to a strong family unit. What instructions should the nurse provide to the parents?
4. During a routine checkup, a 36-year-old unmarried client reveals to the nurse that she is anxious to start a family and have a baby. What are the challenges this client is likely to face?

## SECTION III: GETTING READY FOR NCLEX

**Activity H** *Answer the following questions.*

1. A 25-year-old client who has recently graduated wants to know what he should focus on at this point in his life. Which of the following is the best choice for this client?
   a. Selecting an occupation
   b. Focusing on intimate relationships
   c. Focusing on marriage
   d. Creating a self-identity
2. A housewife in her 30s complains of regular headaches and tells the nurse that she is contemplating a divorce. How should the nurse react?
   a. Inform the client about the risk of financial instability after divorce
   b. Advise the client to compromise with her spouse
   c. Advise the client to consult her in-laws
   d. Encourage the client to concentrate on her career
3. A middle-aged client is contemplating retirement. What advice should the nurse give the client? (Select all that apply.)
   a. Develop interests and hobbies.
   b. Look for part-time work.
   c. Buy a bigger house.
   d. Enroll in university.
   e. Spend your money now while you still can.
4. A 25-year-old client is wondering why people choose to get married. What should the nurse's response include? (Select all that apply.)
   a. Marriage provides a sense of protection.
   b. Marriage is required for sustaining an intimate relationship.
   c. Marriage provides support during sad times.
   d. Marriage is required for prestige.
   e. Marriage indicates maturity.
5. The nurse is caring for a 53-year-old client who is worried that he will not achieve all his professional goals before he dies. What are the consequences of an adult's failure in resolving midlife crisis that the nurse should consider? (Select all that apply.)
   a. Brooding
   b. Physical illness
   c. Rebellion
   d. Criminal tendencies
   e. Chemical dependency
6. A 45-year-old client tells the nurse about struggling with several issues. The nurse knows that a client of this age is typically dealing with which period transition?
   a. Career choice
   b. Self-identity
   c. Settling down
   d. Change of career
7. Concerns for a 30-year-old are commonly very different from younger populations. What concern for a 30-year-old married woman with two children needs to be addressed first at this time?
   a. Financial ability to pay for costs of college for two children
   b. Financial ability to pay for costs of healthcare of children
   c. Emotional concerns for an aging parent
   d. Physical ability to care for a parent who retires in 5 years
8. A client tells the nurse about several choices confronting life. What is a common choice in life that occurs during middle adulthood?
   a. Entering a serious relationship
   b. Choosing to work in a people-oriented occupation
   c. Developing the intellectual self by continuing education
   d. Establishing adult identification

**9.** A young couple have sought out counseling on how to manage their young family to ensure a positive family structure. What would be an appropriate strategy the nurse could provide to this couple? (Select all that apply.)

  **a.** Mother participates in household responsibilities

  **b.** Father participates in household responsibilities

  **c.** Mother is primarily responsible for childcare responsibilities

  **d.** Both parents share childcare responsibilities

**10.** The nurse is addressing a meeting in which college students are being informed about researchers' theories of development as it applies to young and middle adulthood. What information should be included about Erikson's theory in the presentation?

  **a.** Developmental tasks are based on learned behaviors that arise from the financial status of an individual.

  **b.** Development during this stage is connected with the ability to make successful transitions.

  **c.** There are psychosocial challenges that individuals face in young and middle adulthood.

  **d.** Adults want to build a safe structure for the future and have commitments and security.

CHAPTER 13

# Older Adulthood and Aging

## SECTION I: TESTING WHAT YOU KNOW

**Activity A** *Match the terms related to older adulthood in Column A with their definitions in Column B.*

| Column A | Column B |
|---|---|
| ____ **1.** Gerontology | **a.** Study of characteristics and changes that cause balance in a population |
| ____ **2.** Demographics | **b.** Labeling and discrimination against elderly adults; prejudice based on chronological age |
| ____ **3.** Ageism | **c.** Study of the aging process in all dimensions (physical, psychological, economic, sociologic, and spiritual) |

**Activity B** *Mark each statement as either "T" (True) or "F" (False). Correct any false statements.*

**1.** T F Ageism refers to discrimination against individuals as they grow older.

**2.** T F Health, stress, loss, and poverty are significant concerns for older adults.

**3.** T F In many cultural groups, it is considered unthinkable for older relatives to live alone or in nursing homes.

**4.** T F Optimal function for age is the goal for development in older adulthood.

**5.** T F The key elements of maintaining independence in older adulthood are health, financial stability, and social resources.

**Activity C** *Fill in the blanks.*

**1.** A majority of older adults rely on Social Security income, which was originally designed as a ____________ to other income.

**2.** Erikson encourages ____________ while working with older clients in a healthcare facility.

**3.** Groups such as the ____________ and the Gray Panthers are likely to have significant political influence in ensuring quality, convenient, and cost-effective services for older adults.

**4.** Reflecting on one's ____________ is an adaptation to the prospect of death.

**5.** Some people do not adhere to a specific religion but fulfill their ____________ needs by having some quiet, private time to pray or to reflect.

**Activity D** *Briefly answer the following questions.*

1. Why is it important for the nurse to have knowledge about the normal aging process?

______________________________________

______________________________________

2. What are the major physical changes related to the normal aging process taking place in older people?

______________________________________

______________________________________

3. What are the challenges faced by clients in the older adulthood phase?

______________________________________

______________________________________

4. What are the challenges for society to examine in the 21st century related to the rising older population?

______________________________________

______________________________________

5. What are the factors that lead to a loss of independence in older adults?

______________________________________

______________________________________

## SECTION II: APPLYING WHAT YOU KNOW

**Activity E** *Answer the following questions, which involve the nurse's role in caring for older adults.*

The nurse assists older clients during the normal aging process and helps clients understand the developmental tasks that should be accomplished in older adulthood.

1. An elderly client wants to know about the major physical changes related to the normal aging process. What physical changes should the nurse make the client aware of?
2. An elderly client is eager to know about the developmental tasks that should be accomplished in the older adulthood stage. Which developmental tasks should the nurse discuss with the client?
3. A nurse is discussing with a social activist issues related to the growing population of the elderly. What issues should the nurse focus on?
4. An elderly client is confused regarding the activities to be taken up after retirement. How can a nurse help the client?

## SECTION III: GETTING READY FOR NCLEX

**Activity F** *Answer the following questions.*

1. An elderly client believes that developmental tasks related to social changes can be prevented if older adults continue to stay with their families. Based on Erikson's theory, what should the nurse tell the client?
   a. Developmental tasks focus on necessary adjustments to physical change.
   b. Developmental tasks focus on the social changes associated with age.
   c. Developmental tasks relate to career enhancement and finances.
   d. Developmental tasks focus on the review of past decisions.
2. A client complains that her 60-year-old father is no longer "sticking to the day-to-day routine that he has been following for the past 2 decades." How can the nurse help the client, using Levinson's theory?
   a. Explain that her father is choosing modes of living more freely.
   b. Suggest that she explain to her father his social responsibilities.
   c. Advise her to force her father to revert to following his routine.
   d. Advise her to send her father to an extended care facility.

3. A 55-year-old client is anxious about the changes taking place in his body. What are the areas of general physical alteration on which the nurse can focus in this discussion? (Select all that apply.)
   a. Cells
   b. Body organs
   c. Body systems
   d. Height
   e. Body odor
4. A 70-year-old client at an extended care facility asks the nurse for advice on maintaining independence at this stage. What are the psychosocial considerations of maintaining independence?
   a. Sustaining health, social responsibilities, and financial stability
   b. Maintaining mental stability and satisfaction's in one's family
   c. Moving out of the extended care facility to live alone
   d. Working for the poor in the locality
5. A client who has lost his spouse recently is very depressed and needs some consolation. How can the nurse help the client to overcome this situation?
   a. Encourage the client to join a fitness training center.
   b. Talk to the client about the principles of beliefs and spirituality.
   c. Instruct the client to take some voluntary work to occupy his time.
   d. Encourage the client to take up educational opportunities.
6. A 60-year-old client is not ready to accept the physical limitations associated with age. What should the nurse instruct the client to do according to Erikson's theory?
   a. Feel comfortable with life changes to attain dignity.
   b. Avoid breaking out of unsatisfactory life patterns.
   c. Find a new balance of involvement with society and self.
   d. Achieve ego integrity.
7. A nurse is reviewing the characteristics and changes that cause balance in the local older adulthood population. What is the nurse studying?
   a. Demographics
   b. Ageism
   c. Gerontology
   d. Mortality trends
8. A son of an elderly parent asks the nurse about expected age-related physical changes for his father. What are the normal physical changes for older adulthood? (Select all that apply.)
   a. Decreased functioning of organs
   b. Changes in visual and auditory acuity
   c. Increased reaction time
   d. Decreased physical and emotional losses
   e. Increased tactile sensations
9. An elderly client sold the family home and moved into an independent senior center because of an inability to manage alone. What are the key factors that can lead to this individual's further loss of independence? (Select all that apply.)
   a. Financial
   b. Health
   c. Intellectual
   d. Social
10. The nurse is reviewing some key demographics with a daughter of an elderly client. What is a correct demographic to share about the older population and society?
    a. A minority of elderly rely on Social Security income.
    b. Women earn an average of twice the per capita annual income of men.
    c. Most older people live in suburban areas.
    d. About one third of prescription medications are taken by older adults.

CHAPTER 14

# Death and Dying

## SECTION I: TESTING WHAT YOU KNOW

**Activity A** *Match the terms related to death and dying in Column A with their explanations in Column B.*

| Column A | Column B |
|---|---|
| ____ 1. Detachment | a. State in which an individual faces a medical condition that will end in death within a limited period |
| ____ 2. Reactive depression | b. Stage in which an individual gradually separates from the world |
| ____ 3. Terminal illness | c. Stage in which an individual concentrates on past losses |

**Activity B** *Mark each statement as either "T" (True) or "F" (False). Correct any false statements.*

1. T F Basic human needs are a priority for the dying person.
2. T F In the detachment stage of dying, an individual gradually separates from the world.
3. T F All terminally ill people go through the six stages of dying in order.
4. T F The nurse should instruct the family not to cry or express sadness in front of a dying loved one.
5. T F Children who are dying should be told the truth and be allowed to ask questions.
6. T F Spirituality is an outlet that helps individuals to handle death and dying.
7. T F During the detachment stage of dying, nursing care is primarily directed toward the spiritual needs of the client.

**Activity C** *Fill in the blanks.*

1. The process of dying has been compared to the process of ____________.
2. ____________ illness is a state in which an individual faces a medical condition that will end in death within a limited period.
3. A benefit of normal ____________ is being able to gradually adjust to the inevitability of death.
4. ____________ is the final stage of growth and development.
5. ____________ human needs are a priority for the dying person.
6. ____________ often forces people to consider the meaning of life, the existence of the soul, and the possibility of an afterlife.
7. During the ____________ stage of depression, the individual concentrates on past losses.
8. The final stage of dying is ____________.

**Activity D** ***The stages of dying described by Kübler-Ross are given below in random order. Write the correct sequence in which they occur in the boxes provided.***

1. Anger
2. Depression
3. Detachment
4. Denial
5. Bargaining
6. Acceptance

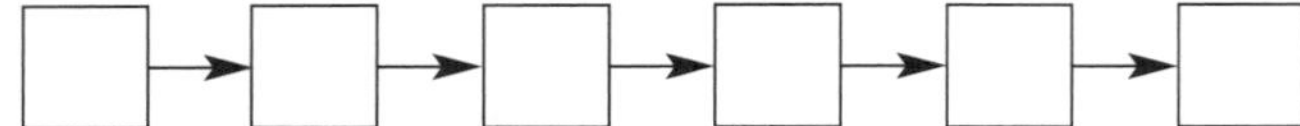

**Activity E** ***Briefly answer the following questions.***

1. How do culture, ethnicity, and religion influence people's attitudes toward death?

_______________

_______________

2. How can the nurse honor the process of dying?

_______________

_______________

3. Why is the concept of death not acceptable to many people?

_______________

_______________

## SECTION II: APPLYING WHAT YOU KNOW

**Activity F** ***Answer the following questions, which involve the nurse's role in management of death and dying.***

The nurse assists clients through the process of dying and helps clients' families to cope with the situation.

1. A young client with a terminal illness expresses anger when his family visits. The client's response has the family upset and disturbed.
   a. Which stage of dying is the client passing through?
   b. How should the nurse care for the client and the family?
2. A nurse is caring for a dying client who belongs to an organized religious group.
   a. How can the nurse help the client to draw strength from his or her religious faith?
   b. Why is spirituality important for individuals faced with death?
3. The family of a young client diagnosed with a terminal illness expresses doubts regarding the medical reports and wants to consult other doctors to get additional opinions.
   a. What does this reaction of the family imply?
4. A nurse is caring for a dying client who does not belong to any organized religious group. The client is dejected and says that life seems meaningless and all the achievements in life useless at this point.
   a. How can the nurse help the client cope with the situation?

## SECTION III: GETTING READY FOR NCLEX

**Activity G** ***Answer the following questions.***

1. A client with a terminal illness shouts at his visitors, who are hurt and upset. Which of the following is a reason for the client's behavior? (Select all that apply.)
   a. The client is angry with the visitors.
   b. The client is envious of healthy young people.
   c. It is a natural behavior for a person facing death.
   d. The client does not want to meet anybody.
   e. The client is expressing his helplessness.
2. A dying client tells the nurse that she hopes to stay alive until the following month to attend her son's wedding. The nurse understands that the client is exhibiting which of the following kinds of behavior?
   a. Denial
   b. Anger
   c. Depression
   d. Bargaining

**3.** A nurse is caring for a client in the depression stage of dying. Which of the following characteristics are peculiar to this stage of dying? (Select all that apply.)

**a.** Severe sense of loss
**b.** Anger and frustration
**c.** Denial of death
**d.** Concentration on previous losses
**e.** Realization of the impact of loss

**4.** A nurse is caring for a dying client who has ceased to be responsive and is gradually separating from the world. Which of the following needs of the client should be addressed in this stage of detachment?

**a.** Spiritual needs
**b.** Physical needs
**c.** Emotional needs
**d.** Ritual needs

**5.** An elderly man is dying, and his family is hesitant about allowing his grandchildren to see him in this condition. Which of the following nursing interventions is most appropriate in this situation?

**a.** Ask the family to be honest with the children about death.
**b.** Agree that it may be a frightening experience.
**c.** Tell them that the presence of the children may disturb the client.
**d.** Agree that children need not be part of grieving.

**6.** A nurse caring for a dying client understands that the person is in the acceptance and peace stage of death. Which of the following behaviors does the client display in this stage?

**a.** Seems devoid of all feeling
**b.** Reacts angrily with visitors
**c.** Tries to bargain for time
**d.** Seeks an acceptable prognosis

**7.** A client diagnosed with terminal illness refuses to accept the diagnosis and insists on seeking advice from other healthcare professionals. Which of the following stage of dying is this behavior related to?

**a.** Anger
**b.** Acceptance
**c.** Detachment
**d.** Denial

**8.** A young client with terminal illness tells the family to get out of the room. The client tells the nurse of being very angry about the family visits. In what stage of grief does this type of behavior typically occur?

**a.** Acceptance
**b.** Anger
**c.** Denial
**d.** Detachment

**9.** An elderly patient has just been told of having bladder cancer that will result in death within 3 months. What term describes this individual's medical condition?

**a.** Terminal illness
**b.** Detachment
**c.** Reactive depression
**d.** Grief

**10.** A client is continually concentrating on sharing with the nurse about losing his wife of 50 years. He talks about the fact that his only son was killed in the war 10 years ago and he is the only one left. What term relates to this individual's concerns?

**a.** Terminal illness
**b.** Detachment
**c.** Reactive depression
**d.** Denial

CHAPTER 15

# Organization of the Human Body

## SECTION I: TESTING WHAT YOU KNOW

**Activity A** *Match the parts of the cell in Column A with their meanings in Column B.*

**Column A**

____ 1. Cell membrane

____ 2. Cilia

____ 3. Cytoplasm

____ 4. Nucleus

**Column B**

a. Control center, responsible for reproduction and coordination of other cellular activities

b. Area of the cell not located in the nucleus

c. Hair-like threads that sweep materials across the cell surface

d. Surrounds the cell's outer boundary and is capable of selective permeability

**Activity B** *Match the cell properties in Column A with their corresponding definitions in Column B.*

**Column A**

____ 1. Anabolism

____ 2. Catabolism

____ 3. Contractility

____ 4. Conductivity

____ 5. Irritability

____ 6. Reproduction

**Column B**

a. Ability of cells to break down, disintegrate, or tear substances into simpler substances

b. Ability of muscle cells to move

c. Ability of cells to duplicate themselves

d. Ability of cells to respond to stimuli

e. Ability of nerve cells to send and receive impulses

f. Ability of cells to build up, assimilate, or convert ingested substances

**Activity C** *Mark each statement as either "T" (True) or "F" (False). Correct any false statements.*

1. T F Transitional epithelium is a type of stratified squamous epithelium that changes shape.

2. T F A mixture is a blend of two or more substances that have been mixed together to form a new compound involving a chemical reaction.

3. T F In meiosis, cell division produces eggs or sperm that contain half (23) the total number of chromosomes.

4. T F Prefixes, roots, and suffixes are the sources of most medical terms.

5. T F Genes contain information about inherited characteristics.

6. T F Chromosomes are composed of RNA molecules that synthesize proteins.

**Activity D** ***Fill in the blanks.***

1. An ____________ is a pure, simple chemical in the body.
2. When atoms of two or more elements react chemically with one another, they form substances called ____________.
3. The study of disorders of functioning is called ____________.
4. The study of body structure is called ____________.
5. The ____________ is a large muscle that separates the ventral cavities in the body.
6. An ____________ is a group of different types of tissues that form in a specific manner to perform a definite function.
7. ____________ are cell fragments that play a major role in the blood-clotting process.

**Activity E** ***Consider the following figure.***

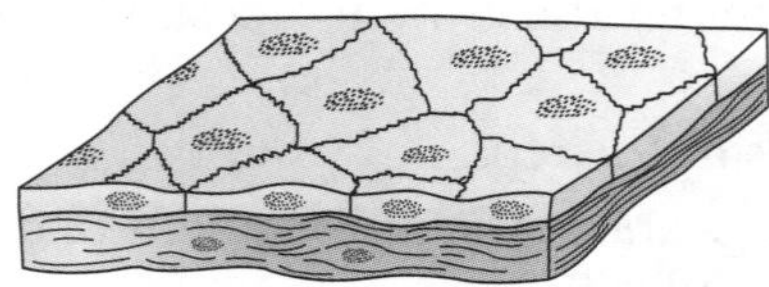

1. What type of tissue does the figure represent?

______________________________________________

______________________________________________

2. Explain the different types of this tissue.

______________________________________________

______________________________________________

3. What are the various functions of this tissue?

______________________________________________

______________________________________________

**Activity F** ***Briefly answer the following questions.***

1. Name the various elements found in the human body.

______________________________________________

______________________________________________

2. What is the difference between a physical reaction and a chemical reaction?

______________________________________________

______________________________________________

3. What are the meanings of the terms anatomy, physiology, and pathophysiology?

______________________________________________

______________________________________________

4. How does the sagittal plane divide the human body?

______________________________________________

______________________________________________

5. How is the abdominal cavity divided into quadrants?

______________________________________________

______________________________________________

6. What are the various parts of a cell?

______________________________________________

______________________________________________

7. What are the functions of a body system?

______________________________________________

______________________________________________

## SECTION II: APPLYING WHAT YOU KNOW

**Activity G** ***Answer the following questions, which involve the nurse's role in the management of such conditions.***

A nurse is required to know and understand body structures, body functions, and disorders of functioning.

1. A nurse attending to athletes should know how muscles function and other characteristics of muscles that help in aiding movement of the body.
   a. How do muscle tissues function?
   b. What are the various types of muscle tissues?

2. A nurse is caring for a client who has lost all sensations in the extremities.
   a. What are nerve tissues composed of?
   b. What are the two main types of neurons?

## SECTION III: GETTING READY FOR NCLEX

**Activity H** *Answer the following questions.*

1. Which of the following is a function of cartilaginous tissue?
   a. Cartilage acts as a shock absorber, reducing friction between moving parts.
   b. Cartilage contains fibers that contract and relax, bringing about movement.
   c. Cartilage anchors and supports the various body structures.
   d. Cartilage provides protection for the various organs in the body.
2. The dorsal cavity is subdivided into which of the following?
   a. Cranial and spinal cavities
   b. The diaphragm
   c. Thoracic and abdominal cavities
   d. Abdominal and pelvic portions of the abdominal cavity
3. The nurse explains to a client with a nose injury that recovery of the cartilaginous tissue after surgery will be slow. Which of the following should the nurse identify as a reason for the slow healing of cartilaginous tissue?
   a. Cartilaginous tissue inhibits the secretion of synovial fluid.
   b. Cartilaginous tissue causes friction between bones.
   c. Cartilaginous tissue is poorly supplied with blood vessels.
   d. Cartilaginous tissue does not have flexible strength.
4. Which of the following tissues is found in the external ear?
   a. Adipose tissue
   b. Elastic connective tissue
   c. Areolar tissue
   d. Fibrous connective tissue
5. How does the frontal plane divide the human body?
   a. Divides the body into equal right and left halves
   b. Divides the body into upper and lower parts
   c. Divides the body into front and back parts
   d. Divides the body into right or left sides
6. Which of the following is considered a form of connective tissue? (Select all that apply.)
   a. Areolar tissue
   b. Nerve tissue
   c. Blood
   d. Muscle tissue
   e. Cartilage
7. What is the importance of the process of cell reproduction in the body? (Select all that apply.)
   a. Brings about the conversion of ingested substances
   b. Brings about and promotes protein synthesis
   c. Promotes the growth of a single fertilized egg
   d. Aids in the repair of wounds
   e. Brings about the replacement of damaged or dead cells
8. Seven elements make up approximately 99% of human body weight. Which of the following elements is one of those elements?
   a. Potassium
   b. Iron
   c. Chromium
   d. Phosphorous
9. In the division of the abdominal cavity based on the costal margins and pubic bones, which region forms the epigastric region?
   a. Central area above costal margins
   b. Central area below pubic bones
   c. Central area between the two dividing lines
   d. Left and right iliac and lumbar regions

**10.** Which of the following are functions of muscle tissue? (Select all that apply.)

**a.** Composed of neurons that respond to stimuli

**b.** Send impulses to and receive impulses from all parts of the body

**c.** Control action as voluntary or involuntary

**d.** Contract or shorten and relax, thereby bringing about movement

**e.** Cover or line surfaces or separate organs

CHAPTER 16

# The Integumentary System

## SECTION I: TESTING WHAT YOU KNOW

**Activity A** *Match the layers of the skin in Column A with their definitions in Column B.*

| Column A | Column B |
|---|---|
| ____ 1. Epidermis | a. Deep thick layer |
| ____ 2. Dermis | b. Layer on top of muscle |
| ____ 3. Hypodermis | c. Thin superficial layer |

**Activity B** *Mark each statement as either "T" (True) or "F" (False). Correct any false statements.*

1. T F Glands made of epithelial tissue provide secretions from the body's internal environment to the external world.
2. T F Skin is responsible for sensations of heat, cold, pain, touch, and pressure.
3. T F Microorganisms cannot penetrate unbroken skin because of keratin.
4. T F Vitamin D along with melanin protects the body from the damaging effects of ultraviolet (UV) light.
5. T F Estrogen contributes to male pattern baldness in men.
6. T F Sudoriferous glands are glands found only in the skin of the external auditory meatus, a passage that leads into the ear.

**Activity C** *Fill in the blanks.*

1. ___________ are patches of melanin clustered together on the skin.
2. The ___________ is the outermost protective layer of the skin.
3. Microorganisms cannot penetrate unbroken skin because of the presence of ___________.
4. Melanin is a brown-black pigment produced by ___________ which are found mostly in the basal layer of the epidermis.
5. ___________ is a skin condition in which the melanocytes stop making melanin, causing distinct, localized areas of white.
6. The integumentary system is responsible for maintaining the body's internal temperature through a process called ___________.
7. ___________ plays a role in absorbing calcium from the body's gastrointestinal tract.

**Activity D** *Consider the following figure.*

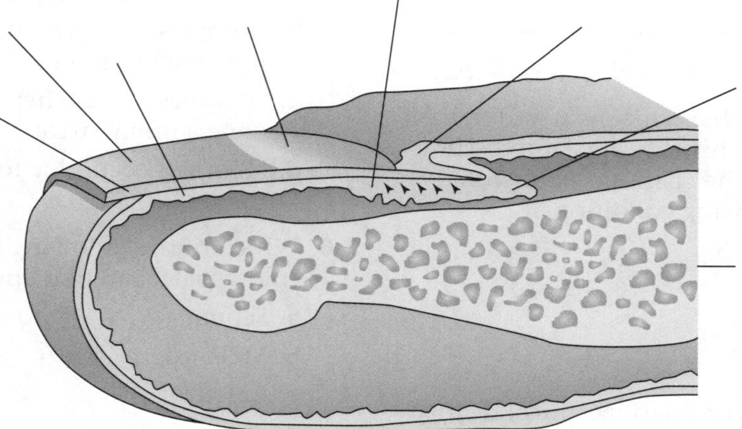

1. What part of the integumentary system is shown in the figure? Label the parts represented in the figure.

___

___

2. Explain the process of growth of this part of the integumentary system.

___

___

**Activity E** *Briefly answer the following questions.*

1. What is the integumentary system composed of?

___

___

2. What is the function of the stratum basale or stratum germinativum?

___

___

3. How are fingerprints formed?

___

___

4. What is the purpose of the subcutaneous tissue?

___

___

5. What are the three types of sudoriferous or sweat glands?

___

___

6. What is the role of nerve endings?

___

___

## SECTION II: APPLYING WHAT YOU KNOW

**Activity F** *Answer the following questions, which involve the nurse's role in the management of the integumentary system.*

The nurse answers a client's questions regarding the integumentary system and helps the client learn about mechanisms of heat loss, heat production, and heat conservation.

1. What should the nurse accurately measure as an indicator of sudden physiologic changes that occur in the client's body?
2. A nurse measures the body temperature of a 25-year-old client with fever and finds that it is increasing rapidly. What can the nurse do to reduce the body temperature of the client?
3. A client whose skin has developed a bluish hue is diagnosed by the physician as having cyanosis. What causes cyanosis, and what should the nurse monitor in such a case?
4. What should the nurse know about vasoconstriction in the extremities?

## SECTION III: GETTING READY FOR NCLEX

**Activity G** *Answer the following questions.*

1. A 4-year-old client has white skin and hair all over his body, and his eyes appear red. The nurse knows that the client probably has which of the following conditions?
   a. Albinism
   b. Freckles
   c. Vitiligo
   d. Liver spots
2. A client working in a pharmaceutical factory has developed thick skin and calluses on the soles of the feet and the palms of the hands. The client visits a clinic and asks the nurse the reason for the development of thick skin. What should the nurse's response include?
   a. "The condition may be caused by oversecretion of melanin."
   b. "The condition may be caused by the separation of epidermis and dermis."
   c. "The condition may be caused by contact with harmful chemicals."
   d. "The condition may be caused by the formation of lipocytes."
3. Which of the following are functions of the integumentary system? (Select all that apply.)
   a. "It helps in retarding the loss of body fluid."
   b. "It helps in the prevention of rashes and allergies."
   c. "It helps in excreting waste products from the skin."
   d. "It prevents the occurrence of hypothermia."
   e. "It helps in preventing invasion into the internal environment."
4. Which of the following hormones is responsible for facial and chest hair growth in men?
   a. Testosterone
   b. Estrogen
   c. Cerumen
   d. Progesterone
5. A 16-year-old female client visits the healthcare facility because she is worried about pimples on her face. What explanation should the nurse offer as the cause of pimples in the client?
   a. "Pimples occur due to a lack of protein supplements."
   b. "Pimples occur when sebum traps bacteria in the skin's pores."
   c. "Pimples occur when apocrine glands secrete a milky sweat."
   d. "Pimples occur due to a lack of iron supplements."
6. Which of the following give skin its natural color? (Select all that apply.)
   a. Sebum
   b. Melanin
   c. Calcitrol
   d. Hemoglobin
   e. Carotene
7. A 45-year-old male client with hair loss is diagnosed with alopecia. Which of the following reasons should the nurse identify as the possible cause for the client's condition?
   a. High secretion of melanin
   b. Sedentary lifestyle
   c. Emotional stress
   d. Use of hair care products
8. Which of the following details can be identified from the study of a hair sample? (Select all that apply.)
   a. Environmental exposure to heavy metals
   b. Cause of hair loss
   c. Nutritional status
   d. DNA for identification purposes
   e. Level of stress
9. What caution should the nurse offer the client who bites her nails?
   a. Nail biting leads to nail bed damage.
   b. Nail biting leads to skin infections.
   c. Nail biting leads to slow growth of nails.
   d. Nail biting leads to calcium deficiency.
10. What instructions should a nurse offer to help a client maintain healthy skin? (Select all that apply.)
    a. Consume a healthy diet.
    b. Drink plenty of fluids daily.
    c. Drink warm water daily.
    d. Limit exposure to the sun.
    e. Use only herbal products on the skin.

CHAPTER 17

# Fluid and Electrolyte Balance

## SECTION I: TESTING WHAT YOU KNOW

**Activity A** *Match the terms in Column A with their definitions in Column B.*

**Column A**

____ 1. Isotonic

____ 2. Hypertonic

____ 3. Hypotonic

____ 4. Edema

**Column B**

a. The excess accumulation of fluid in the interstitial spaces.

b. A solution that exerts equal pressure on opposite sides of a membrane.

c. A solution that is stronger compared to that on the opposite side of a membrane.

d. A solution that is weaker compared to that on the opposite side of a membrane.

**Activity B** *Match the conditions in Column A with their characteristics in Column B.*

**Column A**

____ 1. Ascites

____ 2. Anasarca

____ 3. Diarrhea

____ 4. Hemorrhage

**Column B**

a. Causes frequent and watery bowel movements

b. Causes abnormal, severe internal or external discharge of blood

c. Causes accumulation of serous fluid in the abdominal cavity

d. Causes accumulation of fluid in cellular tissues of the body

**Activity C** *Mark each statement as either "T" (True) or "F" (False). Correct any false statements.*

1. T F A positively charged ion is known as a cation.

2. T F Diffusion is the random movement of molecules from an area of lower concentration to an area of higher concentration.

3. T F A salt is created when the negative ions of a base replace the positive oxygen ions of an acid.

4. T F A vesicle transports large molecules or whole cells across the plasma membrane.

5. T F Oxygen is the main component of the pH system of the body.

6. T F An atom that has gained or lost one or more electrons is called an ion.

7. T F Electrolytes are substances that dissociate in water into ions.

**Activity D** *Fill in the blanks.*

1. ____________ is the dynamic process through which the body maintains balance by constantly adjusting to internal and external stimuli.
2. ____________ feedback occurs when the body reverses an original stimulus to regain physiological homeostasis.
3. Intravascular fluid is the watery fluid of the blood known as ____________.
4. With a decrease in blood volume, ____________ is released by the kidneys.
5. ____________ is an excess of water in the body.
6. A ____________ is the substance dissolved in a solvent.
7. The process of ____________ involves the dissociation of compounds into their respective ions.
8. The ability of a membrane to allow molecules to pass through is known as ____________.

**Activity E** *Consider the following figures.*

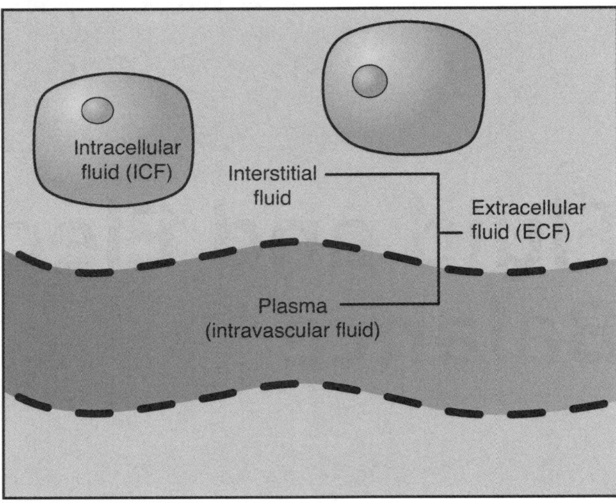


1. What are the two main compartments of body fluid?

____________________________________________

____________________________________________

2. What are the features of extracellular fluid (ECF)?

____________________________________________

____________________________________________

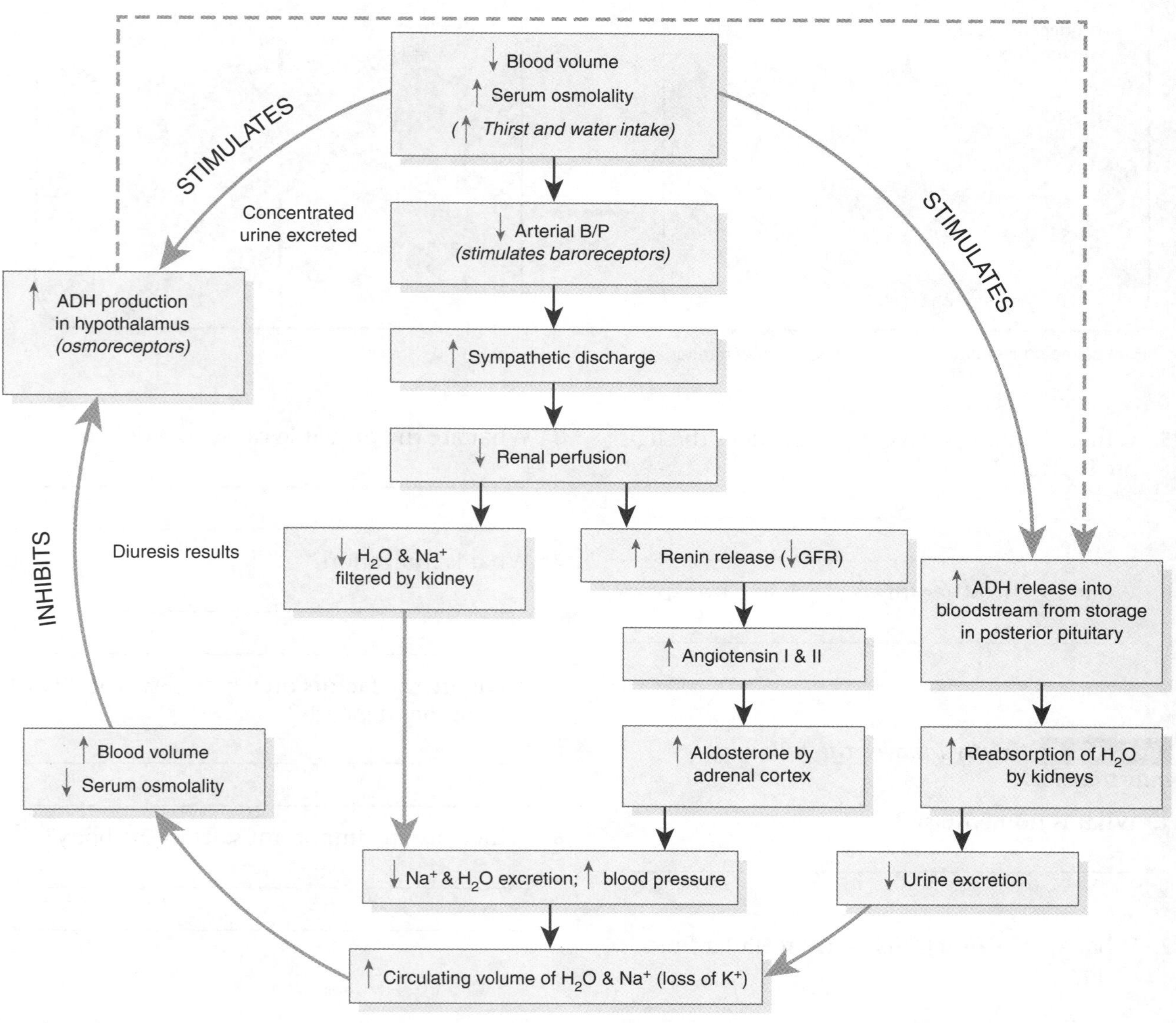


3. When is ADH released from the posterior pituitary gland?

________________________________________

________________________________________

4. What causes renin to be released by the kidneys?

________________________________________

________________________________________

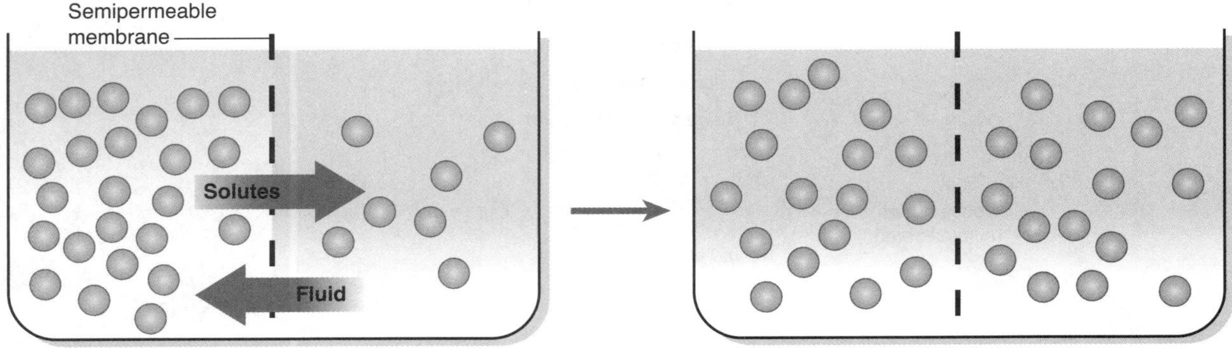


5. Which form of passive transport does the figure indicate?

_______________________________________________

_______________________________________________

6. What are the other forms of passive transport?

_______________________________________________

_______________________________________________

**Activity F** ***Briefly answer the following questions.***

1. What is homeostasis?

_______________________________________________

_______________________________________________

2. What are the functions of intracellular fluid (ICF)?

_______________________________________________

_______________________________________________

3. What are the principle causes of edema?

_______________________________________________

_______________________________________________

4. What is ionization?

_______________________________________________

_______________________________________________

5. What are the factors on which permeability of membranes depends?

_______________________________________________

_______________________________________________

6. Which are the important salts in the body?

_______________________________________________

_______________________________________________

## SECTION II: APPLYING WHAT YOU KNOW

**Activity G** *Answer the following questions, which involve the nurse's role in the management of fluid imbalances.*

Excess water (overhydration), accumulation of fluid in the interstitial spaces (edema), or loss of water (dehydration) in the body are all concerns. The nurse assists clients in the treatment of fluid imbalances and helps clients prevent such symptoms.

1. A nurse is caring for a client with severe dehydration. What are some of the causes of dehydration that the nurse should educate the client about?
2. The nurse is caring for a group of elderly clients.
   a. What are the effects of aging on fluid and electrolyte balance that the nurse should be aware of?
   b. What are the nursing interventions for elderly clients who are at high risk of fluid and electrolyte imbalance?

## SECTION III: GETTING READY FOR NCLEX

**Activity H** *Answer the following questions.*

1. A nurse is monitoring a client who has elevated levels of extracellular fluid (ECF). Which of the following conditions should the nurse monitor?
   a. High blood pressure
   b. Vomiting
   c. Hypovolemic shock
   d. Diarrhea
2. Which of the following causes increased capillary pressure and results in edema?
   a. Neoplastic disease
   b. Extensive burns
   c. Liver disease
   d. Arteriolar dilatation
3. Which of the following symptoms should the nurse assess for when caring for a client with increased levels of electrolytes?
   a. Hypocalcemia
   b. Hypermagnesemia
   c. Anemia
   d. Hyponatremia
4. What is the function of extracellular fluid (ECF)?
   a. Stabilizing agent for the cell
   b. Helps maintain cell shape
   c. Helps maintain normal blood pressure
   d. Assists with transport of nutrients
5. Which of the following factors influence intake of water? (Select all that apply.)
   a. Liquid intake
   b. Food metabolism
   c. Medication
   d. Exercise
   e. Cellular respiration
6. In which part of the body is synovial fluid found?
   a. In the brain
   b. In the joint cavities
   c. In the spinal cord
   d. In the eyes
7. A client is admitted to the hospital with overhydration. Which of the following instructions might the nurse provide the client before discharge that might help to prevent the condition from recurring?
   a. Instruct the client to urinate frequently.
   b. Instruct the client to lower the level of sodium in the diet.
   c. Instruct the client to increase the level of calcium in the diet.
   d. Instruct the client to avoid drinking fruit juices.

**8.** Which of the following electrolytes are intracellular? (Select all that apply.)

**a.** Potassium

**b.** Sodium

**c.** Magnesium

**d.** Chloride

**e.** Phosphate

**9.** Which of the following factors place adolescents at an increased risk for fluid and electrolyte imbalances? (Select all that apply.)

**a.** Increased sexual activity

**b.** Excessive exercise

**c.** High-sodium soft drinks

**d.** Increased stress levels

**e.** Improper fad diets

**10.** A client has been admitted to the unit with an excess amount of serous fluid in the abdominal cavity. For what condition should the nurse monitor?

**a.** Anasarca

**b.** Ascites

**c.** Pleural effusion

**d.** Pericardial effusion

CHAPTER 18

# The Musculoskeletal System

## SECTION I: TESTING WHAT YOU KNOW

**Activity A** ***Match the bones in Column A with their functions in Column B.***

| Column A | Column B |
|---|---|
| ____ 1. Long bones | a. Facilitate movement; transfer forces |
| ____ 2. Short bones | b. Provide broad surfaces for muscle attachment and for protection |
| ____ 3. Flat bones | c. For attachment of other structures or articulations |
| ____ 4. Irregular bones | d. Act as levers; support frame |

**Activity B** ***Match the classification of synovial joints in Column A with their range of movement in Column B.***

| Column A | Column B |
|---|---|
| ____ 1. Ginglymus | a. Moves within a cup-shaped depression in the other bone |
| ____ 2. Spheroidal | b. Slide against each other |
| ____ 3. Arthrodial | c. Allows movement in only one plane |

**Activity C** ***Mark each statement as either "T" (True) or "F" (False). Correct any false statements.***

1. T F The bones of adults are more pliable than those of children.
2. T F Infants have a wide-based gait.
3. T F Bones are classified according to their mass.
4. T F Any prominence or projection of bone is called a bony process.
5. T F A ligament is said to arise or originate in the bone or structure that is more stationary.

**Activity D** ***Fill in the blanks.***

1. The ___________ ("cross-shaped") ligaments of the knee arise from the femur and attach to the tibia at the knee.
2. The hollow inner part of the bone is filled with a soft substance called ___________.
3. The end of a long bone, the ___________ is sponge-like and covered by a shell of harder bone.
4. The greater ___________ of the femur is a large bony process.
5. A ___________ is a type of fibrous joint in which a conical process is inserted into a socket type of structure.

6. Strong fibrous bands called ____________ hold bones together.
7. ____________ is a type of connective tissue that is organized into a system of fibers or embedded into a ground substance or matrix.

**Activity E** *Consider the following figure.*

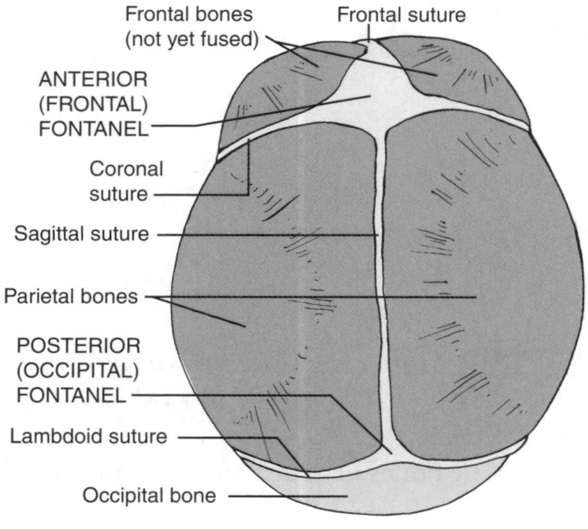

1. What is a fontanel?

______________________________________________

______________________________________________

2. What is the function of fontanels?

______________________________________________

______________________________________________

**Activity F** *Briefly answer the following questions.*

1. What are isotonic exercises?

______________________________________________

______________________________________________

2. What is muscle tone?

______________________________________________

______________________________________________

3. What are the consequences of long-term inactivity of muscles?

______________________________________________

______________________________________________

4. What are the musculoskeletal changes caused by lack of mobility?

______________________________________________

______________________________________________

5. What are clavicles?

______________________________________________

______________________________________________

## SECTION II: APPLYING WHAT YOU KNOW

**Activity G** *Answer the following questions based on the musculoskeletal system.*

A nurse needs to have a thorough understanding of the musculoskeletal system to be able to care for clients with disorders of the musculoskeletal system.

1. What are the musculoskeletal changes caused by lack of mobility?
2. What are the major bones that form the hand and wrist?

## SECTION III: GETTING READY FOR NCLEX

**Activity H** *Answer the following questions.*

1. The nurse observes that a client, who has been prescribed a week of complete bed rest and a regimen of isometric exercises, prefers to lie in a fetal position. Which of the following are possible serious long-term consequences of maintaining this posture for prolonged periods?
   a. Bone density will gradually decrease.
   b. Muscles may remain contracted.
   c. The client may develop a sore back.
   d. Muscles may atrophy completely.
2. Which of the following muscles initiates movement?
   a. Antagonist
   b. Synergistic
   c. Prime mover
   d. Intercostal

**3.** Which of the following is the strongest bone in the human body?

**a.** Humerus

**b.** Tibia

**c.** Scapula

**d.** Femur

**4.** Which of the following is the major difference between the skull of a newborn infant and that of an adult?

**a.** Three pairs of bones of the middle ear are missing in newborns.

**b.** The lower mandible is incapable of movement in the infant.

**c.** Sutures are not rigid and permit movement of cranial muscles in the infant.

**d.** The newborn's cranium has several fontanels located between the cranial bones.

**5.** Which of the following is a characteristic of a synovial joint?

**a.** Allows movement in only one plane

**b.** Allows bones to slide against each other

**c.** Allows all movements except axial rotation

**d.** Allows movements in several directions

**6.** Which of the following conditions is termed as a "slipped" disk?

**a.** An intervertebral disk that has shifted out of position

**b.** A protrusion in the walls of the disk

**c.** Abnormal lateral curvature of the spine

**d.** Exaggeration of the normal lumbar spine curve

**7.** Which of the following interventions should the nurse perform when caring for a client on bed rest? (Select all that apply.)

**a.** Adjust the client's body to positions that do not cause strain.

**b.** Instruct the client to lie in a fetal position.

**c.** Encourage the client to perform isometric exercises.

**d.** Ensure that the client does not change positions frequently.

**e.** Support the client on his or her first time out of bed.

**8.** What are the effects of aging on the musculoskeletal system? (Select all that apply.)

**a.** Osteoporosis

**b.** Osteoarthritis

**c.** Kyphosis

**d.** Osteomalacia

**e.** Lordosis

**9.** A client is on bed rest following a knee replacement. What is the specific musculoskeletal change that can result in blood clots in the legs?

**a.** Decreased joint flexibility

**b.** Decreased muscle tone

**c.** Decreased muscle strength

**d.** Decreased muscle activity

**10.** A client who is pregnant has been ordered to be on complete bed rest for 2 weeks. What type of exercise should the nurse encourage the client to do?

**a.** Isometric

**b.** Isotonic

**c.** Aerobic

**d.** Anaerobic

CHAPTER 19

# The Nervous System

## SECTION I: TESTING WHAT YOU KNOW

**Activity A** *Match the parts of the neuron in Column A with their functions in Column B.*

| Column A | Column B |
|---|---|
| ____ 1. Axon | a. A junction or space between the axon of one neuron and dendrites of the next |
| ____ 2. Dendrites | b. Allows nerve impulses to cross the synapse and reach the dendrites |
| ____ 3. Synapse | c. Carries impulses away from the neuron cell body |
| ____ 4. Neurotransmitter | d. Short, highly branched extensions that receive impulses from the axons of other neurons and transmit these impulses toward the cell body |

**Activity B** *Match the cranial nerves in Column A with their functions in Column B.*

| Column A | Column B |
|---|---|
| ____ 1. Olfactory | a. Enervates the sternocleidomastoid |
| ____ 2. Trochlear | b. Carries impulses for the sense of smell |
| ____ 3. Abducent | c. Controls an extraocular muscle |
| ____ 4. Accessory | d. Enervates a muscle that moves the eyeball |

**Activity C** *Mark each statement as either "T" (True) or "F" (False). Correct any false statements.*

1. T F Motor (efferent) neurons receive and transmit messages from the central nervous system to all parts of the body.
2. T F The homeostatic mechanism that balances the parasympathetic nervous system is the sympathetic nervous system (SNS).
3. T F The left hemisphere of the brain controls the muscles of, and receives sensory information from, the left side of the body.
4. T F The axon is the basic structural and functional cell of the nervous system.
5. T F Visual and auditory reflexes are integrated in the midbrain.
6. T F The number of neuroglia found in the body is five times greater than the number of neurons found in the body.
7. T F An axon surrounded by a myelin sheath is said to be myelinated.

**Activity D** *Fill in the blanks.*

1. The ____________ is the basic structural and functional cell of the nervous system.
2. A/an ____________ is an extension that carries impulses away from the neuron cell body.
3. ____________ are short, often highly branched extensions of the cell body.
4. ____________ axons conduct impulses more rapidly than unmyelinated axons.

**5.** A ____________ is a chemical that an axon releases to allow nerve impulses to cross the synapse and therefore reach the dendrites.

**6.** The thalamus is located in the ____________ portion of the brain, between the hemispheres and the brain stem.

**7.** Eighty percent of the brain's volume is the ____________ which fills the upper part of the skull cavity.

**Activity E** *Consider the following figures.*

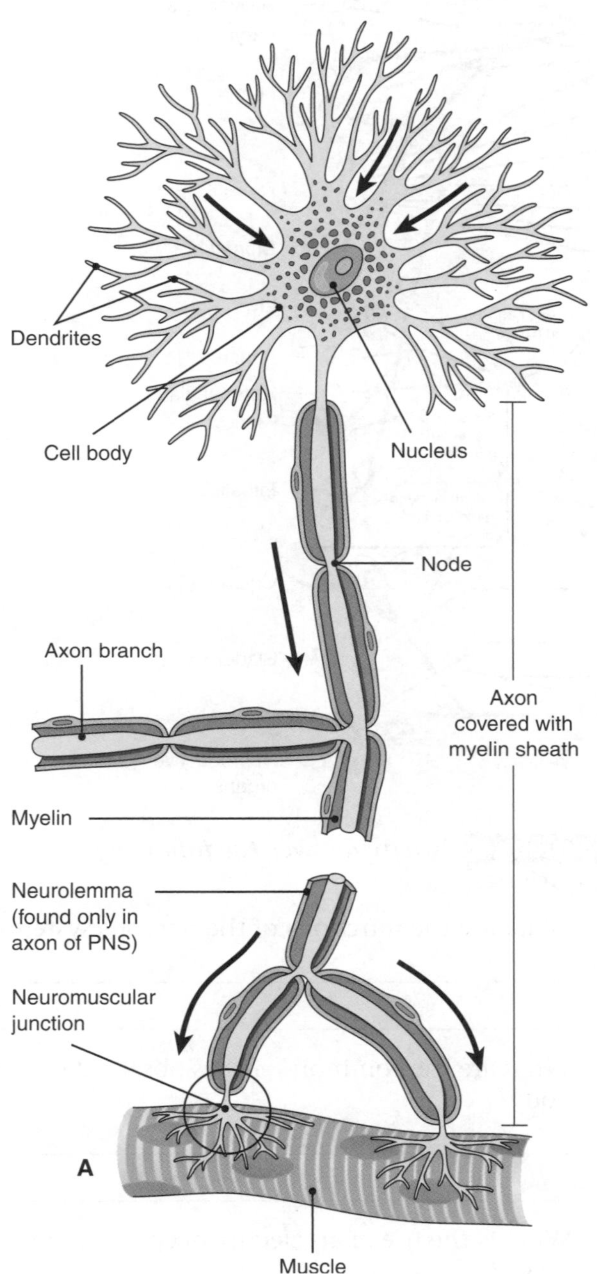


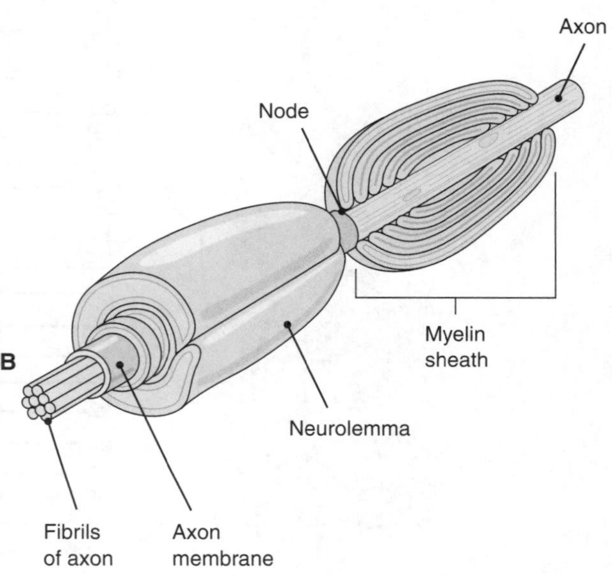


**1.** Identify the type of neuron.

______________________________________

______________________________________

**2.** What are its functions?

______________________________________

______________________________________

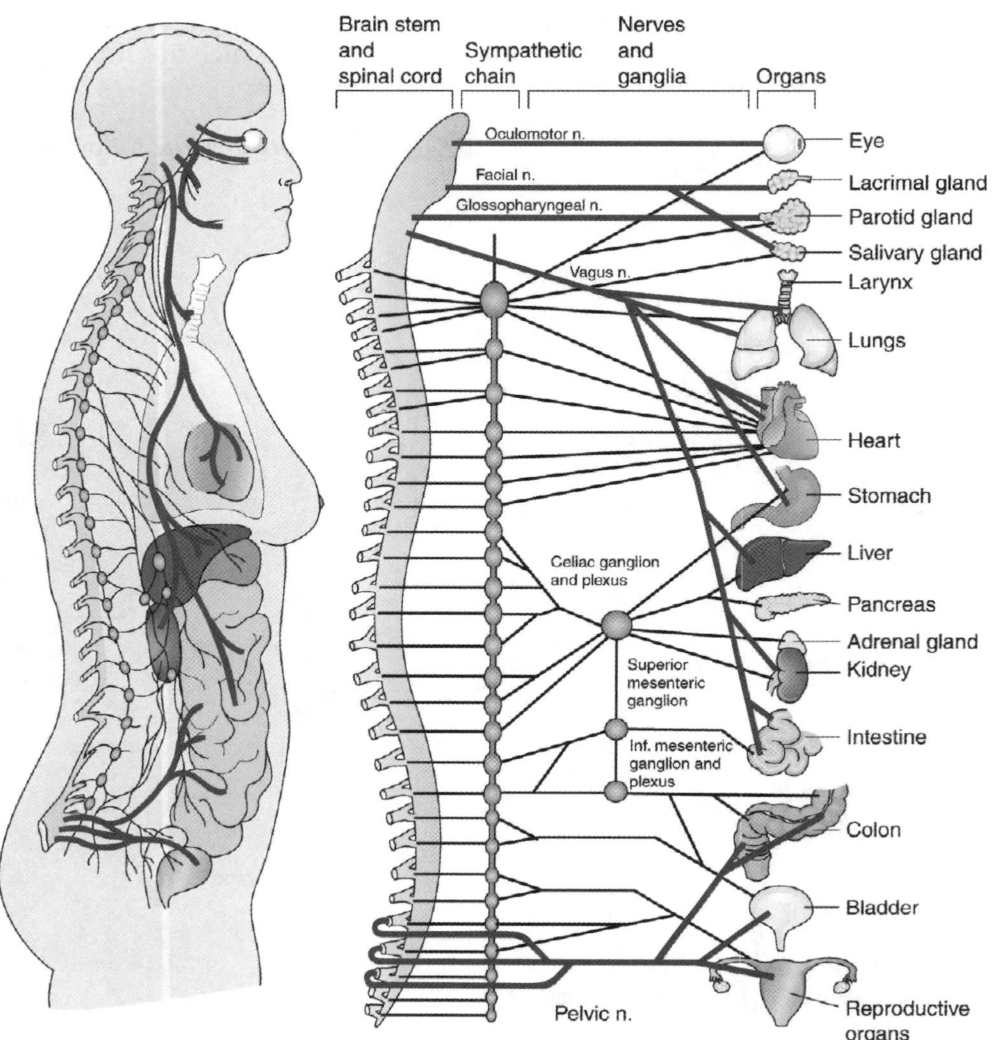


3. Distinguish between the parasympathetic and sympathetic nervous systems.

_______________________________________________

_______________________________________________

4. When does the sympathetic division of the autonomic nervous system (ANS) produce a response?

_______________________________________________

_______________________________________________

5. What are the effects of the parasympathetic division of the ANS on the organs of the body?

_______________________________________________

_______________________________________________

**Activity F** ***Briefly answer the following questions.***

1. What are the functions of the nervous system?

_______________________________________________

_______________________________________________

2. What are the common reflexes observed in the body?

_______________________________________________

_______________________________________________

3. What is the use of an electroencephalogram (EEG)?

_______________________________________________

_______________________________________________

4. What are the functions of pons in the nervous system?

_______________________________________________

_______________________________________________

5. What does increased intracranial pressure (ICP) signify?

_______________________________________________

_______________________________________________

## SECTION II: APPLYING WHAT YOU KNOW

**Activity G** *Answer the following questions based on the nervous system.*

The nurse assists and educates clients about the structure and function of the nervous system and the components of the brain.

1. A nurse is caring for a client who is diagnosed with an injury to the cervical plexus.
   a. What consequences of an injury to the plexuses should the nurse monitor for in the client?
   b. What effect of an injury to the cervical plexus should the nurse be aware of?
2. A nurse is caring for a client with an injured spinal cord.
   a. What effects of spinal cord injuries should the nurse monitor for in the client?
   b. What adverse effect should the nurse be aware of if an injury is caused close to where the brain and spinal cord connect?

## SECTION III: GETTING READY FOR NCLEX

**Activity H** *Answer the following questions.*

1. A nurse is caring for a client who is being treated for a nervous system disorder. What clinical assessment should the nurse conduct to see whether the nervous system is working properly?
   a. The nurse should test the cerebrospinal fluid.
   b. The nurse should check for deep tendon reflexes.
   c. The nurse should test the fluid leaking from the nose.
   d. The nurse should check for reflex control of the heart rate.
2. For which of the following effects should the nurse monitor the client who has had a stroke?
   a. Slower heart rate
   b. Damage to the respiratory center
   c. Paralysis of the body
   d. Constriction of the pupil
3. Which of the following is the function of the myelin sheath around an axon?
   a. To provide a link between sensory and motor neurons
   b. To transmit impulses toward the cell body
   c. To prevent continuous responses to the receiving cell
   d. To electrically insulate the nerve cell
4. A nurse is caring for a client with a head injury caused by a bicycle accident. Which of the following could be the consequence of an injury close to where the brain and spinal cord connect?
   a. Damage to the respiratory center
   b. Temporary or permanent paralysis
   c. Fracture or the dislocation of vertebrae
   d. Heavy bleeding in the central gray matter
5. A nurse is caring for a client with a neurologic problem who has been advised to have an electroencephalogram (EEG). What information should the nurse provide the client and family regarding the use of an EEG?
   a. It records the electrical activity of neurons.
   b. It electrically insulates the nerve cells.
   c. It receives and transmits messages to the central nervous system.
   d. It enables the association of impressions and information.
6. Which of the following conditions are the effects of aging on the nervous system? (Select all that apply.)
   a. Electrolyte imbalances
   b. True dementia
   c. Loss of equilibrium
   d. Respiratory arrest
   e. Temporary paralysis

7. A nurse is caring for a client who is diagnosed with increased intracranial pressure (ICP). What condition might increased ICP indicate?
   a. Atherosclerosis
   b. Herniation of the brain
   c. Hydrocephalus
   d. Alzheimer's disease

8. Which of the following nursing interventions should the nurse implement when caring for elderly clients? (Select all that apply.)
   a. Treat the clients as normal and intelligent.
   b. Educate the clients about the various illnesses.
   c. Evaluate any changes in the personality of the clients.
   d. Encourage the clients to take herbal or folk remedies.
   e. Caution the clients against excessive use of sleep aids.

9. Which of the following is a function of the nervous system?
   a. It monitors information from internal stimuli.
   b. It acts as a shock absorber for the brain and spinal cord.
   c. It connects the brain to the spinal cord.
   d. It carries messages between the cerebrum and medulla.

10. Which of the following is a function of the thalamus?
   a. It regulates body temperature.
   b. It adjusts to impulses from the proprioceptors.
   c. It integrates sensations.
   d. It regulates visceral activities.

CHAPTER 20

# The Endocrine System

## SECTION I: TESTING WHAT YOU KNOW

**Activity A** ***Match the glands associated with the endocrine system in Column A with their corresponding hormones in Column B.***

| Column A | Column B |
|---|---|
| ____ 1. Pineal gland | a. Catecholamines |
| ____ 2. Adrenal gland | b. Glycoproteins |
| ____ 3. Thyroid gland | c. Melatonin |
| ____ 4. Pituitary gland | d. Calcitonin |

**Activity B** ***Match the hormone secreting sites in Column A with their corresponding hormonal functions in Column B.***

| Column A | Column B |
|---|---|
| ____ 1. Placenta | a. Stimulates the gastric glands to secrete gastric juice |
| ____ 2. Kidney | b. Maintains fluid homeostasis |
| ____ 3. Heart | c. Maintains pregnancy |
| ____ 4. Stomach | d. Assists in blood pressure control |

**Activity C** ***Mark each statement as either "T" (True) or "F" (False). Correct any false statements.***

1. T F Endocrine glands secrete hormones, which are transported to target tissues through the nervous system.
2. T F The adrenal medulla secretes hormones that mimic the action of the sympathetic nervous system.
3. T F Oxytocin stimulates the uterus to contract during delivery and helps to keep it contracted after delivery.
4. T F The parathyroids regulate the amount of iron in the blood.
5. T F Glucocorticoids have an important influence on the synthesis of glucose, amino acids, and fats during metabolism.
6. T F The thyroid is responsible for controlling the body's rate of metabolism and the rate at which cells work.

**Activity D** ***Fill in the blanks.***

1. ____________ hormones are active in emergencies or in stressful situations.
2. The disorder that originates from an insufficient dietary intake of iodine is called ____________.
3. As an endocrine gland, the pancreas secretes ____________ which lowers blood sugar.
4. ____________ the hormone secreted by the pineal gland, helps regulate the sleep–wake cycle.
5. ____________ hormone-like substances whose effects are localized to the area in which they are produced, influence blood pressure, respiration, digestion, and reproduction.

**Activity E** *Consider the following figure.*

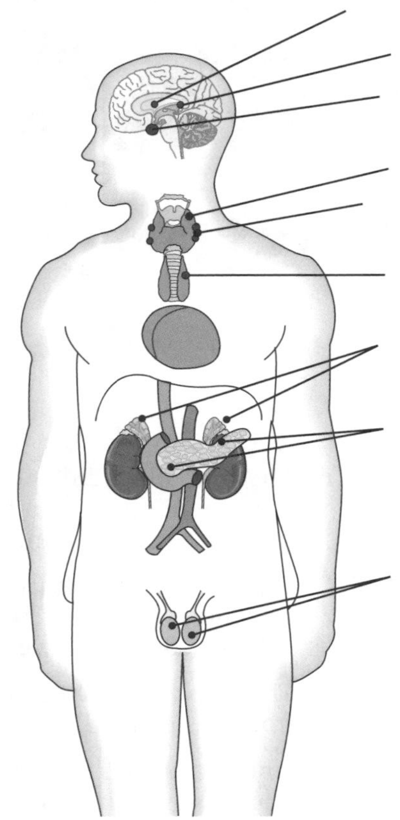

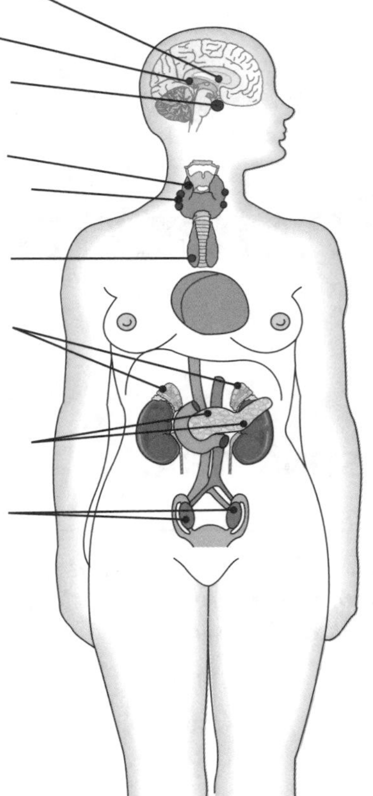

1. Identify the locations of the major endocrine glands in the body on the figure.

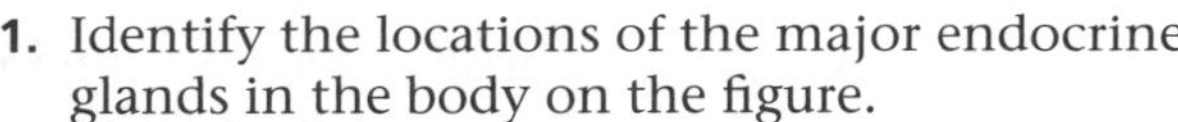

**Activity F** *Briefly answer the following questions.*

1. What is the effect of epinephrine on the body?

_______________________________________________

_______________________________________________

2. What is the function of somatostatin on the human body?

_______________________________________________

_______________________________________________

3. What is the function of hormones secreted by the placenta?

_______________________________________________

_______________________________________________

4. What is the function of parathormone or parathyroid hormone (PTH)?

_______________________________________________

_______________________________________________

5. What is the function of T cells?

_______________________________________________

_______________________________________________

6. What is the function of melanocyte-stimulating hormone (MSH)?

_______________________________________________

_______________________________________________

## SECTION II: APPLYING WHAT YOU KNOW

**Activity G** *Answer the following questions, which involve understanding of the endocrine system.*

The nurse educates clients about the structure and function of the endocrine system and treatment of endocrinologic disorders.

1. A client with diabetes mellitus is prescribed insulin. The client is eager to know how insulin will help to control his glucose level.
   a. What information should the nurse provide the client regarding the action of insulin in controlling the glucose level?
   b. What is the consequence if there is a lack of insulin or if the insulin is not working as it should?
2. A nurse caring for elderly clients in an extended healthcare facility is required to educate the clients on the effects of aging on the endocrine system.
   a. What are the factors that affect the endocrine system as a result of aging?
   b. What are the special problems for older adults related to the endocrine system?
   c. What measures should the nurse take to prevent/minimize these problems?

## SECTION III: GETTING READY FOR NCLEX

**Activity H** *Answer the following questions.*

1. Which of the following is the function of hormones secreted by the lining of the upper part of the small intestine?
   a. Stimulate the pancreas to release pancreatic juice
   b. Release digestive enzymes into the duct system
   c. Control the blood's glucose level
   d. Inhibit the release of insulin and glucagon
2. A nurse observes which of the following conditions in a client with diminished T-cell count?
   a. Low blood pressure
   b. Diminished immune response
   c. Decreased metabolic rate
   d. Muscle twitching and spasms
3. Which of the following are influenced by the prostaglandins? (Select all that apply.)
   a. Blood pressure
   b. Body temperature
   c. Pulse rate
   d. Respiration
   e. Reproduction
4. When educating a client with high blood pressure, the nurse identifies which of the following hormones as assisting in blood pressure control?
   a. Erythropoietin
   b. Renin
   c. Prostaglandins
   d. Glucagon
5. Which of the following special problems for older individuals are related to the endocrine system? (Select all that apply.)
   a. Decrease in voluntary movements
   b. Lack of dexterity
   c. Hirsutism in women
   d. Loss of pubic hair
   e. Decreased metabolic rate
6. When educating a postpartum client, the nurse identifies which of the following hormones as responsible for lactation?
   a. Prolactin
   b. Vasopressin
   c. Calcitonin
   d. Calcitriol

7. Which of the following is a hormone that stimulates reabsorption of sodium into the plasma, resulting in increased water reabsorption and, therefore, an increase in blood volume?
   a. Androgen
   b. Estrogen
   c. Progestin
   d. Aldosterone
8. Which of the following hormones is secreted when the blood calcium level is too low?
   a. Parathormone
   b. Calcitonin
   c. Vasopressin
   d. Aldosterone
9. Which of the following signs should a nurse monitor for when caring for clients taking glucocorticoids? (Select all that apply.)
   a. Moon face
   b. Hirsutism
   c. Large abdomen
   d. Convulsions
   e. Buffalo hump
10. Which of the following are functions of growth hormone? (Select all that apply.)
    a. Stimulates red blood cell production
    b. Stimulates growth in all body tissues
    c. Aids in the release of fatty acids from adipose
    d. Helps to regulate blood nutrient levels after eating
    e. Stimulates the breakdown of fats and proteins

CHAPTER 21

# The Sensory System

## SECTION I: TESTING WHAT YOU KNOW

**Activity A** *Match the conditions associated with the visual system in Column A with their possible causes in Column B.*

| Column A | Column B |
|---|---|
| ____ 1. Myopia | a. The eyeball is too short and one cannot see close objects clearly. |
| ____ 2. Presbyopia | b. An irregularity in the curvature of the cornea and lens, which cannot bring horizontal and vertical lines into focus, causing blurry vision. |
| ____ 3. Hyperopia | c. Lens muscles contract too tightly, making distant objects blurry. |
| ____ 4. Astigmatism | d. Gradual age-related loss of accommodation. |

**Activity B** *Match the organs of the sensory system in Column A with their functions in Column B.*

| Column A | Column B |
|---|---|
| ____ 1. Iris | a. Focuses the light rays on the retina |
| ____ 2. Eustachian tube | b. Gathers and guides sound waves |
| ____ 3. Pinna | c. Communicates with the nasopharynx |
| ____ 4. Lens | d. Gives the eye its specific color and is known as the pigmented section |

**Activity C** *Mark each statement as either "T" (True) or "F" (False). Correct any false statements.*

1. T F The lacrimal glands, which produce tears, keep the eye's surface moist and lubricated.
2. T F Presbycusis is the gradual loss of the function of accommodation.
3. T F The lens adjusts the light rays to facilitate projection of the rays on the central fovea.
4. T F Bitter tastes are sensed at the back of the tongue.
5. T F A greater number of tactile receptors are located in some areas, such as the fingertips and around the lips.
6. T F In myopia, the focal point of the light rays is behind, instead of directly on, the retina.
7. T F The replacement of taste buds with connective tissue, as a person ages, results in the person's not feeling hungry.

**Activity D** *Fill in the blanks.*

1. The ____________ of the eye is the transparent, tough section over the front of the eyeball.

2. ___________ receptors are located in the areas such as the fingertips and around the lips, constantly receiving nerve impulses with regard to pain and pleasure.
3. ___________ is the high-pitched, buzzing sound or ringing in the ear that often accompanies vertigo.
4. The adjustment of light rays by the lens to make a sharp, clear image is called ___________.
5. Pain that is located in an internal organ system could be described as ___________ pain.

**Activity E** *Consider the following figure.*

1. Label each of the following parts on the figure, and state one function for each.
   a. Iris ___________
   b. Lens ___________
   c. Optic nerve ___________

**Activity F** ***The steps in the path taken by sound waves to reach the brain are given next in random order. Arrange the steps in the correct sequence in the boxes provided.***

1. Sound waves enter through the ear's external auditory canal and strike the tympanic membrane.
2. The stapes vibrates against this membrane, setting the fluid of the cochlea in motion, which in turn passes on to the hair-like nerve ending in the organ of Corti.
3. The tympanic membrane vibrates at various speeds in response to various pitches of sounds.
4. The ossicles within the middle ear act as a movable bridge to transmit these vibrations to the oval window, which amplifies the sound waves.
5. The stimuli from the nerve endings in the organ of Corti are sent to the vestibulocochlear nerve and then to the temporal lobe in the cerebral cortex, where the sounds are interpreted.

☐ → ☐ → ☐ → ☐ → ☐

**Activity G** ***Briefly answer the following questions.***

1. What is the function of the sensory organs in the human body?

___________

___________

2. What is vitreous humor?

___________

___________

3. What is the function of the external ear?

___________

___________

4. What are the factors upon which vision is dependent?

___________

___________

5. What are the effects of aging on the senses of smell and taste?

___________

___________

## SECTION II: APPLYING WHAT YOU KNOW

**Activity H** ***Answer the following questions, which involve understanding of the functioning of the body's sensory system and its various components.***

The nurse assists and educates clients about the structure and function of the sensory system.

1. A nurse is required to teach a group of students about the various parts of the eye and how they protect the eye.
   a. What information should the nurse provide about eyelids and their function?
   b. How will the nurse explain the function of the lacrimal gland?
2. A nurse is caring for a client who has been admitted for a corneal transplant. As part of client education, the nurse is required to explain the function of the cornea. What information should the nurse provide the client?
3. A client complains to the nurse that she often feels dizzy and nauseated and there is a high-pitched, buzzing sound in her ear. What condition is the client most likely experiencing? What may be the cause of this condition?
4. A nurse is required to care for a 65-year-old client with presbycusis.
   a. What is the clinical manifestation of this condition?
   b. What is its common cause?
   c. What are the other causes of impaired hearing in older people?
5. A client who had recently suffered a heart attack had complained about pain in the left arm prior to the attack. How does this pain help in diagnosing a medical condition?
6. A nurse is caring for a child with an inner ear infection. The child's mother is worried because her child is having recurrent ear infections. What information should the nurse provide the mother?

## SECTION III: GETTING READY FOR NCLEX

**Activity I** ***Answer the following questions.***

1. The perception of light, dark, and color takes place in which part of the eye?
   a. Iris
   b. Retina
   c. Pupil
   d. Lens
2. Which of the following nerves is responsible for carrying the sensations of pain in the eye and temperature to the brain?
   a. Optic nerve
   b. Oculomotor nerve
   c. Trochlear nerve
   d. Ophthalmic nerve
3. A nurse is caring for a child with an ear infection. What information should the nurse provide the mother, who wants to know about the function of the hair and wax in the external ear?
   a. They separate the external ear from the middle ear.
   b. They guide the sound waves into the auditory canal.
   c. They transmit vibrations to the fluid-filled inner ear at the oval window.
   d. They protect the ear from foreign objects.
4. Which of the following parts of the eye is responsible for sharpest vision?
   a. Lens
   b. Retina
   c. Central fovea
   d. Iris
5. A 45-year-old client arrives at the community clinic complaining of blurry vision when looking at objects at a distance. Which of the following conditions is the client most likely experiencing?
   a. Hyperopia
   b. Myopia
   c. Astigmatism
   d. Presbyopia

6. Which of the following is the effect of aging on the senses of smell and taste?
   a. Connective tissues replace the taste buds.
   b. Tear formation decreases.
   c. There is an increased buildup of cerumen.
   d. Depth perception decreases.
7. Which of the following is the function of the lens in providing a clear image?
   a. It carries stimuli for vision from each eye.
   b. It regulates the amount of light that enters the eye.
   c. It adjusts light rays to facilitate their projection on the central fovea.
   d. It maintains intraocular pressure.
8. Which of the following could be the cause of impaired hearing in an older person? (Select all that apply.)
   a. Decreased cochlear function
   b. Fusing of the ossicles in the middle ear
   c. Lifelong exposure to loud noises
   d. Gradual loss of the function of accommodation
   e. Replacement of the taste buds with connective tissue
   f. Clouding of the lens
9. Which of the following is a likely consequence of the tympanic membrane's not being able to vibrate freely?
   a. Impaired hearing
   b. Feeling of vertigo
   c. Ringing sounds in the ear
   d. Presbycusis
10. Which of the following parts of the ear is considered the true organ of hearing?
   a. Vestibules
   b. Semicircular canals
   c. Organ of Corti
   d. Labyrinths

CHAPTER 22

# The Cardiovascular System

## SECTION I: TESTING WHAT YOU KNOW

**Activity A** ***Match the layers of the heart in column A with their description in column B.***

| Column A | Column B |
|---|---|
| ____ 1. Endocardium | a. Thick, strong muscles making up the middle layer |
| ____ 2. Myocardium | b. The thin outer layer of the cardiac wall |
| ____ 3. Epicardium | c. A membrane lining the heart's interior wall |
| ____ 4. Fibrous pericardium | d. The outermost layer anchoring the heart |

**Activity B** ***Mark each statement as either "T" (True) or "F" (False). Correct any false statements.***

1. T F Cardiac output is the amount of blood the ventricles pump out in 3 minutes.
2. T F Events in the cardiac cycle create normal and sometimes extra heart sounds.
3. T F Blood pressure is the force exerted by the blood against the walls of the heart.
4. T F The valves of the heart allow unidirectional blood flow through the heart.
5. T F A cardiac cycle consists of the contraction and relaxation of the ventricles, followed by the atria.
6. T F The right and left coronary arteries supply the heart muscle with blood.

**Activity C** ***Fill in the blanks.***

1. The cardiovascular system consists of the heart and the blood ____________.
2. ____________ heartbeats that increase with age should not automatically be considered an indicator of disease.
3. To adapt to the body's metabolic needs, the heart can alter its ____________ output.
4. ____________ is the amount of pressure or resistance the ventricles must overcome to empty their contents.
5. The rhythmic expansion of the arterial wall as the blood flows through it is the ____________.

**Activity D** ***The steps that occur during the process of blood flow through the body are given below in random order. Write the correct sequence in the boxes provided.***

1. It travels through the mitral valve and into the left ventricle.
2. Blood then passes through the tricuspid valve into the right ventricle.
3. Blood then enters the pulmonary artery and lungs, where it receives oxygen.
4. It moves on through the pulmonic valve during ventricular contraction.

5. The right atrium receives *deoxygenated* blood from the superior and inferior vena cava and the coronary sinus.
6. It then returns to the left atrium via the pulmonary veins.

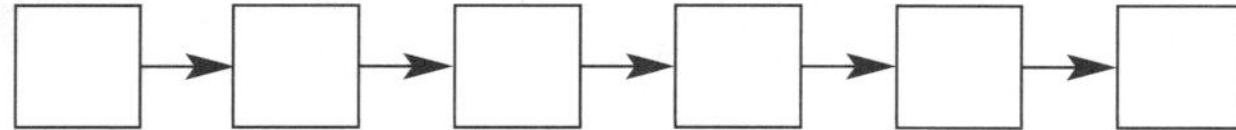

**Activity E** ***Briefly answer the following questions.***

1. What path does blood travel in the body?

_______________________________________________

_______________________________________________

2. What do the cells located at the tips of the toes receive and send?

_______________________________________________

_______________________________________________

3. What are the functions of the cardiovascular system?

_______________________________________________

_______________________________________________

4. What is the function of the pericardial fluid?

_______________________________________________

_______________________________________________

5. Which are the centers for receiving blood?

_______________________________________________

_______________________________________________

## SECTION II: APPLYING WHAT YOU KNOW

**Activity F** ***Answer the following questions, which involve understanding of the functioning of the cardiovascular system.***

The nurse assists and educates clients about the structure and function of the cardiovascular system and its components.

1. A nurse is required to educate a group of students about the structure of the heart.
   a. What information should the nurse provide regarding the three major layers of the heart wall?
   b. What information should the nurse provide regarding how the layers of the heart relate to the pericardium?
2. The nurse is educating a group of students about the heart's chambers and the muscular septum wall.
   a. What information can she give about the division of the heart into right and left sides?
   b. What information can she give about the four chambers into which the heart is divided?
3. How are the pulmonary arteries and pulmonary veins different from other arteries and veins?
4. A nurse is explaining the physiology of the heart with reference to heartbeats and pumping.
   a. What makes the implantation of an electronic pacemaker necessary?
   b. What activities occur before a heartbeat?

## SECTION III: GETTING READY FOR NCLEX

**Activity G** ***Answer the following questions.***

1. What is the function of the pericardial cavity?
   a. Acts as a lubricant and reduces friction between the layers of the heart
   b. Makes up the pericardium's visceral layer and adheres to the heart's surface
   c. Anchors the heart in the mediastinum and prevents overfilling
   d. Acts as a sac that surrounds and protects the heart as a whole
2. What is the function of the fibrous pericardium?
   a. Makes up the pericardium's visceral layer and adheres to the heart's surface
   b. Anchors the heart in the mediastinum and prevents overfilling
   c. Acts as a lubricant and reduces friction between the layers of the heart
   d. Acts as a sac that surrounds and protects the heart as a whole

3. What is the function of the cardiac valves?
   a. Contract with sufficient force to pump blood
   b. Act as receiving centers for blood
   c. Divide the heart into right and left sides
   d. Allow blood to flow in one direction only
4. Which of the following is the primary function of the capillary walls in the circulation system?
   a. Draining of blood from the anterior surface of the heart
   b. Branching out to supply blood to the inferior septum
   c. Exchanging of oxygen and nutrition that takes place
   d. Supplying heart tissue with oxygen and nourishment
5. Why does the heart muscle need its own blood supply?
   a. To exit into the aorta and out to the systemic circulation
   b. To fill the semilunar cusps and cause the valves to close
   c. To prevent the valve cusps from everting (turning inside out)
   d. To provide oxygen and nourishment to the heart tissue
6. How does the oxygenated blood enter the systemic circulation?
   a. During ventricular contraction, the blood exits into systemic circulation through the aorta.
   b. During ventricular contraction, the papillary muscles contract to pump blood.
   c. The LAD descends along the anterior intraventricular groove to provide oxygenated blood.
   d. During ventricular contraction, the blood moves to enter the pulmonary artery and lungs.
7. A client with a cardiovascular disorder has an order for an electronic pacemaker. The nurse knows that the electronic pacemaker is used for what condition?
   a. Lipid accumulation
   b. Poor functioning of the SA node
   c. Increased incidence of heart block
   d. Calcification of vessel walls
8. The daughter of a 78-year-old client diagnosed with increased incidence of heart blockage asks the nurse why this may have happened. The nurse explains that older adults are at an increased risk for heart blocks related to which of the following?
   a. Lipid accumulation
   b. Decreased number of pacemaker cells in the SA node
   c. Calcification of vessel walls
   d. Decreased fibers in the bundle of His
9. The nurse is educating the client about the heart. Which of the following is an accurate description of the endocardium?
   a. Thick strong muscles making up the middle layer
   b. The thin outer layer of the cardiac wall
   c. A membrane lining the heart's interior wall
   d. The outermost layer anchoring the heart
10. The nurse is teaching the client about the four chambers of the heart. Which is the thickest chamber?
    a. Left ventricle
    b. Right ventricle
    c. Left atrium
    d. Right atrium

CHAPTER 23

# The Hematologic and Lymphatic Systems

## SECTION I: TESTING WHAT YOU KNOW

**Activity A** ***Match the terms associated with the hematologic and lymphatic system in Column A with their descriptions in Column B.***

| Column A | Column B |
|---|---|
| ____ 1. Phagocytosis | a. Formation of red blood cells |
| ____ 2. Pinocytosis | b. Consist of the basophils, neutrophils, and eosinophils |
| ____ 3. Erythropoiesis | c. Engulfing of particulate matter |
| ____ 4. Agranulocytes | d. Engulfing of extracellular fluid materials |
| ____ 5. Granulocytes | e. Consist of the monocytes and lymphocytes |

**Activity B** ***Match the blood cells in Column A with their average lifespans in Column B.***

| Column A | Column B |
|---|---|
| ____ 1. Red blood cells | a. 12 hours to 3 days |
| ____ 2. Eosinophils | b. 10 hours |
| ____ 3. Neutrophils | c. 100 to 300 days |
| ____ 4. Monocytes and lymphocytes | d. 120 days |

**Activity C** ***Mark each statement as either "T" (True) or "F" (False). Correct any false statements.***

1. T F Hematopoiesis refers to the destruction of blood cells.
2. T F Erythropoietin is secreted by the kidneys in adults.
3. T F Lymph nodes produce red blood cells.
4. T F Blood is composed of plasma and red blood cells, white blood cells, and platelets.
5. T F Blood plasma consists of 60% water and 40% primarily plasma proteins.
6. T F Platelets are the smallest of the blood's formed elements essential for clotting.

**Activity D** ***Fill in the blanks.***

1. ____________ a glycoprotein-type hormone, stimulates the stem cells of bone marrow to produce the red blood cells.
2. The functions of the ____________ system include transportation of nutrients and oxygen to the cells, blood volume regulation, and production of blood cells and antibodies.
3. The formation of blood cells originating in ____________ cells in red bone marrow is called hematopoiesis or hemopoiesis.
4. Vitamin ____________ is necessary for the formation of prothrombin and other clotting factors.

5. A bacterial infection would most likely produce an increase in ___________ which are considered to be first in the line of defense against bacteria.

**Activity E** ***The steps that occur during the process of production and circulation of blood through the body are given below in random order. Write the correct sequence in the boxes provided.***

1. Blood carries out the transportation of oxygen, carbon dioxide, nutrients, heat, waste products, and hormones.
2. Blood is carried through a closed system of vessels pumped by the heart.
3. Lymph nodes, spleen, and thymus contribute to additional production and maturation of agranular white blood cells.
4. Blood in the general (systemic) circulation returns to the right atrium of the heart.
5. The red bone marrow manufactures all blood cells.

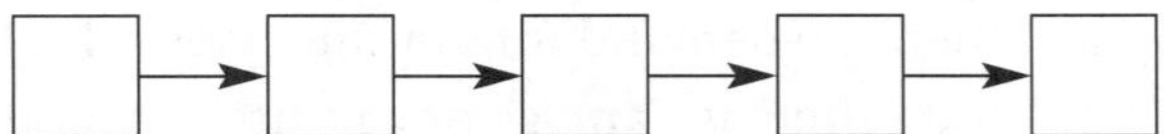

**Activity F** ***Briefly answer the following questions.***

1. Differentiate between the hematologic system and the lymphatic system.

_______________________________________________

_______________________________________________

2. What are antibodies?

_______________________________________________

_______________________________________________

3. What is the function of the iron in hemoglobin?

_______________________________________________

_______________________________________________

4. Differentiate between white blood cells (WBCs) and red blood cells (RBCs).

_______________________________________________

_______________________________________________

5. What is hemostasis?

_______________________________________________

_______________________________________________

## SECTION II: APPLYING WHAT YOU KNOW

**Activity G** ***Answer the following questions, which involve understanding of the functioning of the body's hematologic and lymphatic systems and their various components.***

Blood is a versatile vascular fluid that maintains homeostasis via its viscosity (thickness), its ability to carry dissolved substances, and its ability to move to all body parts.

1. A client visiting a healthcare clinic for a complete blood count test seeks information on the composition and function of blood.
   a. What is the primary objective of blood?
   b. What are the components of blood?
2. A nurse is educating a client on the difference between blood and other connective tissues.
   a. Why is blood considered a connective tissue?
   b. How is blood different from other connective tissues?
3. During a lecture on the lymphatic system, the nurse explains to student nurses the constituents of lymph and the networking of lymphatic vessels.
   a. What are lymphatic vessels?
   b. What is known as the lymph?
   c. How does the lymphatic fluid move through the body?
4. A nurse is caring for a client with an injury. The blood along the wound has already clotted. The nurse explains to the client the importance of clotting.
   a. Why is the clotting of blood important?
   b. Explain the process of the clotting of blood.

## SECTION III: GETTING READY FOR NCLEX

**Activity H** *Answer the following questions.*

1. Which of the following is a function of blood?
   a. To destroy old used red blood corpuscles
   b. To filter and destroy pathogens
   c. To develop antibodies against antigens
   d. To regulate pH and body temperature
2. Which of the following is a function of albumin?
   a. To absorb the salts from food for use by body cells
   b. To maintain fluid volume and blood pressure
   c. To contribute to the body's chemical and fluid balance
   d. To protect against blood loss and foreign body invasion
3. Which of the following is a description of the structure or function of antibodies?
   a. They are insoluble threads that entrap red blood cells and platelets.
   b. They decrease the release of chemical mediators during allergic reactions.
   c. They are materials synthesized by the body in response to antigens.
   d. They are involved in phagocytosis and defense against bacteria.
4. Which of the following describes hematopoiesis or hemopoiesis?
   a. Clumping of cells
   b. Engulfing and devouring of invaders
   c. Process of forming fibrin
   d. Formation of blood cells
5. Which of the following factors controls the chemical and acid–base balance of the blood?
   a. Maintenance of the electrolytic salts within the plasma
   b. Volume of circulating blood with individual body size
   c. Manufacturing of formed elements of the blood
   d. Removal of the hematologic waste products
6. Which of the following promotes the clotting of blood?
   a. Albumin
   b. Globulin
   c. Prothrombin
   d. Heparin
7. Which of the following is a characteristic of erythrocytes?
   a. They contain nuclei and move in an ameboid fashion.
   b. They are heavier and more viscous than water.
   c. They are the largest group of plasma proteins.
   d. They are the most numerous of the blood cells.
8. Under which of the following conditions is histamine released in the body?
   a. When there is a foreign invader in the body
   b. When hemoglobin is saturated with oxygen
   c. When the demand for granulocytes is high
   d. When there is damage or rupture to blood vessels
9. The nurse is educating a group of high school biology students about the lifespan of blood cells. What is the average lifespan of red blood cells?
   a. 10 hours
   b. 12 hours to 3 days
   c. 200 to 300 days
   d. 120 days
10. A client has developed a bacterial infection. What cells will be increased and are considered the first line of defense against bacteria?
    a. Granulocytes
    b. Agranulocytes
    c. Neutrophils
    d. Pinocytosis

CHAPTER 24

# The Immune System

## SECTION I: TESTING WHAT YOU KNOW

**Activity A** *Match the different types of antibodies in Column A with their functions in Column B.*

| Column A | Column B |
|---|---|
| ____ 1. IgD | a. Helps in defense against invasion of microbes via nose, eyes, lungs, and intestines |
| ____ 2. IgE | b. Protects fetus before birth against antitoxins, viruses, and bacteria |
| ____ 3. IgA | c. Functions as an antigen receptor |
| ____ 4. IgG | d. Stimulates complement activity |
| ____ 5. IgM | e. Helpful in the developing world in fighting against parasitic infections |

**Activity B** *Match the type of immunity in Column A with its related occurrence in Column B.*

| Column A | Column B |
|---|---|
| ____ 1. Artificially acquired passive immunity | a. Occurs between a mother and her infant |
| ____ 2. Naturally acquired active immunity | b. Occurs through injection of a causative agent into the person's system |
| ____ 3. Naturally acquired passive immunity | c. Occurs when a child is exposed to, or develops, a disease |
| ____ 4. Artificially acquired active immunity | d. Occurs with the injection of ready-made antibodies into the person's system |

**Activity C** *Mark each statement as either "T" (True) or "F" (False). Correct any false statements.*

1. T F The immune system in humans consists only of specific immune system responses.
2. T F Clones of B cells that do not become plasma cells disintegrate.
3. T F IgA protects the fetus before birth against antitoxins, viruses, and bacteria.
4. T F B lymphocytes are responsible for antibody production.
5. T F Natural killer cells produce humoral immunity.
6. T F Persons exposed to latex allergies develop autoimmune disorders.

**Activity D** *Fill in the blanks.*

1. ____________ is the body's ability to recognize and destroy specific pathogens and to prevent infectious diseases.
2. An ____________ is any foreign substance or molecule entering the body that stimulates an immune response.
3. An ____________ is a protein substance that the body produces in response to an antigen.

4. Along with the bone marrow, the ___________ is considered a central or primary lymphoid organ.

5. T lymphocytes produce an immunity called ___________ immunity.

**Activity E** ***Steps that occur during the process of complement fixation for antigen destruction are given below in random order. Write the correct sequence in the boxes provided.***

1. Complements help in the formation of highly specialized antigen–antibody complexes.
2. Sodium and water flow into cell, causing it to burst open.
3. Complexes cause holes to develop in the cell membrane.
4. Complements become active.
5. Specific cells are targeted.

☐ → ☐ → ☐ → ☐ → ☐

**Activity F** ***Briefly answer the following questions.***

1. What are the two types of immune responses?

___________________________________

___________________________________

2. What is immunity?

___________________________________

___________________________________

3. What kind of differentiation in lymphocytes must occur before detection of foreign invaders begin?

___________________________________

___________________________________

4. What are antigens? Where are they found?

___________________________________

___________________________________

5. What is the function of IgA?

___________________________________

___________________________________

6. Why are some cells called natural killer cells?

___________________________________

___________________________________

7. What are the peripheral organs?

___________________________________

___________________________________

## SECTION II: APPLYING WHAT YOU KNOW

**Activity G** ***Answer the following questions, which involve understanding of the functioning of the body's immune system and its various components.***

The nurse assists and educates clients about the structure and function of the immune system.

1. A nurse is required to educate a group of students about lymphocytes and their importance in the immune system.
   a. What information should the nurse give on the formation of lymphocytes in the immune system?
   b. What information should the nurse give on the importance of lymphocytes in the immune system?
2. A nurse is caring for a client who has undergone organ transplant surgery.
   a. How are T cells responsible for tissue and organ rejection after organ transplantation?
   b. What medications should be given by the nurse when a client's body rejects transplanted tissue and organs?
3. A nurse is caring for a 14-year-old client with measles. The client has studied about non-specific defense mechanisms in school and wants to know more about them. What information does the nurse provide the client on the various non-specific defense mechanisms in the body?
4. A nurse is addressing a group of PN students about caring for a client with an immune system disorder. The nurse is required to communicate the importance of the thymus in the immune system.

a. What is the importance of the thymus in the immune system?
b. What are the hormones produced by the thymus? What are their functions?

## SECTION III: GETTING READY FOR NCLEX

**Activity H** *Answer the following questions.*

1. A nurse caring for a client with measles understands that which of the following defense mechanisms has occurred in the client's immune system?
   a. Humoral immunity
   b. Complement fixation
   c. Immunologic memory
   d. Cell-mediated immunity
2. Which of the following times in the life cycle is marked by atrophy of the thymus?
   a. Early in life
   b. Middle age
   c. Old age
   d. Puberty
3. Which of the following causes scleroderma?
   a. Immunodeficiency
   b. Specific immunity
   c. Autoimmune reaction
   d. Latex allergy
4. Which of the following provides the type of antibody generated by a tetanus booster?
   a. IgM
   b. IgD
   c. IgA
   d. IgE
5. Which part of the immune system produces antibodies?
   a. B cells
   b. T cells
   c. Natural killer cells
   d. Phagocytes
6. Which of the following is the effect of chickenpox on the immune system?
   a. It will build naturally acquired passive immunity.
   b. It will build naturally acquired active immunity.
   c. It will build artificially acquired passive immunity.
   d. It will build artificially acquired active immunity.
7. A mother passes the necessary immunity on to her infant. What type of immunity does this represent?
   a. Artificially acquired passive immunity
   b. Naturally acquired active immunity
   c. Naturally acquired passive immunity
   d. Artificially acquired active immunity
8. The nurse is educating a client about how the immune system functions. What term should the nurse tell the client is used to describe any foreign substance or molecule entering the body that stimulates an immune response?
   a. Antibody
   b. Antigen
   c. Cell-mediated
   d. Humoral
9. The nurse is reviewing the organs involved in the body's immune system. What are the functions of T cells? (Select all that apply.)
   a. Help protect against viral infections.
   b. Can detect and destroy some cancer cells.
   c. Produce antibodies.
   d. Produce plasma cells.
   e. Create antigens
10. The nurse is educating a group of students about different types of white blood cells. What types of cells are agranular white blood cells? (Select all that apply.)
   a. Neutrophils
   b. Basophils
   c. Eosinophils
   d. Monocytes
   e. Lymphocytes

CHAPTER 25

# The Respiratory System

## SECTION I: TESTING WHAT YOU KNOW

**Activity A** *Match the part of the respiratory system in Column A with its function in Column B.*

| Column A | Column B |
|---|---|
| ____ 1. Olfactory nerve | a. Providing resonance for the voice |
| ____ 2. Sinuses | b. Guarding the entrance of the larynx |
| ____ 3. Auditory tubes | c. Carrying nerve impulses to the brain |
| ____ 4. Epiglottis | d. Connecting the nasopharynx to the middle ear |

**Activity B** *Mark each statement as either "T" (True) or "F" (False). Correct any false statements.*

1. T F The enlargement of the adenoids causes snoring or obstruction of the upper airway.
2. T F The esophagus transports air from the pharynx to the stomach.
3. T F The parietal pleura covers the lungs.
4. T F Breathing air in is called inhalation or inspiration.
5. T F Normal respiration is called dyspnea.
6. T F Coughing is needed to dislodge material from the respiratory passage.

**Activity C** *Fill in the blanks.*

1. The ____________ is a dome-shaped muscle that separates the thoracic and abdominal cavities.
2. The ____________ is the part of the pharynx that extends from the uvula to the epiglottis.
3. A lid or cover of cartilages called the ____________ guards the entrance to the larynx.
4. The function of the ____________ is to allow the lungs to move without causing pain or friction against the chest walls.
5. The exchange of oxygen for carbon dioxide within the alveoli of the lungs is called ____________ respiration.

**Activity D** *Consider the following figure.*

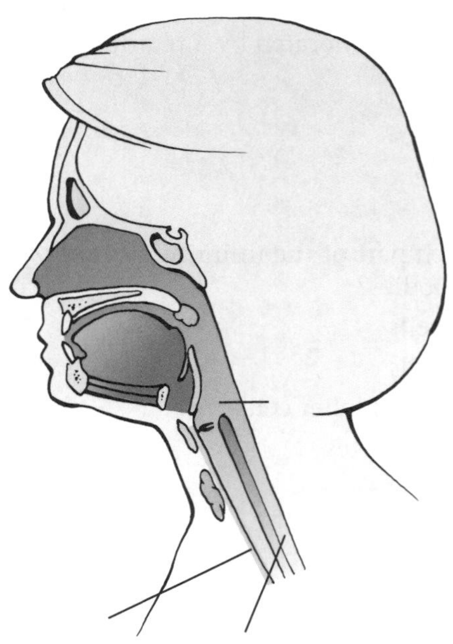

1. Label each of the following parts of the figure; then list the functions for each.
   a. Esophagus

      ______________________________

      ______________________________

   b. Trachea

      ______________________________

      ______________________________

   c. Larynx

      ______________________________

      ______________________________

**Activity E** ***The organs of the respiratory system are given below in random order. Write the correct sequence in which they function during respiration, from the nose to the lungs, in the boxes provided.***

1. Trachea
2. Larynx
3. Epiglottis
4. Nasal cavity
5. Alveolar sac
6. Nasopharynx

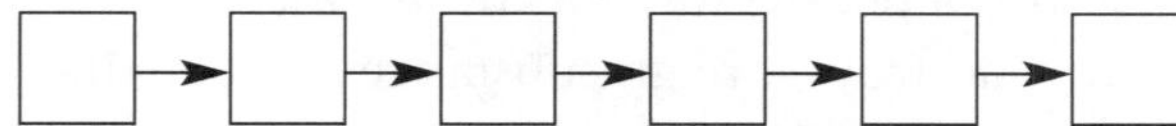

**Activity F** ***Briefly answer the following questions.***

1. What are the processes of respiration?
2. What are the effects of aging on the respiratory system?
3. What are the two types of respiration?
4. What is the nasal septum, and what is its function?
5. How many sets of tonsils can be found in the oropharynx, and where are they located?

## SECTION II: APPLYING WHAT YOU KNOW

**Activity G** ***Answer the following questions, which involve understanding of the functioning of the respiratory system and its components.***

The nurse assists and educates clients about the structure and function of the immune system.

1. A client has been admitted to the healthcare center with a sinus problem. What are the sinuses, and how do they get infected?
2. A client who had been involved in a serious accident has suffered a puncture wound to the chest. Why is it important that this wound be closed immediately?
3. A nurse is conducting a session on the respiratory system for a group of students. How will she explain what inhalation is? What are the percentages of oxygen and carbon dioxide in exhaled air?
4. A nurse on his rounds notices that a patient who had been eating her food rather hastily has begun to cough. What could the reason be for her cough?

## SECTION III: GETTING READY FOR NCLEX

**Activity H** ***Answer the following questions.***

1. Which of the following describes the function of the diaphragm?
   a. It separates the thoracic from the abdominal cavity.
   b. It divides the internal nose into two sides or cavities.
   c. It connects the nasopharynx to the middle ear.
   d. It aids in warming and moistening the air before it enters the lungs.

2. What is surfactant?
   a. A sticky membrane that lines the nasal cavity
   b. Four cavities found on each side of the nasal area
   c. The tube-shaped passage for food and air
   d. A chemical that lines the walls of the alveoli
3. While describing the exchange of gases in the body, how will the nurse explain the formation of carbonic acid ($H_2CO_3$)?
   a. Reaction of carbon dioxide with water
   b. Combination of hydrogen ions
   c. Combination of bicarbonate ions
   d. A waste product of metabolism
4. Which of the following are protective respiratory reflexes? (Select all that apply.)
   a. Coughing
   b. Sneezing
   c. Yawning
   d. Tracheotomy
   e. Expiration
5. Why should a nurse encourage clients to perform deep-breathing exercises?
   a. To improve oxygen delivery to the lungs and tissues
   b. To increase the level of carbon dioxide in the body
   c. To make speech louder and clearer
   d. To break up the surface tension in the pulmonary fluid
6. Which of the following are causes of respiratory acidosis? (Select all that apply.)
   a. Emphysema
   b. Asthma
   c. Hyperventilation
   d. Severe pneumonia
   e. Pleurisy
7. What is the function of the pleura?
   a. To allow the lungs to move without causing any pain or friction against the chest walls
   b. To increase the chest space by contracting and flattening
   c. To carry food to the esophagus and air to the trachea
   d. To guard the entrance of the larynx
8. How is homeostasis maintained during respiration?
   a. Reaction of carbon dioxide with water
   b. Interaction between the respiratory and renal systems
   c. Combination of hydrogen ions
   d. Combination of bicarbonate ions
9. What is the function of the hairs in the nostril?
   a. To aid in warming and moistening the air before it enters the lungs
   b. To filter the air and remove foreign particles to prevent them from entering the lungs
   c. To trap dust particles, dirt, and microorganisms from the air
   d. To divide the internal nose into two cavities
10. What is the function of the oropharynx?
   a. It permits air to enter or to leave the middle ear.
   b. It is a passageway for the air only.
   c. It destroys foreign substances that are inhaled or ingested.
   d. It carries food to the esophagus and air to the trachea.

CHAPTER 26

# The Digestive System

## SECTION I: TESTING WHAT YOU KNOW

**Activity A** *Match the organs of the digestive tract in Column A with their functions in Column B.*

**Column A**

____ **1.** Pharynx

____ **2.** Salivary gland

____ **3.** Stomach

____ **4.** Tongue

**Column B**

**a.** It senses the temperature and texture of food and is also involved with the mixing of the food with saliva.

**b.** Within this organ, food is mixed with gastric juices and churned until it is in a semiliquid form called chyme.

**c.** The contraction of this organ results in continuation of the act of swallowing and pushes the food into the esophagus.

**d.** Its secretion helps in the moistening of the food, making it easier to swallow, and in preventing oral infections.

**Activity B** *Match the processes involved during digestion in Column A with their definitions in Column B.*

**Column A**

____ **1.** Mastication

____ **2.** Peristalsis

____ **3.** Deglutition

____ **4.** Absorption

**Column B**

**a.** Alternate contraction and relaxation of muscles that sends the food down through the digestive tube

**b.** The act of chewing

**c.** The process of transferring broken-down food elements into the circulation for transport

**d.** The process of swallowing

**Activity C** *Mark each statement as either "T" (True) or "F" (false). Correct any false statements.*

**1.** T F Contractions of the pharynx continue the act of swallowing and push the food into the muscular duodenum.

**2.** T F Bile is a greenish-brown liquid that is produced in the liver and stored within the gallbladder.

**3.** T F The lower esophageal sphincter, or cardiac sphincter, guards the opening of the stomach and prevents food from entering into the jejunum.

**4.** T F The liver is involved in the function of formation of plasma proteins.

**5.** T F Cholecystokinin activates the gallbladder to release bile.

**Activity D** ***Fill in the blanks.***

1. The system of passageways for the transport of bile from the liver to the gallbladder to the intestine is known as ___________ apparatus.
2. ___________ digestion is the breakdown of chemical bonds in food with the addition of enzymes, acids, and water.
3. ___________ cells in the stomach mucosa secrete pepsinogen (breakdown proteins) and gastric lipase.
4. A small, finger-like projection of the cecum is the vermiform ___________.
5. In the stomach, all foods mix with gastric juices and churn until they are in a semiliquid form called ___________.

**Activity E** ***Consider the following figure.***

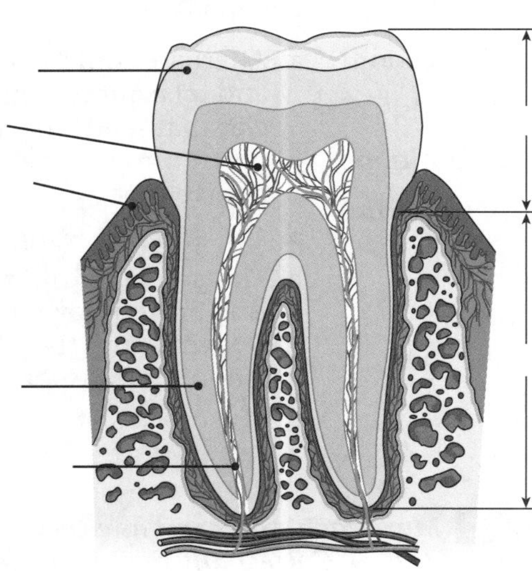

1. Label the various parts of a tooth. Then list the different types of teeth and where each type is located.

___________________________________________

___________________________________________

2. What is the main function of teeth?

___________________________________________

___________________________________________

**Activity F** ***The steps involved in digestion are given below in random order. Write the correct sequence in the boxes provided.***

1. The process of churning the food takes place in the pylorus of the stomach.
2. Absorption of the dissolved molecules occur in the small intestine. The molecules are then taken into circulation.
3. The physical breakdown of food is accomplished by the process of mastication.
4. Chemical breakdown of food occurs by the release of various enzymes.
5. Dilution of the food entering the digestive tract is accomplished by water and various enzymes.

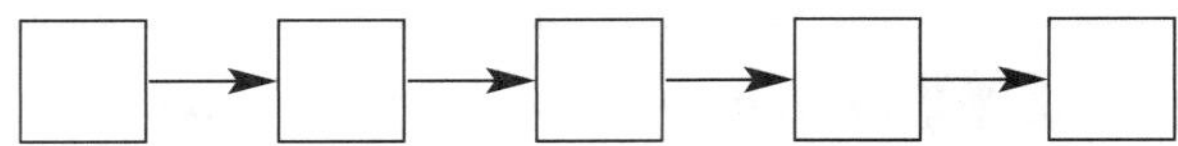

**Activity G** ***Briefly answer the following questions.***

1. Define metabolism. What is the difference between basal metabolism, catabolism, and anabolism?

___________________________________________

___________________________________________

2. Describe the digestive process that takes place in the stomach.

___________________________________________

___________________________________________

3. What is the role of the gallbladder in fat digestion?

___________________________________________

___________________________________________

## SECTION II: APPLYING WHAT YOU KNOW

**Activity H** *Answer the following questions, which involve understanding of the digestive system.*

To be able to provide optimal care to clients with problems involving digestion, a nurse needs to understand the functions performed by various organs of the digestive system.

1. A nurse is undertaking a general assessment of a 3-year-old client who has been brought in because of speech difficulty. She notes that the client is tongue-tied. The mother of the client wants to know more about it.
   a. How would the nurse describe the function of the frenulum to the mother and the complications that can occur with the tongue?
   b. What are the functions of the tongue?
2. A 38-year-old client informs the nurse that he has been experiencing a burning sensation in the chest for 2 days. Assessment reveals heartburn.
   a. What is the cause of heartburn? What is its consequence? Write a note on its treatment.
   b. What is the function of the lower esophageal sphincter (LES)?
3. What are the various functions of the liver that the nurse needs to know to help explain the pathology of the liver to a client?
4. A nurse is assessing a 65-year-old client who complains of constipation. What are the effects of aging on the digestive system that a nurse needs to know in treating such a client?

## SECTION III: GETTING READY FOR NCLEX

**Activity I** *Answer the following questions.*

1. Which of the following should a nurse consider as a cause of achalasia?
   a. Partial closure of the pyloric sphincter
   b. Inadequate relaxation of the external anal sphincter
   c. Non-relaxation of the lower esophageal sphincter
   d. Impaired closure of the ileocecal valve
2. Which of the following is the mechanism for vomiting?
   a. Decrease in the process of peristalsis
   b. Reverse peristaltic wave within the stomach
   c. Propulsive peristaltic wave occurring in the small intestine
   d. Weak peristaltic wave occurring in the esophagus
3. Which of the following are the end-products produced during catabolism? (Select all that apply.)
   a. Oxygen
   b. Energy
   c. Glycogen
   d. Carbon dioxide
   e. Water
4. Which of the following lead to the development of appendicitis?
   a. Retained bolus
   b. Dislodged chyme
   c. Overflowing chyle
   d. Impacted feces
5. Which one of the following would be affected after an impairment of the liver?
   a. Formation of vitamin D
   b. Absorption of fat-soluble vitamins
   c. Synthesis of urea
   d. Digestion of starch
6. Which of the following are enzymes secreted by the pancreas? (Select all that apply.)
   a. Pepsin
   b. Amylase
   c. Trypsin
   d. Ptyalin
   e. Lipase
7. Which of the following would be the cause of a client's speech difficulty?
   a. Short frenulum
   b. Long rugae
   c. Expanded fundus
   d. Small mesentries

8. Which of the following is the function of the salivary gland?
   a. It senses the temperature and texture of food and is also involved with the mixing of the food with saliva.
   b. Within this organ, food is mixed with gastric juices and churned until it is in a semiliquid form called chyme.
   c. The contraction of this organ results in continuation of the act of swallowing and pushes the food into the esophagus.
   d. Its secretion helps in the moistening of the food, making it easier to swallow, and in preventing oral infections.

9. The nurse is reviewing the amount of energy used by the body at rest to sustain a client's life. What is this called?
   a. Metabolism
   b. Basal metabolism
   c. Catabolism
   d. Anabolism

10. Which enzyme is secreted by the salivary glands?
    a. Ptyalin
    b. Pepsin
    c. Amylase
    d. Trypsin

CHAPTER 27

# The Urinary System

## SECTION I: TESTING WHAT YOU KNOW

**Activity A** *Match the organs in Column A with their functions in Column B.*

| Column A | Column B |
|---|---|
| ____ 1. Urinary bladder | a. Extracts wastes from the blood, balances body fluids, and forms urine |
| ____ 2. Ureter | b. Conducts urine from the bladder to the outside of the body for elimination |
| ____ 3. Kidney | c. Serves as a reservoir for urine |
| ____ 4. Urethra | d. Conducts urine from the kidneys to the urinary bladder |

**Activity B** *Match the hormones in Column A with their functions in Column B.*

| Column A | Column B |
|---|---|
| ____ 1. Renin | a. Increases the reabsorption of water by the kidney tubules |
| ____ 2. Aldosterone | b. Stimulates the formation of angiotensin I |
| ____ 3. Atrial natriuretic peptide | c. Increases kidney filtration and blood flow when blood volume increases |
| ____ 4. Antidiuretic hormone | d. Promotes sodium and water retention |

**Activity C** *Mark each statement as either "T" (True) or "F" (False). Correct any false statements.*

1. T F The left kidney is slightly lower than the right kidney.
2. T F The renal papillae of the renal pyramids point laterally toward the renal cortex.
3. T F The juxtaglomerular apparatus lies at the point where the distal convoluted tubule contacts the afferent arteriole.
4. T F Aldosterone stimulates excretion of sodium ions and reabsorption of potassium ions.
5. T F The antidiuretic hormone is secreted by the posterior pituitary gland.

**Activity D** *Fill in the blanks.*

1. The functional units of the kidney are called ____________.
2. Angiotensin II stimulates the adrenal cortex to secrete ____________.
3. At one end of each microscopic nephron the ____________ are partially enclosed in a funnel-shaped structure called Bowman's capsule.
4. The male urethra passes through the ____________ gland.
5. Involuntary micturition is called urinary ____________.

**Activity E** *Consider the following figure.*

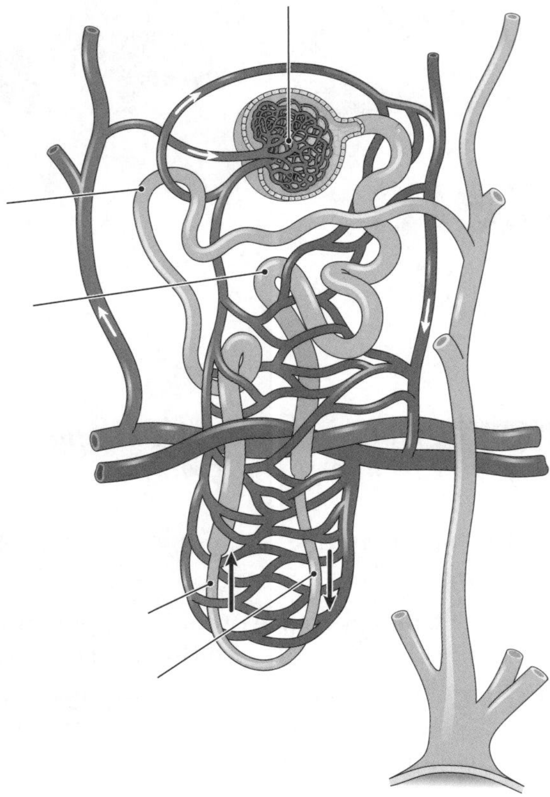

1. Identify the following structures of the nephron in the figure. Then discuss the function of each.
   a. Glomerulus

   ______________________________________

   ______________________________________

   b. Proximal convoluted tubule

   ______________________________________

   ______________________________________

   c. Loop of Henle

   ______________________________________

   ______________________________________

   d. Distal convoluted tubule

   ______________________________________

   ______________________________________

**Activity F** *The stages involved in the renin-angiotensin-aldosterone (RAA) mechanism for raising the blood pressure are given below in random order. Write the correct sequence in which they occur in the boxes provided.*

1. Constriction of blood vessels
2. Formation of angiotensin I
3. Secretion of aldosterone
4. Formation of angiotensin II
5. Sodium and water retention
6. Secretion of renin
7. Increase in cardiac output
8. Increase in peripheral resistance

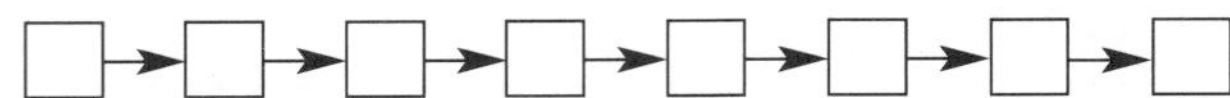

**Activity G** *Briefly answer the following questions.*

1. What is the trigone?

   ______________________________________

   ______________________________________

2. Describe the blood supply of the kidney.

   ______________________________________

   ______________________________________

3. Discuss the differences between the male and the female urethra.

   ______________________________________

   ______________________________________

## SECTION II: APPLYING WHAT YOU KNOW

**Activity H** *Answer the following questions, which involve understanding of the urinary system.*

To be able to effectively administer care for clients with disorders of the urinary tract, a nurse needs to understand the functions performed by the various organs of the urinary tract.

1. An 85-year-old client complains of a frequent urge to void.
   a. What factors bring about change in the urinary tract due to aging?
   b. What are results of the effect of aging on the urinary tract?
2. What are the functions of the urinary system that a nurse should be aware of?
3. What are the nursing interventions that should be performed when caring for an elderly client?
4. A client complains of a decreased amount of micturition. When his urine is examined, it is found to be dark yellow or amber in color.
   a. What does this indicate?
   b. What factors affect the quantity of urine produced?

## SECTION III: GETTING READY FOR NCLEX

**Activity I** *Answer the following questions.*

1. Which of the following is the function of the ureter?
   a. Conducts urine to the urinary bladder
   b. Acts as a reservoir for urine before elimination
   c. Conducts urine to the outside for elimination
   d. Extracts wastes from the blood and from urine
2. Which of the following are the functions of the kidneys? (Select all that apply.)
   a. They balance the pH of the body fluids.
   b. They eliminate alkalis into the urine.
   c. They control the volume of body fluids.
   d. They help in control of the blood pressure.
   e. They secrete the hormone aldosterone.
3. Which of the following hormones is produced by the kidneys?
   a. Aldosterone
   b. Erythropoietin
   c. Atrial natriuretic peptide
   d. Antidiuretic hormone
4. What is the function of the hormone erythropoietin?
   a. It helps in the maintenance of blood pressure.
   b. It helps in the formation of red blood cells.
   c. It helps in promoting water retention.
   d. It helps in the formation of white blood cells.
5. What substance, when present in the urine, would indicate a disease or malfunction of the urinary system?
   a. Urea
   b. Pigments
   c. Protein
   d. Sodium
6. A laboratory analysis of a client's urine sample shows a pH of 3. What food in the client's diet should the nurse consider to be a possible cause of this abnormal pH?
   a. Dairy products
   b. Meat
   c. Citrus fruits
   d. Legumes
7. Which of the following is a function of the urethra?
   a. Extracts wastes from the blood, balances body fluids, and forms urine.
   b. Conducts urine from the bladder to the outside of the body for elimination.
   c. Serves as a reservoir for urine.
   d. Conducts urine from the kidneys to the urinary bladder.
8. An elderly client needs assistance with frequent urges to void. What are nursing interventions that should be performed when caring for the client? (Select all that apply.)
   a. Watch for bladder infection.
   b. Allow for bathroom visits once every 6 hours.
   c. Administer diuretics carefully.
   d. Monitor the fluid intake and output every shift.
   e. Perform straight catheterization every shift.

**9.** The nurse is reviewing the structures of the nephron. What is the function of the Loop of Henle?

**a.** Filters water, wastes (urea), glucose, and salts (electrolytes) out of blood.

**b.** Reabsorbs some needed electrolytes (potassium, chloride) water, and glucose, as well as some amino acids and bicarbonate.

**c.** Reabsorbs water and additional electrolytes.

**d.** Reabsorbs sodium, water, and the remainder of glucose.

**10.** The nurse is reviewing the similarities and differences between a male and female urethra. What is the length of the female urethra?

**a.** 1.5 inches

**b.** 3 inches

**c.** 5.5 inches

**d.** 8 inches

CHAPTER 28

# The Male Reproductive System

## SECTION I: TESTING WHAT YOU KNOW

**Activity A** ***Match the organs of the male reproductive tract in Column A with their functions in Column B.***

| Column A | Column B |
|---|---|
| ____ 1. Testes | a. Location of final stages of maturation of sperm cells |
| ____ 2. Epididymis | b. Produce spermatozoa and secrete sex hormones |
| ____ 3. Seminal vesicles | c. Transports sperm from the epididymis to the ejaculatory duct |
| ____ 4. Ductus deferens | d. Produce semen, the fluid medium for sperm |

**Activity B** ***Mark each statement as either "T" (True) or "F" (False). Correct any false statements.***

1. T F The purpose of the reproductive system is to work to continue the species and to pass genetic information from parents to child.
2. T F A woman's ability to reproduce depends only on sexual excitement.
3. T F In men, orgasm is acompanied by the ejaculation of semen.
4. T F Urine and semen can pass simultaneously through the urethra during intercourse.
5. T F Before puberty, the blood concentrations of androgens and estrogens are the same in every person.

**Activity C** ***Fill in the blanks.***

1. Surgical removal of the foreskin on the penis is called ____________.
2. During puberty, the ____________ gland stimulates the secretion of both interstitial cell–stimulating hormone (ICSH) and follicle-stimulating hormone (FSH).
3. The formation of mature and functional spermatozoa is called ____________.
4. The tip of the head of the sperm cell, called the ____________ contains enzymes that can dissolve the tough cell wall of the ovum.
5. Sperm can live for a maximum of ____________ days after ejaculation.
6. The process of ____________ in men is sometimes called andropause.
7. ____________ is the forceful expulsion of semen from the ejaculatory ducts, through the urethra.

**Activity D** *Consider the following figure.*

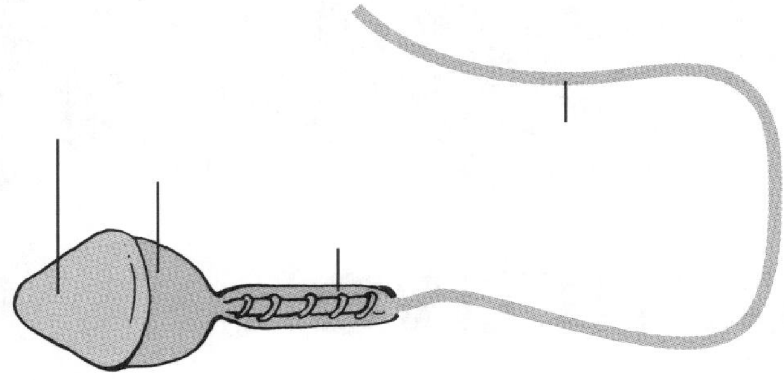

1. Identify the following divisions of a sperm cell in the figure. Then state the purpose of each:
   a. Acrosome
   ______________________________
   ______________________________
   b. Head
   ______________________________
   ______________________________
   c. Body
   ______________________________
   ______________________________
   d. Tail
   ______________________________
   ______________________________

**Activity E** *The stages of the male sex act are given below in random order. Write the correct sequence in which they occur in the boxes provided.*

1. Ejaculation
2. Erection
3. Emission
4. Secretion

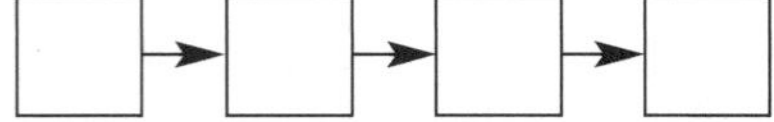

**Activity F** *Briefly answer the following questions.*

1. Which are the three organs that produce hormones to influence the male reproductive system?
   ______________________________
   ______________________________
2. What are the functions of the scrotum?
   ______________________________
   ______________________________
3. Why is seminal fluid alkaline?
   ______________________________
   ______________________________
4. What is the effect of age on sperm production?
   ______________________________
   ______________________________
5. Where is the epididymis located?
   ______________________________
   ______________________________
6. What is the process by which spermatogonia develop into spermatozoa?
   ______________________________
   ______________________________

## SECTION II: APPLYING WHAT YOU KNOW

**Activity G** *Answer the following questions, which involve understanding of the male reproductive system.*

To be able to effectively administer care for clients with disorders of the male reproductive tract, a nurse needs to understand the functions performed by the various organs of the male reproductive tract.

1. A 34-year-old male client who has four children is eager to learn more about the vasectomy procedure because he and his wife do not want to have any more children.
   a. What is a vasectomy?
   b. What is the role of the ductal system in the male reproductive process?

2. A nurse is conducting a session on sex education in a high school and explaining the role of the sexual organs in the reproductive process. What are the characteristics and functions of the penis, scrotum, and testes that the students should be informed about?
3. A mother of a 17-year-old boy informs the nurse that her son is experiencing delayed puberty. She wants to know about the normal age of puberty in boys and the biological causes that trigger puberty.
   - **a.** What is the normal age of puberty in boys?
   - **b.** What are the major hormones that precipitate changes during puberty, and what effects do they have?
   - **c.** What are the secondary sexual characteristics displayed by boys during puberty?

## SECTION III: GETTING READY FOR NCLEX

**Activity H** *Answer the following questions.*

1. The results of a urology test for a 28-year-old client reveal that his sperm count is 7 million sperm cells per milliliter. What information should the nurse give to the client regarding the results of the test?
   - **a.** The client's sperm cells have a very low degree of motility.
   - **b.** The client's sperm count will gradually increase with age.
   - **c.** The client's semen may have difficulty fertilizing an ovum.
   - **d.** An increased amount of ejaculatory fluid will lead to a better sperm count.
2. Which of the following is a function of the ductus deferens?
   - **a.** It transports sperm to the ejaculatory duct.
   - **b.** It is the location where sperm cells are produced and mature.
   - **c.** It secretes testosterone and other androgens.
   - **d.** It is the source of semen production.
3. Which of the following is the function of testosterone?
   - **a.** It triggers the development of secondary sexual characteristics.
   - **b.** It stimulates the formation of sperm cells.
   - **c.** It stimulates the production of follicle-stimulating hormone (FSH).
   - **d.** It regulates the temperature of the scrotum.
4. A client has been diagnosed with low sperm count. Which of the following instructions should the nurse give him to increase his sperm count?
   - **a.** Take hot baths and saunas.
   - **b.** Eat a protein-rich diet.
   - **c.** Perform regular exercises.
   - **d.** Avoid wearing tight underpants.
5. Which of the following are the effects of an enlarged prostate? (Select all that apply.)
   - **a.** Difficulty in urination
   - **b.** Incontinence
   - **c.** Difficulty in defecation
   - **d.** Pain in the testes
   - **e.** Inability to have an erection
6. A mother of a teenage boy is concerned about whether her son is experiencing delayed puberty. What is the normal age of puberty in boys?
   - **a.** 9 to 12 years
   - **b.** 10 to 13 years
   - **c.** 11 to 14 years
   - **d.** 12 to 16 years
7. What is the function of follicle-stimulating hormone during puberty?
   - **a.** Regulates the temperature of the scrotum.
   - **b.** Triggers the development of secondary sex characteristics.
   - **c.** Stimulates the formation of sperm.
   - **d.** Stimulates production of testosterone.
8. A client asks the nurse about the functions of various parts of the sperm cell. What is the purpose of the tail of the sperm cell?
   - **a.** Contains 23 chromosomes.
   - **b.** Contains enzymes that can dissolve the tough cell wall of the ovum.
   - **c.** Provides energy necessary for locomotion.
   - **d.** Propels sperm with lashing movement.

9. A client has been diagnosed with a low sperm count. What temperature is necessary in the testes to facilitate sperm production?
   a. 35 degrees C
   b. 37 degrees C
   c. 39 degrees C
   d. 41 degrees C

10. A school nurse is reviewing the role of sex organs in the reproductive system. Which of the following is the function of the testes?
   a. Deposit sperm in the vagina.
   b. Produce sperm cells.
   c. Secrete growth hormone.
   d. Support and protect testes.

CHAPTER 29

# The Female Reproductive System

## SECTION I: TESTING WHAT YOU KNOW

**Activity A** *Match the internal organs of the female reproductive system in Column A with their functions in Column B.*

**Column A**

____ **1.** Oviduct

____ **2.** Uterus

____ **3.** Ovary

____ **4.** Vagina

**Column B**

**a.** Receives sperm, provides an exit for menstrual flow, and serves as the birth canal

**b.** Produces female gametes or ova and secretes female sex hormones

**c.** Catches the ovum that has burst from the ovary in structures called fimbriae

**d.** Receives the fertilized ovum and provides housing and nourishment for a fetus

**Activity B** *Match the phase of the ovarian cycle in Column A with its process in Column B.*

**Column A**

____ **1.** Luteal phase

____ **2.** Ovulation phase

____ **3.** Follicular phase

**Column B**

**a.** Under the influence of follicle-stimulating hormone (FSH), several follicles begin to ripen, and the ovum within each begins to mature.

**b.** The empty, ruptured graafian follicle becomes the corpus luteum and begins to secrete progesterone and estrogen.

**c.** About day 14, a surge of hormones causes the ovum to burst through the ovary.

**Activity C** *Mark each statement as either "T" (True) or "F" (False). Correct any false statements.*

**1.** T F Menarche is the first menstrual period and marks the onset of puberty.

**2.** T F In women, progesterone hormones stimulate the formation of ova and the secretion of hormones from the sex organs.

**3.** T F At the start of meiosis, the oogonium is called a secondary follicle.

4. T F Women experience sharp pains or cramps when ovulation occurs, known as endometrium.

5. T F All the ova that an individual woman will produce in her lifetime are present as oocytes at her birth.

6. T F The mammary glands are modified sweat glands located in the breasts, anterior to the pectoralis major muscles.

7. T F As the ovum bursts from the ovary into the pelvic cavity, the oviduct catches it in structures called zygotes.

**Activity D** *Fill in the blanks.*

1. The female ___________ is the space between the vaginal orifice and the anus.
2. A fertilized ovum is called a ___________ and becomes embedded in the uterine lining.
3. ___________ is the flow of blood and other materials from the uterus through the vagina.
4. The female climacteric is called ___________.
5. A ___________ is a physician who specializes in treating disorders unique to women.
6. Maturation of a/an ___________ occurs during the ovarian cycle.
7. The external structure of the female reproductive system consists of components of the ___________.

**Activity E** *Consider the following figures.*

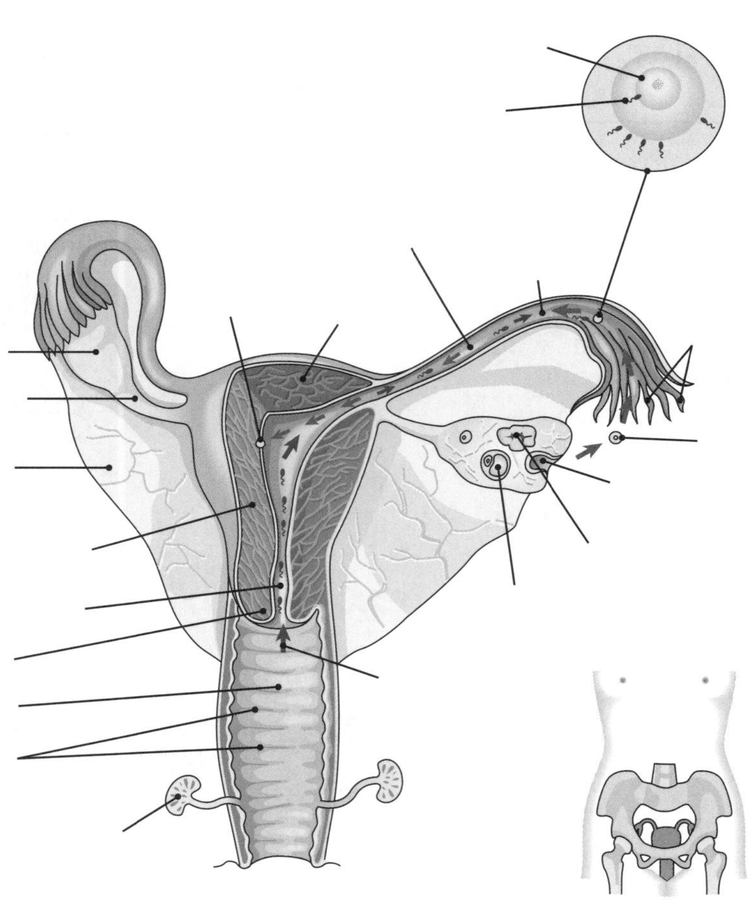

1. Label the different parts of the uterus. Then list and describe them.

_______________________________________________

_______________________________________________

2. Describe the three layers of the uterus.

_______________________________________________

_______________________________________________

3. Label the parts of the breast and ducts of the mammary glands. Then list and describe them.

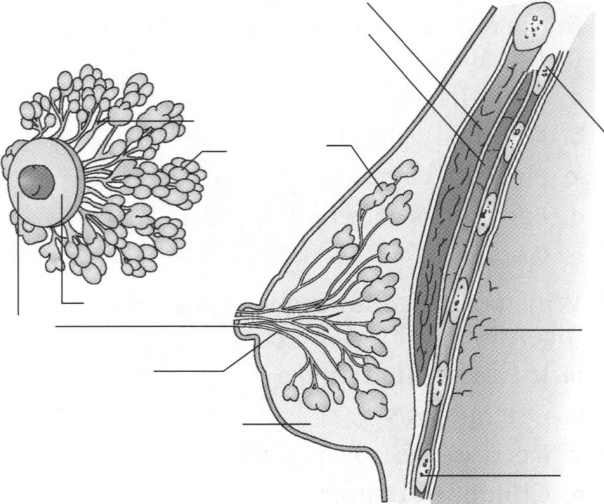

**Activity F** ***Stages of oocyte development throughout a woman's life are given below in random order. Write the correct sequence in which each oocyte develops in the boxes provided.***

1. Graafian follicle
2. Ovum
3. Primary oocyte
4. Oogonia
5. Secondary follicle

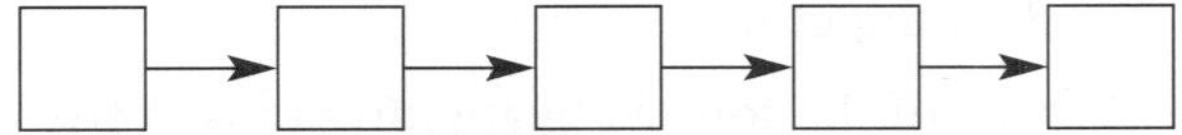

**Activity G** ***Briefly answer the following questions.***

1. What are the hormones secreted by the ovaries?

2. What is a graafian follicle?

3. What is mons pubis?

4. What are the two interrelated cycles of menstruation? Which secretions control these cycles?

5. What are fornices?

6. What is the clitoris?

7. What happens during the proliferative phase of the uterine cycle?

## SECTION II: APPLYING WHAT YOU KNOW

**Activity H** ***Answer the following questions, which involve the nurse's role in the management of such situations.***

The nurse helps clients manage problems concerning the female reproductive system; provides information about the various changes in the reproductive system; and cares for female clients during menstruation, pregnancy, labor, childbirth, and menopause.

1. A mother visits the healthcare clinic with her daughter, who is experiencing menstrual cramps. The daughter asks the nurse for information on menstruation.
   a. What information should the nurse give to the client about the menstrual cycle?
   b. What information should the nurse give about the physical changes caused by secretion of the hormones estrogen and progesterone?

2. A nurse is caring for a client with an ectopic pregnancy. The client wants to know how her condition is different from that of a normal pregnancy.
   a. How does an ectopic pregnancy take place?
   b. What capacity changes take place in the pregnant uterus?
3. A nurse is caring for a 45-year-old female client experiencing menopause.
   a. What symptoms of menopause should the nurse assess the client for?
   b. What are the possible problems that the client could encounter during menopause?

## SECTION III: GETTING READY FOR NCLEX

**Activity I** *Answer the following questions.*

1. What describes the movement of the ovum from the ovaries to the uterus? (Select all that apply.)
   a. The ovum enters the abdominal cavity.
   b. The oviduct catches the ovum in the fimbriae.
   c. Cilia help the ovum to move toward the uterus.
   d. The ovum embeds in the uterine lining in preparation for growth.
   e. Muscles of the oviducts propel the ovum.
2. Which of the following is a sign of a non-pregnant uterus?
   a. Weighs about 120 g
   b. Tips forward
   c. Holds about 100 mL
   d. Falls into the vagina
3. A 48-year-old client informs the nurse that she has not menstruated for the last 2 months. What symptoms of menopause should the nurse assess for in the client?
   a. Sensation of heat
   b. Deepening of voice
   c. Unique fatty deposits
   d. Hair in pubic and axillary areas
4. Which of the following is the cause of menstruation?
   a. Ovaries stop producing estrogen.
   b. Eggs do not mature.
   c. The endometrium sloughs off.
   d. The activity of the ovaries decreases.
5. Which of the following glands are involved in the regulation of the reproductive system? (Select all that apply.)
   a. Hypothalamus
   b. Mammary glands
   c. Pituitary gland
   d. Bartholin's glands
   e. Gonads
6. Which of the following is a cause of urinary incontinence in women?
   a. Increased fluid intake
   b. Osteoporosis
   c. Decreased estrogen level
   d. Childbirth trauma
7. Where are the ovaries located?
   a. Within the brim of the pelvis, on either side of the uterus
   b. Within the pelvis, between the urinary bladder and rectum
   c. At either side of the uterus
   d. Behind the pectoralis major muscle
8. Which of the following is the major cause of osteoporosis in menopausal women?
   a. Reduced intake of calcium
   b. Loss of estrogen
   c. Reduced activity of ovaries
   d. Poor appetite
9. Which of the following are functions of the uterus? (Select all that apply.)
   a. It receives the fertilized ovum.
   b. It serves as the birth canal.
   c. It provides housing and nourishment for the fetus.
   d. It expels the fetus at the end of gestation.
   e. It secretes mucus to assist in transport of the ovum.

**10.** Which of the following is part of the uterine cycle?

**a.** Maturation of the ovum

**b.** Expulsion of the ovum into the oviduct

**c.** Formation of the graafian follicle

**d.** Preparation for implantation of the ovum

CHAPTER 30

# Basic Nutrition

## SECTION I: TESTING WHAT YOU KNOW

**Activity A** ***Match the nutrients in Column A with their functions in Column B.***

| Column A | Column B |
|---|---|
| ____ 1. Proteins | a. Help to provide energy |
| ____ 2. Minerals | b. Help to build and repair tissue |
| ____ 3. Fats | c. Help to synthesize body compounds such as bone and blood |
| ____ 4. Vitamins | d. Help maintain muscle tone, regulate body processes, and maintain acid–base balance |

**Activity B** ***Match the B-complex vitamins in Column A with their roles in Column B.***

| Column A | Column B |
|---|---|
| ____ 1. Thiamine ($B_1$) | a. Release of energy from carbohydrate, fat, and protein |
| ____ 2. Niacin ($B_3$) | b. Synthesis of DNA and RNA, and the formation of red and white blood cells |
| ____ 3. Folate/folic acid ($B_9$) | c. Folate metabolism and blood cell formation |
| ____ 4. Cobalamin ($B_{12}$) | d. Growth, cell metabolism, appetite, and neurologic functioning |

**Activity C** ***Mark each statement as either "T" (True) or "F" (False). Correct any false statements.***

1. T F A severe deficiency of thiamine leads to pellagra, the signs and symptoms of which include dermatitis, diarrhea, dementia, and death.
2. T F Enzymes are biological catalysts made of proteins.
3. T F The term *hypoglycemia* means abnormally high blood sugar.
4. T F Saturated fatty acids are solid at room temperature.
5. T F Proteins are complex molecules composed of at least 100 individual units known as amino acids.
6. T F Glycogen is formed as an intermediate in starch digestion by the action of enzymes or heat.

**Activity D** ***Fill in the blanks.***

1. A marked deficiency of vitamin D causes a childhood condition known as ____________ in which the bones do not harden as they should, but instead bend into deformed positions, such as bowlegs.
2. Cholesterol is a member of a large group of compounds called ____________.
3. ____________ nutrients are those that a person must obtain through food because the body cannot make them in sufficient quantities to meet its needs.

4. A nurse should emphasize foods with nutrient ___________ that is, foods that provide significant amounts of key nutrients per volume consumed.
5. A recently recognized type of fatty acid called ___________ fat is created when a polyunsaturated fatty acid, such as vegetable oil, is hydrogenated to make it solid at room temperature.
6. ___________ fats have fewer essential fatty acids than the original oil, because the unsaturated fat content is lowered.

**Activity E** *Briefly answer the following questions.*

1. What are the recommendations made by the MyPlate Food Guidance System?

   ________________________________________

   ________________________________________
2. What are phytochemicals, and what is their function in nutrition?

   ________________________________________

   ________________________________________
3. What are the six classes of nutrients?

   ________________________________________

   ________________________________________
4. How and where does the body store glycogen?

   ________________________________________

   ________________________________________
5. What is REE?

   ________________________________________

   ________________________________________
6. What are "empty calorie" foods and why are they harmful?

   ________________________________________

   ________________________________________
7. What are fat-soluble vitamins?

   ________________________________________

   ________________________________________
8. What is the role of cobalamin in the body?

   ________________________________________

   ________________________________________

## SECTION II: APPLYING WHAT YOU KNOW

**Activity F** *Answer the following questions, which involve understanding of nutrition.*

A nurse's role in managing clients with nutritional deficiencies involves assisting the clients in learning about the importance of nutritious food.

1. A nurse is assigned to care for a client with an enlarged thyroid gland. What condition is the client experiencing, and what has been the cause of this condition?
2. A client with dehydration is admitted to a healthcare facility. During the assessment of the client, the nurse observes that the client does not drink an adequate amount of water.
   a. What is the importance of water in the body?
   b. What is the average daily requirement of water for an adult?
3. A nurse is caring for a pregnant client. What instructions should the nurse offer the client to prevent rickets in her baby?

## SECTION III: GETTING READY FOR NCLEX

**Activity G** *Answer the following questions.*

1. Which concept should the nurse use when teaching clients about the interrelationships among nutrition, activity, and diet therapy?
   a. Recommended Dietary Allowances
   b. MyPlate
   c. Tolerable Upper Intake Level
   d. Adequate Intake
2. Which of the following conditions should the nurse monitor for in a client with thiamine deficiency?
   a. Glossitis
   b. Poor appetite
   c. Diarrhea
   d. Headaches
3. Which of the following would you expect in a client with hyperglycemia?
   a. High levels of low-density lipoproteins
   b. Abnormally high cholesterol levels
   c. Abnormally high blood sugar level
   d. Abnormally high levels of sodium

4. A client has been instructed to increase the fiber in his diet by including fibrous foods such as oats, legumes, apples, and citrus fruits. What reason should the nurse provide the client for the prescribed diet?
   a. It increases stool bulk.
   b. It lowers the transit time of food through the intestines.
   c. It helps prevent constipation.
   d. It slows gastric emptying time.

5. What symptoms should the nurse monitor for in a client with a fatty acid deficiency?
   a. Bleeding gums
   b. Dermatitis
   c. Stiff joints
   d. Tiny hemorrhages

6. What instructions should the nurse offer a client with diabetes that would encourage her to eat less sugar? (Select all that apply.)
   a. Replace soft drinks with fruit juice or low-fat milk.
   b. Cook food in very small amounts of oil.
   c. Rely on natural sugars in fruit to satisfy a "sweet tooth."
   d. Cut sugar in home-baked products, if possible.
   e. Do not overcook food, and serve it at once.

7. A nurse is assessing a client with retarded growth. Which of the following vitamin deficiencies should the nurse identify as responsible for the client condition?
   a. Deficiency of vitamin $B_3$
   b. Deficiency of vitamin $B_{12}$
   c. Deficiency of vitamin $B_6$
   d. Deficiency of vitamin $B_1$

8. Which of the following conditions should the nurse monitor for in the client with a high dietary sodium intake? (Select all that apply.)
   a. Hypertension
   b. Cardiovascular disease
   c. Glossitis
   d. Impaired nerve function
   e. Osteoporosis

9. A nurse is caring for a client with high cholesterol. The client is administered a megadose of niacin. Which of the following side effects of niacin should the nurse monitor for in the client? (Select all that apply.)
   a. Flushing of skin
   b. Confusion
   c. Seizures
   d. Liver damage
   e. Hypotension

10. Which instruction to a client by the nurse offers a recommendation made by the MyPlate Food Guidance System?
   a. Increase intake of saturated fat, trans fat, and cholesterol.
   b. Avoid varying foods in your diet.
   c. Eat more fruits, vegetables, and whole grains.
   d. Decrease intake of low-fat dairy products.

CHAPTER 31

# Transcultural and Social Aspects of Nutrition

## SECTION I: TESTING WHAT YOU KNOW

**Activity A** *Match the type of vegetarian diet in Column A with the foods eaten in Column B.*

| Column A | Column B |
|---|---|
| ____ 1. Vegan | a. Plant foods and eggs but no dairy products |
| ____ 2. Lacto-vegetarian | b. Only plant foods and no animal foods |
| ____ 3. Ovo-vegetarian | c. Plant foods, eggs, and dairy products |
| ____ 4. Lacto-ovo-vegetarian | d. Plant foods plus dairy products |

**Activity B** *Match the ethnic group in Column A with the common dietary practices in Column B.*

| Column A | Column B |
|---|---|
| ____ 1. Black Americans from the Caribbean | a. May eat every mouthful of food with a bite of bread |
| ____ 2. Vietnamese Americans | b. Believe that a balance of "hot" and "cold" food is required for health |
| ____ 3. Hispanic Americans | c. May consume cooked starchy tubers and tropical fruits |
| ____ 4. Middle Eastern Americans | d. Eat poultry, pork, and fermented fish and consume beef occasionally |

**Activity C** *Mark each statement as either "T" (True) or "F" (False). Correct any false statements.*

1. T F A belief in a yin-yang theory of diet can be found within Japanese American culture.
2. T F The Chinese American diet is very low in sodium and high-sodium seasonings.
3. T F Vegans are vegetarians who eat only plant and dairy products.
4. T F A vegetarian diet may offer some protection against lung and breast cancer.
5. T F A diet high in proteins is associated with heart disease.

**Activity D** *Fill in the blanks.*

1. ____________ food refers to both a cooking style (fried, barbecued) and particular foods (eg, black-eyed peas, collard greens) that people living in the southeastern United States commonly eat.
2. Persons who eat plant and dairy products but no eggs are called ____________.
3. Tofu is a good source of ____________ and calcium.
4. Mexican Americans often serve ____________ with all meals, along with rice and refried beans.
5. Jews who follow a ____________ diet do not eat pork products, shellfish, or scavenger fish.

**Activity E** *Briefly answer the following questions.*

1. Why should a nurse assess the dietary beliefs of clients?

_______________________________________________

_______________________________________________

2. What are the eating habits of Cambodian Americans?

_______________________________________________

_______________________________________________

3. What is the yin-yang theory of diet?

_______________________________________________

_______________________________________________

## SECTION II: APPLYING WHAT YOU KNOW

**Activity F** *Answer the following questions, which involve the nurse's role in effective dietary planning.*

Proper assessment of a client's personal food preferences or aversions helps the nurse to adjust the client's diet without disregarding his or her dietary beliefs.

1. A nurse is assessing an Orthodox Jewish client in a healthcare facility. During assessment, what should the nurse keep in mind about the diet of such a client?
2. A nurse is assessing a client in a healthcare facility. The client states that she is vegetarian. What dietary advice should the nurse give to such a client for obtaining a balanced diet?
3. An obese client reads about a weight loss scheme in a newspaper. He plans to enroll himself in the program. What criteria should a nurse advise the client to look for before enrolling in the program?
4. What should a nurse keep in mind regarding clients following ethnic diets?

## SECTION III: GETTING READY FOR NCLEX

**Activity G** *Answer the following questions.*

1. A nurse is assessing a South American client regarding her dietary practices. What food is the nurse more likely to notice in the diet of such a client, compared with a client from North America?
   a. Bread
   b. Fruits
   c. Beer
   d. Milk
2. Which of the following are conditions that are more likely to occur in Black American clients? (Select all that apply.)
   a. Hypertension
   b. Renal disease
   c. Obesity
   d. Gout
   e. Diabetes
3. A nurse has been asked to plan the diet for a lacto-vegetarian client. What can the nurse include in the diet plan of such a client?
   a. Plant products only
   b. Plant and dairy products
   c. Plant products, dairy products, and eggs
   d. Plant products and eggs
4. A nurse is assessing a 30-year-old client of Cuban origin. Which of the following is the nurse most likely to notice when assessing this client's diet?
   a. Limited intake of milk
   b. Highly spiced food
   c. Extensive use of meat
   d. Limited use of rice and beans
5. A Puerto Rican woman is admitted to a healthcare facility in her 38th week of pregnancy. Being culturally sensitive, what food should the nurse omit from the client's diet chart?
   a. Sweet food
   b. Sour food
   c. Bitter food
   d. Spicy food

6. Which of the following vitamins is most likely to be deficient in a vegan client?
   a. Vitamin A
   b. Vitamin $B_{12}$
   c. Vitamin C
   d. Vitamin D

7. Which of the following statements indicates a correct dietary response to the condition listed?
   a. Decreased fluid intake for hypertension
   b. Increased fluid intake for fever
   c. Limited salt intake for malabsorption
   d. Large, frequent meals for anorexia

8. A nurse has to help an elderly client feel comfortable during his meals and provide for a secure and safe environment. Which of the following mealtime interventions are most appropriate for the nurse to perform when caring for this client? (Select all that apply.)
   a. Allow the client to eat his meal alone.
   b. Visit the client for a few minutes.
   c. Encourage the client to telephone home.
   d. Stop visitors from coming during mealtimes.
   e. Turn on the television or radio.

9. Ethnic dietary practices may play different roles in the health and illness of a client. What potential health problems can occur with a diet with low intake of milk and dairy products?
   a. Rickets or osteoporosis
   b. Hypertension and cardiac disease
   c. Atherosclerosis and gallbladder disease
   d. Diabetes and obesity

10. During the assessment of an Orthodox Jewish client, the nurse should keep in mind that most people of this religious group follow a Kosher diet. What is requirement of this diet?
    a. Meat and dairy products are served at the same meal.
    b. Only the hind quarter of the animal may be eaten.
    c. Only foods such as pork products, rabbit, and shell fish may be eaten.
    d. Food is not cooked during the Sabbath, which is sundown Friday to sundown Saturday.

CHAPTER 32

# Diet Therapy and Special Diets

## SECTION I: TESTING WHAT YOU KNOW

**Activity A** ***Match the enteral tube feeding devices used for nutritional support in Column A with their placement sites in Column B.***

| Column A | Column B |
|---|---|
| ____ 1. Nasogastric tube | a. Inserted into the stomach |
| ____ 2. Gastrostomy tube | b. Placed through the skin |
| ____ 3. Percutaneous tube | c. Inserted into the small intestine |
| ____ 4. Jejunal tube | d. Inserted through the nose into the stomach |

**Activity B** ***Match the category of diet in Column A with the related health condition in Column B.***

| Column A | Column B |
|---|---|
| ____ 1. Bland diet | a. Diabetes mellitus |
| ____ 2. Carbohydrate-controlled diet | b. Seizure disorder in a child |
| ____ 3. Fat-controlled diet | c. Gastroesophageal reflux disease |
| ____ 4. Ketogenic diet | d. Before and after intestinal surgery |
| ____ 5. Low-residue diet | e. Hyperlipidemia |

**Activity C** ***Mark each statement as either "T" (True) or "F" (False). Correct any false statements.***

1. T F Soluble fiber helps increase stool bulk and stimulates peristalsis.
2. T F A high-potassium diet is given to clients who are taking diuretics.
3. T F Low-fat diets are prescribed if anticonvulsant drugs and a balanced diet have failed to control seizures.
4. T F A controlled-gluten diet is suggested for clients with kidney or liver disorders.
5. T F Edema is an excess accumulation of water and salts in tissues, especially in the lower extremities.
6. T F High sodium intake is indicated for both the prevention and treatment of osteoporosis.
7. T F Tube feeding is a means of providing liquid nourishment through a tube into the gastrointestinal tract.
8. T F Intravenous therapy involves injecting sterile solutions into a vein.

**Activity D** *Fill in the blanks.*

1. ____________ is the medical term for a swallowing disorder.
2. A ____________ soft diet is recommended for people with difficulty in chewing or swallowing.
3. A high-____________ diet is often ordered as part of the treatment for constipation and diverticulosis.
4. The goal of a ____________ diet is to limit foods that stimulate the production of gastric acid.
5. A ____________ diet is extremely low in carbohydrates and can contain as much as 80% to 90% fat.
6. Allergic reactions to certain food substances are caused by an autoimmune response to ____________ in these foods.
7. Total parenteral nutrition is used when the ____________ tract is functioning improperly.

**Activity E** *Consider the following figure.*

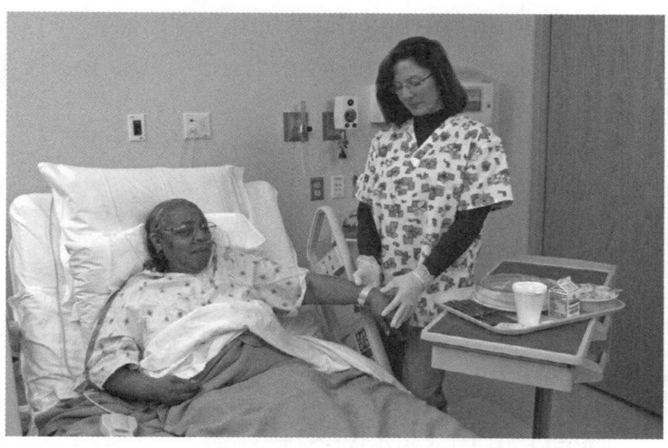

1. What should the nurse check for before handing over the food tray to the client?

____________________________________________

____________________________________________

2. What care should the nurse take when the client has NPO status?

____________________________________________

____________________________________________

**Activity F** *The steps for continuous feeding using the feeding pump are given below in random order. Write the correct sequence in which the steps are to be performed in the boxes provided.*

1. Open the clamp and prime the tubing.
2. Attach the end of the setup to the gastric tube.
3. Open the clamp and turn on the pump.
4. Flush the tube every 6 to 8 hours (if mandated by doctor's order or hospital policy).
5. Clamp the feeding setup and hang it on the pole.
6. Add the feeding solution to the bag.
7. Thread the tubing through or load the tubing into the pump.
8. Set the prescribed rate and volume according to the manufacturer's directions.
9. Stop the feeding every 4 to 8 hours to assess the residual. (Check hospital policy before stopping any feeding.)

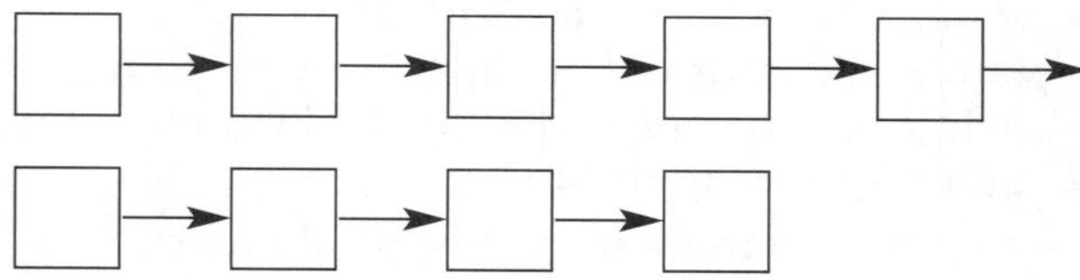

**Activity G** *Briefly answer the following questions.*

1. In what cases does a physician order fluid restriction?

____________________________________________

____________________________________________

2. What are the types of soft diets?

____________________________________________

____________________________________________

3. What food items should be avoided on a bland diet?

____________________________________________

____________________________________________

4. What is the goal of diabetes mellitus treatment?

____________________________________________

____________________________________________

5. What is lactose intolerance?

______________________________________

______________________________________

6. What kinds of clients require tube feeding?

______________________________________

______________________________________

## SECTION II: APPLYING WHAT YOU KNOW

**Activity H** *Answer the following questions, which involve the nurse's role in assisting clients to eat.*

A nurse encourages clients to eat by serving food attractively, providing assistance at mealtimes, and ensuring that eating is easy and safe. If the nurse has to feed the client the entire meal, he should take time to make the client feel comfortable and encourage her to eat as much as she desires.

1. A nurse is caring for a client who needs assistance with eating. The client is a very young, helpless, and confused individual who requires special attention.
   a. What are the nursing responsibilities to make sure that the young client ingests nutrients?
   b. What should the nurse's assessment include when caring for a young client?
2. A nurse is assisting a client who is temporarily blinded due to eye surgery.
   a. What are the nurse's responsibilities when helping this client eat his meal?
   b. How can the nurse help the client to learn to locate the food on the plate?
3. A nurse is caring for a client with dysphagia.
   a. What should the nurse do to determine appropriate diet consistency in a client with dysphagia?
   b. What are the nursing interventions to prevent choking in clients with dysphagia?

## SECTION III: GETTING READY FOR NCLEX

**Activity I** *Answer the following questions.*

1. What should the nurse keep in mind when serving food to a client in a healthcare facility?
   a. Present food that includes at least a dessert
   b. Ensure that the food includes calcium-rich items
   c. Present the food in an attractive and appetizing manner
   d. Ensure that the food is cold when served
2. What type of diet is prescribed for a client with pancreatic and gallbladder diseases?
   a. Gluten-restricted diet
   b. Fat-controlled diet
   c. Low-fat diet
   d. High-protein diet
3. What nursing interventions should the nurse perform for a client who is receiving nutritional support through tube feedings? (Select all that apply.)
   a. Position the bed flat when feeding
   b. Prepare and administer the formula food while it is cold
   c. Administer water in case of inadequate hydration
   d. Replace the feeding bag according to hospital policy
   e. Check for signs such as dry mouth or fever
4. A client with gastric ulcer has been prescribed a bland diet by the physician. What instructions should the nurse provide to this client? (Select all that apply.)
   a. Increase intake of fatty foods
   b. Eat smaller, more frequent meals
   c. Avoid lying down for 1 hour after a meal
   d. Avoid the intake of milk-based foods
   e. Drink plenty of water along with food

**5.** A client with constipation is prescribed a high-fiber diet. What are the problems associated with a high-fiber diet?

- **a.** Cramping and diarrhea
- **b.** Iron deficiency
- **c.** Calcium deficiency
- **d.** Reduced intake of minerals

**6.** A nurse is caring for an elderly client in a home care setting. What is the nurse's responsibility during routine nutritional care in this case?

- **a.** Ensuring that the client has food served by tray
- **b.** Ensuring that the family is preparing and serving food
- **c.** Conducting nutritional screenings and counseling
- **d.** Making the client follow a rigid meal schedule

**7.** Which type of diet should the nurse order for a client with oral problems?

- **a.** High-protein diet
- **b.** Mechanical soft diet
- **c.** Digestive soft diet
- **d.** Bland diet

**8.** What precautions should a nurse take while using food trays to help a client meet nutritional needs in a healthcare setting? (Select all that apply.)

- **a.** Ensure that the food tray is labeled with the client's age
- **b.** Ensure that the client's name band matches the name on the food tray
- **c.** Ensure that the client's information is checked against the posted diet list
- **d.** Ensure that the tray is labeled with the client's name and room number
- **e.** Ensure that the food tray strictly contains the client's choice diet

**9.** A client who is recovering from surgery has been prescribed supplemental nourishment. When should the nurse provide supplemental nourishment?

- **a.** Along with the meal
- **b.** Just before the meal
- **c.** Just after the meal
- **d.** Between meals

**10.** A nurse is caring for a client with end-stage renal disease. Fluid intake is restricted in this client. Which of the following is the most important factor that should be monitored by the nurse?

- **a.** Poor appetite
- **b.** Fluid intake and output
- **c.** Supplementary meals
- **d.** Calories consumed

CHAPTER 33

# Introduction to the Nursing Process

## SECTION I: TESTING WHAT YOU KNOW

**Activity A** ***Match the terms related to the nursing process in Column A with their descriptions in Column B.***

| Column A | Column B |
|---|---|
| ____ 1. Trial and error | a. Based on previously proven facts |
| ____ 2. Scientific problem-solving | b. Mix of inquiry, knowledge, intuition, logic, experience, and common sense |
| ____ 3. Critical thinking | c. Experimental approach to problem-solving |

**Activity B** ***Match the nursing process steps in Column A with their meanings in Column B.***

| Column A | Column B |
|---|---|
| ____ 1. Nursing assessment | a. Measurement of effectiveness of nursing care |
| ____ 2. Nursing diagnosis | b. Providing actual nursing care |
| ____ 3. Planning | c. Systematic and continuous collection of data |
| ____ 4. Implementation | d. Development of goals for care and activities to meet them |
| ____ 5. Evaluation | e. Statement of the client's actual or potential problem |

**Activity C** ***Mark each statement as either "T" (True) or "F" (False). Correct any false statements.***

1. T F Scientific problem-solving is an experimental approach to problem-solving.
2. T F Trial and error enables a person to grasp the meaning of multiple clues and find quick answers to difficult problems.
3. T F As a critical thinker, you become an open-minded person, flexible to alternatives.
4. T F As a nurse, you use the trial and error method to care for your clients.
5. T F The nursing care plans are a set of guidelines that ensure consistency among all nursing staff.
6. T F The nursing process focuses on performing specific skills or tasks.
7. T F Clients having the same medical problem will follow the same nursing plan.

**Activity D** ***Fill in the blanks.***

1. ____________ is the basic skill of identifying a problem and taking steps to resolve it.
2. The ____________ process is the method used by the nurse to identify and treat client care problems.
3. ____________ nurses are more likely to develop nursing diagnoses, set overall goals, and plan care.

4. The ___________ step in the nursing process involves measurement of the effectiveness of nursing care.
5. The nursing process provides measurable ___________ indicating the effectiveness of the nursing care given in any setting.
6. When thinking critically, the nurse examines ___________ and compares them with available information.

**Activity E** ***The stages of scientific problem-solving are given below in random order. Write the correct sequence in the boxes provided.***

1. Test solution
2. Formulate another tentative solution
3. Identify the problem
4. Formulate tentative solutions; describe possible solutions; choose preferred solution
5. Gather information relative to the problem
6. Plan action to test suggested solution
7. Evaluate the solution; evaluate the results

☐ → ☐ → ☐ → ☐ → ☐ → ☐ → ☐

**Activity F** ***Briefly answer the following questions.***

1. What is the primary goal of nursing?

___________________________________________

___________________________________________

2. What is critical thinking?

___________________________________________

___________________________________________

3. Briefly describe the nurse's role in each step of the nursing process.

___________________________________________

___________________________________________

4. Explain how and why the nursing process can be dynamic in nature.

___________________________________________

___________________________________________

5. What is a nursing care plan?

___________________________________________

___________________________________________

## SECTION II: APPLYING WHAT YOU KNOW

**Activity G** ***Answer the following questions, which involve the use of these tools.***

Critical thinking skills, the nursing process, and the nursing care plan are important tools to use when caring for a client.

1. A nurse is assigned to care for a client in a healthcare facility who has acute diarrhea. The nurse is expected to apply critical thinking skills when providing care.
   a. What does critical thinking in problem-solving involve? How does it help the nurse?
   b. What are the advantages of critical thinking?
2. A client undergoing treatment for diabetes in a healthcare facility will soon be going home. The nurse prepares a client-oriented nursing care plan to meet the long-term goals.
   a. What are the advantages of using the nursing care plan?
   b. How can the nurse ensure that the client will meet the long-term goals?
3. A client with severe dehydration has been admitted to the healthcare facility. The nurse is to follow a nursing care plan in caring for the client.
   a. How does the nursing process help the nurse to take charge of the situation?
   b. Explain the actions of the nurse at each step of the nursing process.
4. The nurse is asked to monitor the vital signs of a client recovering from surgery every 2 hours.
   a. Why should the nurse document the measurements of vital signs?
   b. How will such documentation help in the course of the treatment?

## SECTION III: GETTING READY FOR NCLEX

**Activity H** *Answer the following questions.*

1. A nurse is assigned to assess the condition of a client with hypertension. Which of the following steps of the nursing process should the nurse perform before she develops goals for care and possible activities to meet them?
   a. Evaluation
   b. Planning
   c. Diagnosis
   d. Implementation
2. When caring for a client with pneumonia, a nurse follows the nursing care plan; however, the client is not progressing according to the plan. Which of the following is the most appropriate nursing intervention in this situation?
   a. Reassess, reevaluate, and revise the nursing care plan
   b. Use the trial and error method with another plan
   c. Care for the client symptomatically without a care plan
   d. Experiment and observe the results
3. As part of the care for a client in a healthcare facility, the nurse needs to obtain the client's medical history. This activity comprises which step in the nursing process?
   a. Nursing diagnosis
   b. Implementation
   c. Nursing assessment
   d. Evaluation
4. A nurse develops nursing care plans for two clients diagnosed with diabetes. One client has a medical history of hypertension. Which of the following is the single most appropriate reason for the nurse to prepare two different nursing care plans?
   a. The nursing care plan is client-oriented.
   b. The nursing care plan identifies potential problems.
   c. The nursing care plan averts complications.
   d. The nursing care plan is dynamic.
5. A client is brought to the community health center in an emergency. Using the nursing process, the nurse has to perform an intervention while evaluating its effect and at the same time assessing another factor and planning priorities of what to do next. This method of functioning indicates which aspect of the nursing process?
   a. Its dynamic nature
   b. Its continuous nature
   c. Its systematic nature
   d. Its experimental nature
6. When caring for a client, the nurse analyzes the client's responses. This action of scientific problem-solving is related to which of the following steps in the nursing process?
   a. Implementation
   b. Nursing diagnosis
   c. Evaluation
   d. Planning
7. A nurse who is caring for a particular client in a healthcare facility is leaving for the day. She is confident that the nurse on the next shift will not overlook any detail in the care of the client. Which of the following factors makes the nurse so confident?
   a. Nurses rely on the physician when caring for the client.
   b. Nurses seek advice from the team leader.
   c. Nurses refer to the same care plan when providing care.
   d. Nurses care for clients symptomatically.
8. Which of the following are advantages of adopting a nursing care plan? (Select all that apply.)
   a. Helps the nurse avert painful complications for the client
   b. Allows the nurse to develop critical thinking skills
   c. Allows the nurse to have a single care plan that applies to all clients
   d. Helps the nurse evaluate the nursing care provided
   e. Provides the nurse with beneficial results for related problems

**9.** Why is critical thinking important in healthcare? (Select all that apply.)

**a.** It helps the nurse grasp the meaning of multiple clues.

**b.** It helps the nurse examine and compare facts with available information.

**c.** It provides an experimental approach to help the nurse solve problems.

**d.** It helps the nurse find quick answers when facing difficult problems.

**e.** It helps the nurse test ideas to decide which methods work and which do not.

**10.** Which of the following steps from the scientific problem-solving method relate to planning?

**a.** Analyze the client's responses

**b.** Formulate tentative solutions

**c.** Gather problem-related information

**d.** Identify the problem

CHAPTER 34

# Nursing Assessment

## SECTION I: TESTING WHAT YOU KNOW

**Activity A** *Match the components of the nursing history in Column A with the information that belongs to the relevant component in Column B.*

| Column A | Column B |
|---|---|
| ____ 1. Biographical data | a. Symptoms of recent disease |
| ____ 2. Recent health history | b. Sexual relationships |
| ____ 3. Important medical history | c. Name, age, birth date |
| ____ 4. Pertinent psychosocial information | d. Family history of disease |
| ____ 5. Activities of daily living | e. Involves how well the client is able to meet basic needs |

**Activity B** *Mark each statement as either "T" (True) or "F" (False). Correct any false statements.*

1. T F Subjective data consist of the client's opinions or feelings about what is happening.
2. T F A client's opinion that she has high blood pressure is an example of objective data.
3. T F Palpation of the skin to assess muscle strength is an example of tactile observation.
4. T F The interview conducted by a physician when a client is admitted to a healthcare facility is known as an admission interview.
5. T F The client should be informed that the purpose of an admission interview is to arrange for the necessary administrative facilities.

**Activity C** *Fill in the blanks.*

1. Nursing ____________ is the systematic and continuous collection and analysis of information about the client.
2. Listening to the heart, lung, or bowel sounds with a stethoscope is known as ____________.
3. ____________ observation refers to the use of the sense of smell to identify odors.
4. Data that are similar or have a pattern can be grouped together to form a ____________.
5. ____________ is an assessment tool that relies on the use of the five senses to discover information about the client.

**Activity D** *The steps to be taken during a nursing assessment are given below in random order. Write the correct sequence in the boxes provided.*

1. Analyze data to reach conclusions
2. Recognize significant data
3. Collect data about the client
4. Recognize patterns or clusters
5. Identify assessment priorities related to the purpose of the interview
6. Identify strengths and problems
7. Validate observations

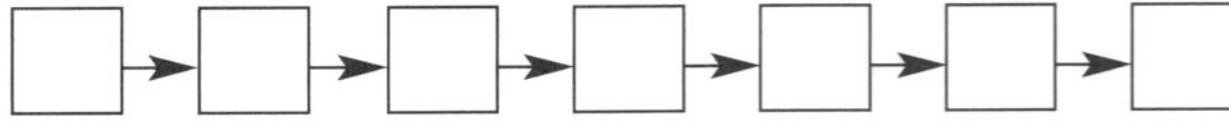

**Activity E** *Briefly answer the following questions.*

1. What is the purpose of the nursing assessment?

   ______________________________

   ______________________________

2. What are the methods used for data collection when assessing a client?

   ______________________________

   ______________________________

3. What are the skills a nurse should have to obtain subjective data from a client?

   ______________________________

   ______________________________

4. What are the elements of visual observation that a nurse should use to collect data when assessing a client?

   ______________________________

   ______________________________

5. What are the ways in which a nurse can validate observations?

   ______________________________

   ______________________________

## SECTION II: APPLYING WHAT YOU KNOW

**Activity F** *Answer the following questions, which involve data collection.*

A nurse's role in providing effective care to clients involves gathering complete and accurate information about the client.

1. A client has just arrived at a healthcare center complaining of a sharp pain in the area near the kidneys. The nurse is preparing for the admission interview of the client.
   a. When collecting data, what information should the nurse classify as objective data?
   b. What information will the nurse classify as subjective data?
2. A nurse is preparing to interview a client. What are the components of the nursing history that the nurse should obtain from the client?
3. A nurse is caring for a client in a healthcare facility. What are the types of observations that a nurse must use when collecting data on the basis of observation?
4. A nurse has conducted the admission interview of a client and has analyzed the data in the nursing history. What are the four possible conclusions that the nurse may arrive at?

## SECTION III: GETTING READY FOR NCLEX

**Activity G** *Answer the following questions.*

1. During the nursing assessment, the client complains of a lower abdominal pain. Which of the following is the most appropriate nursing action in this situation?
   a. Determine whether the client has the necessary strength to cope with the problem.
   b. Base assessment questions on a predefined format.
   c. Ignore any possible risk factors and concentrate on the actual problems.
   d. Conceal the true extent of the problems from the client.
2. A nurse is collecting data on a client's health history. The client's family members are also present. Which of the following interventions should the nurse perform when collecting data regarding the client's medical history?
   a. Concentrate on obtaining only objective data regarding the condition.
   b. Do not ask questions of family members, because they may give conflicting answers.
   c. Confirm the information obtained from the client with family members.
   d. Consult other members of the healthcare team for their analysis of client data.
3. A client arrives at a community healthcare center with a wound on his leg as a result of an accident. Which of the following information about the client's condition should the nurse classify as objective data?
   a. Anxiety felt by client
   b. Size and color of the wound
   c. Pain felt by the client
   d. Client's complaint of feeling nauseated

4. A nurse is monitoring the progress of an Asian client on drug therapy. Which of the following points should the nurse consider when collecting subjective data regarding the client and her response to the therapy?
   a. Assess the client's body language and gestures.
   b. Ignore the presence of any charms or amulets.
   c. Avoid asking the client any direct questions.
   d. Insist on the presence of a family member.

5. A nurse is assessing a client who has undergone surgery. During the assessment, the nurse observes that the client's skin feels warm; therefore, the nurse measures the client's body temperature. Which of the following types of observation did the nurse make before taking the client's temperature with a thermometer?
   a. Visual observation
   b. Tactile observation
   c. Auditory observation
   d. Olfactory observation

6. A nurse is caring for a client who appears to have responded well to the treatment but is looking pale as a result of being confined indoors for the duration of the treatment. When the nurse asked the client how she feels, the client grimaces slightly and responds with an "OK." On further questioning, the nurse finds out that the client is feeling nauseated and has abdominal pain. Which of the following aspects of visual observation did the nurse employ in this case?
   a. Body movements
   b. General appearance
   c. Facial expression
   d. Skin color

7. Which of the following are responsibilities of the registered nurse during the admission interview of a client being admitted to a healthcare facility?
   a. Assign a nursing student to take an admission interview.
   b. Avoid questions on the medical condition of client, which will be covered by the physician.
   c. Work with the team to formulate a nursing diagnosis and plan of care.
   d. Conduct the interview only in the presence of a physician.

8. A nurse is collecting data about a client who has been admitted with an ear infection. Which of the following questions should the nurse ask himself as part of the critical thinking skills used to collect objective data? (Select all that apply.)
   a. What do the client's vital signs reveal about the client's condition?
   b. What is the client's psychological state of mind during the assessment?
   c. What do the physician's history and progress notes indicate about the client's condition?
   d. What do the current and previous laboratory reports reveal about the client's condition?
   e. Does the client believe in the effectiveness of the therapy?

9. A nurse is caring for a client with gastrointestinal problems. Which of the following questions should the nurse ask herself to obtain subjective data about the client? (Select all that apply.)
   a. Do the client's words and behaviors say the same thing?
   b. How did the client's family react about news of the client?
   c. What kind of relationship exists between the client and his or her spouse?
   d. How is the client coping with the immediate environment?
   e. What does the client say is the reason for coming to the healthcare facility?

10. A nurse has conducted the health interview of a client. Which of the following types of information forms a part of the activities of daily living (ADL) section of the nursing history? (Select all that apply.)
    a. Typical diet of the client
    b. Emotional stability of the client
    c. Symptoms of any recent diseases
    d. Exercise regimen followed by the client
    e. Sleep patterns of the client

CHAPTER 35

# Nursing Diagnosis and Planning

## SECTION I: TESTING WHAT YOU KNOW

**Activity A** *Match the components of the nursing diagnostic statement in Column A with their descriptions in Column B.*

| Column A | Column B |
|---|---|
| ____ **1.** Nursing Assessment | **a.** Identifying the nursing care problem based on analysis of data |
| ____ **2.** Nursing Diagnosis | **b.** Collecting data related to client's condition |
| ____ **3.** Planning | **c.** Formulating necessary arrangements for client care |

**Activity B** *Mark each statement as either "T" (True) or "F" (False). Correct any false statements.*

**1.** T F Practical nurses must understand the meaning of a nursing diagnosis and how it is used to plan and to implement nursing care.

**2.** T F A nursing care plan is not necessary if the client's condition is not serious.

**3.** T F NANDA International maintains a list of acceptable nursing diagnoses.

**4.** T F The nursing diagnosis focuses on identifying the cause of the disease.

**5.** T F All nursing diagnoses have equal priority.

**6.** T F While establishing the client's expected outcome, the nurse should ensure that it is a measurable client behavior.

**7.** T F The nurse who has made the nursing assessment independently formulates the nursing care plan.

**Activity C** *Fill in the blanks.*

**1.** A medical ___________ provides a basis for prognosis and medical treatment decisions.

**2.** The ___________ part of the diagnostic statement mentions the cause of the problem.

**3.** A ___________ is a flip-file with card slots, or a notebook, for each client being treated by a unit or nursing care team.

**4.** A ___________ objective is an outcome that the client ultimately hopes to achieve but that requires a longer period of time to accomplish.

**5.** A ___________ problem is one on which the nurses work together with the physician or other healthcare providers.

**Activity D** *A nursing diagnosis is given in the form of a diagnostic statement. Components of a diagnostic statement are given below in random order. Write the correct sequence in which the components would appear in the boxes provided.*

1. Etiology
2. Problem
3. Signs and symptoms

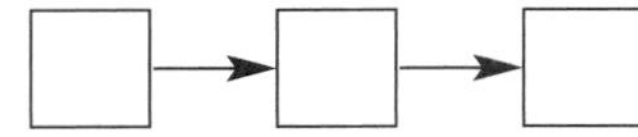

**Activity E** *Briefly answer the following questions.*

1. What is a collaborative problem?

______________________________

______________________________

2. What is NANDA, and what is its contribution to the nursing diagnosis process?

______________________________

______________________________

## SECTION II: APPLYING WHAT YOU KNOW

**Activity F** *Answer the following questions, which concern the nurse's role in the nursing diagnosis process.*

The nursing diagnosis process involves identifying the nursing care problem and planning client care based on the problems or diagnoses identified.

1. A nurse has collected data relating to a new client who was admitted 6 hours ago. The nurse has been assigned the task of writing the nursing care plan. What are the points the nurse must keep in mind while writing the nursing care plan?
2. A student nurse is assisting a registered nurse in the process of data collection and formulation of the nursing diagnosis. What are the purposes of the nursing diagnosis that the registered nurse should explain to the nursing student?
3. A nurse is planning the care of a client. What factors should the nurse keep in mind when setting priorities for the client by ranking nursing diagnoses in terms of importance?
4. A nurse has been caring for a client in a healthcare facility. The nurse must establish the client's expected outcome to measure whether the client has achieved the expected benefit of nursing care and how successfully the client's short- and long-term goals have been met. What are the points the nurse should keep in mind when formulating the expected outcome?

## SECTION III: GETTING READY FOR NCLEX

**Activity G** *Answer the following questions.*

1. When caring for a client, a nurse has analyzed data regarding the client's chief concern. Which of the following would the nurse include in the diagnosis?
   a. Identification of the disease
   b. The medical treatment plan
   c. Identification of the nursing care problem
   d. The cause of the disease
2. A nurse is preparing a two-part diagnostic statement for a client with renal failure. Which of the following is the most appropriate way of phrasing the problem in the diagnostic statement?
   a. Impaired urinary elimination
   b. Chronic renal disorder
   c. Problems in voiding
   d. Caused by diabetes
3. A nurse is formulating the diagnostic statement for a client who had a bicycle accident. The healthcare facility where the nurse works uses a three-part diagnostic statement. The client has multiple lacerations and bruises on her right arm and is unable to make movements using that arm. Which of the following is an example of a correct diagnostic statement?
   a. Impaired mobility of right arm R/T multiple lacerations, bruises, and swelling AEB biking accident
   b. Impaired mobility of right arm R/T biking accident AEB multiple lacerations, bruises, and swelling
   c. Impaired mobility of right arm AEB multiple lacerations, bruises, and swelling
   d. Impaired movement of the client's right arm related to a bike accident

**4.** Which of the following facts must the nurse keep in mind when creating a nursing care plan to meet the requirements of agencies such as the Joint Commission, nursing home regulators, and Medicare?

**a.** All data relating to clients have to be computerized.

**b.** No changes should be made to the original nursing care plan.

**c.** The nursing care plan should be written only on Kardex files.

**d.** The nursing care plan should be available within 12 to 24 hours after admission.

**5.** A nurse is planning the care of a client with severe diarrhea. The nurse knows that which of the following diagnostic results should assume the highest priority?

**a.** Significant water loss

**b.** Abdominal pain

**c.** Fever

**d.** Nausea

**6.** A nurse is caring for a client with multiple fractures in his leg and arms. Which of the following should the nurse plan as the client's long-term objective?

**a.** Walk around the room after 2 days

**b.** Resume playing for college football team

**c.** Absence of any pain or discomfort after discharge

**d.** Perform light exercises with the injured limbs

**7.** A nurse is preparing the care plan for an 8-year-old child with asthma. Which of the following nursing interventions should the nurse perform to help the client meet the treatment goals?

**a.** Interact with client regularly to prevent loneliness

**b.** Change dosage if client's condition worsens

**c.** Set long-term goals to motivate the client

**d.** Administer corticosteroids as ordered by the physician

**8.** A nurse is preparing the nursing diagnosis for a client who has just been admitted to the healthcare facility. The nurse knows that a nursing diagnosis is prepared for which of the following reasons? (Select all that apply.)

**a.** Determining the cause and nature of the disease

**b.** Identifying the client care problems

**c.** Stating the prognosis or projected client outcome

**d.** Directing interventions for the client's priority needs

**e.** Providing a common platform for the entire healthcare team

**9.** A nurse is preparing the goal of the nursing plan. Which of the following points should the nurse keep in mind when formulating the expected outcome statements? (Select all that apply.)

**a.** Ensure that the outcome is client-oriented.

**b.** Generalize the statement to include any new outcome.

**c.** The outcome should be within the client's capacity and abilities.

**d.** The outcome should include whether or not client is feeling better.

**e.** The outcome should be observable and measurable.

**10.** A nurse is required to plan the care of a client. In what order should the following steps be performed when planning care?

**a.** Establishing expected outcomes

**b.** Setting priorities

**c.** Writing a nursing care plan

**d.** Selecting nursing interventions

CHAPTER 36

# Implementing and Evaluating Care

## SECTION I: TESTING WHAT YOU KNOW

**Activity A** ***Match the types of skills used in implementing nursing care in Column A with their examples in Column B.***

| Column A | Column B |
|---|---|
| ____ 1. Technical skills | a. Client encounters promoting development of a trusting relationship |
| ____ 2. Intellectual skills | b. Administering an injection |
| ____ 3. Interpersonal skills | c. Basic sciences |

**Activity B** ***Mark each statement as either "T" (True) or "F" (False). Correct any false statements.***

1. T F It is important to encourage client participation in planning the timetable listing the client activities that need to be performed.
2. T F To enable continuing collection of data, it is important for the nurse to encourage maximum participation from the client's family.
3. T F Planning for discharge begins when the client is prepared to leave the healthcare facility and is ready for continued care when living at home.
4. T F Observing clients and monitoring their vital signs closely enables a nurse to make the safest and most helpful choices for each of her clients.

**Activity C** ***Fill in the blanks.***

1. A nurse is responsible for all the actions that he performs—dependent, interdependent, or independent. This responsibility is also called ____________.
2. ____________ planning is the process by which the client is prepared for continued care outside the healthcare facility or for independent living at home.
3. ____________ is the fourth step in nursing care, after assessment, diagnosis, and planning.
4. ____________ is measuring the effectiveness of assessment, diagnosis, planning, and implementation.

**Activity D** ***Given below are the steps involved in evaluating nursing care. Write the correct sequence in the boxes provided.***

1. Identifying factors contributing to success or failure related to achievement of goals
2. Analyzing the client's response
3. Planning future nursing care

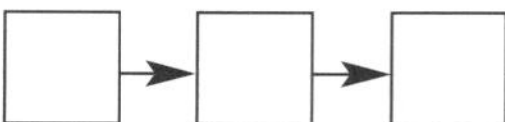

**Activity E** *Briefly answer the following.*

1. What does the action phrase "share it" in nursing implementation mean?

 ______________________________________

 ______________________________________

2. What are dependent, interdependent, and independent nursing actions?

 ______________________________________

 ______________________________________

3. What are the basic skills required in implementing nursing care?

 ______________________________________

 ______________________________________

4. How is the client's response analyzed when evaluating nursing care?

 ______________________________________

 ______________________________________

## SECTION II: APPLYING WHAT YOU KNOW

**Activity F** ***Answer the following questions, which involve the nurse's role in implementing and evaluating care given to the client.***

The step of carrying out the nursing care plan is called implementation.

1. A nurse is accompanied by young students as she does her hospital rounds. The students are asked to observe the nurse at work as she provides care to the clients. The nurse has to address the group and educate them on the implementation of nursing care.
   a. What information should the nurse provide on adequate communication and documentation in continuity of care?
   b. What information should the nurse provide on dependent, interdependent, and independent nursing actions?
   c. What information should the nurse provide on basic skills used in giving care?
2. A nurse is required to care for a client who is admitted in a healthcare facility. The nurse has to prepare a nursing care plan for the client and determine the effectiveness of the plan. The nurse also has to collect adequate data in the continuing care of the client.
   a. What factors should a nurse keep in mind when reviewing a care plan?
   b. What nursing interventions should a nurse perform to effectively collect data in the continuing care of the client?
3. A nurse is assigned to care for a client for whom the nurse has prepared a nursing care plan. The nurse has to evaluate the care plan by following certain steps.
   a. What steps should a nurse follow when evaluating the nursing care?
   b. How can the nurse analyze the client's response?
   c. What steps should a nurse take to plan future nursing care?
4. A nurse has been caring for a client who is now going to be discharged from the healthcare facility. The nurse is required to prepare a discharge plan for the client.
   a. What important steps should a nurse take for discharge planning?
   b. What components of discharge planning should the nurse include in the client's discharge plan?

## SECTION III: GETTING READY FOR NCLEX

**Activity G** *Answer the following questions.*

1. Which of the following factors should a nurse keep in mind when reviewing a client's care plan?
   a. Involve the client actively in the plan.
   b. Develop the plan based only on critical thinking skills.
   c. Encourage family participation.
   d. List nursing orders to meet the nurse's ability.
2. Which of the following steps should the nurse take to plan discharge planning? (Select all that apply.)
   a. Suggest revisions for unmet goals.
   b. Set new goals if earlier goals are met.
   c. Analyze the responses of the client.
   d. Note the goals resolved by the client.
   e. Closely monitor the client's behavior.

3. A nurse has worked on the care plan for a client and now must collect relative data for his continuing care. Which of the following factors will help the nurse effectively collect data in the continuing care of the client?
   a. Refrain from involving the client in planning the activities timetable.
   b. Gather information from the client's family during care.
   c. Observe the client carefully when providing care.
   d. Use logic to determine the effectiveness of nursing orders.
4. A nurse caring for a client in a healthcare facility has prepared a client care plan. Which of the following steps should the nurse take to evaluate the nursing care? (Select all that apply.)
   a. Plan future nursing care for the client.
   b. Analyze the responses of the client.
   c. Assess each client regularly according to the timeline.
   d. Prepare the client for care outside the healthcare facility.
   e. Identify factors contributing to the success and failure of goals.
5. A nurse is required to document information when caring for a client. The client and the client's family wish to know how communication and documentation facilitate the provision of care. Which of the following is the appropriate explanation a nurse should provide?
   a. They help the nurse to analyze the responses of the client.
   b. They allow the next healthcare provider to act with purpose and understanding.
   c. They allow the client's family to actively participate in client care.
   d. They help identify factors contributing to success or failure in meeting goals.
6. Which of the following components should the nurse include in a client's discharge plan? (Select all that apply.)
   a. Focus on the achievement of short-term goals
   b. Special diet with documentation by the dietitian
   c. Documentation of supplies needed by the client's family
   d. Appointment for the next visit to the physician
   e. Instructing the client to monitor his vital signs
7. The nurse is assisting a client with bathing and getting dressed for a scheduled appointment in an hour. What type of nursing action does this represent?
   a. Dependent
   b. Interdependent
   c. Collaborative
   d. Independent
8. The nurse has to administer a daily insulin injection to a client. What type of skill is required for safe and competent performance?
   a. Interpersonal
   b. Intellectual
   c. Critical thinking
   d. Technical
9. A nurse is assigned to care for a client for whom the nurse prepared a nursing care plan 2 days ago. The nurse needs to evaluate the nursing care plan. What should the nurse do for an unresolved goal?
   a. Note on the care plan or care path that it is unresolved and state the reason why.
   b. Delete the current goal and write a new goal.
   c. Make revisions to the nursing care plan.
   d. Mark what problems are resolved on the care plan.
10. The nurse is evaluating the client nursing care plan received during hospitalization. What questions assist the nurse in evaluating the nursing care? (Select all that apply.)
    a. Was each goal met by the client?
    b. Has nursing care helped the client realize self-care goals?
    c. Does this plan protect the client's safety?
    d. Is the care plan based on sound medical knowledge?

CHAPTER 37

# Documenting and Reporting

## SECTION I: TESTING WHAT YOU KNOW

***Match the types of progress records in Column A with their meanings in Column B.***

| Column A | Column B |
| --- | --- |
| ____ 1. Medication administration record (MAR) | a. Handwritten in ink in the manual record |
| ____ 2. Flow sheet | b. Records large amount of information collected at intervals over a specified period in brief, concise entries |
| ____ 3. Nursing progress notes | c. Lists all the medication that the physician has ordered for the client |

**Activity B** ***Mark each statement as either "T" (True) or "F" (False). Correct any false statements.***

1. T F When documenting client-related information, the nurse should directly quote the client and should differentiate the client's words from the observations.
2. T F In case of an error in documentation in a manual health record, the nurse can correct the error under "late entries."
3. T F A nurse should not discuss his or her clients "over coffee."
4. T F The purpose of the plan for care is to list all medications that the physician has ordered for the client.
5. T F A clinical care path specifies expected outcomes and treatments at specified times for all members of a healthcare team.
6. T F The nursing care plan is usually developed by the physician after a thorough assessment of the client's health status has been conducted.
7. T F Healthcare facilities use the medical information system (MIS) for diet, laboratory, pharmacy orders, billing, and statistical data collection.

**Activity C** ***Fill in the blanks.***

1. ____________ reporting is a means of exchanging information between the outgoing and incoming staff on each shift.
2. A ____________ sheet is a graph or form that records large amounts of information collected at intervals over a specified period in brief, concise entries.

3. A ____________ note is entered at regular intervals to summarize the client's condition or response to treatment.
4. ____________ means that conversations with clients, nursing observations, and assessments are shared only with the appropriate caregivers in the proper setting.
5. A ____________ record is a manual or electronic account of a client's relationship with a healthcare facility.
6. In ____________ rounds, caregivers move from client to client discussing pertinent information.

**Activity D** *Consider the following figure.*

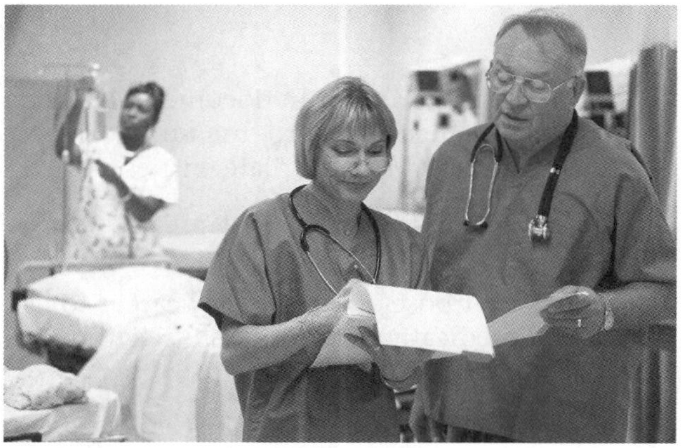

1. Identify the activity being conducted.

______________________________________

______________________________________

2. What are the different forms of the activity depicted in the figure that are generally used?

______________________________________

______________________________________

**Activity E** *Briefly answer the following questions.*

1. What is a health record? What is it used for?

______________________________________

______________________________________

2. What is the importance of a health record?

______________________________________

______________________________________

3. How can a health record be considered a legal document?

______________________________________

______________________________________

4. What is the advantage of electronic recording over manual recording?

______________________________________

______________________________________

5. What information do assessment documents record?

______________________________________

______________________________________

6. What are the different systems for data entry?

______________________________________

______________________________________

7. What is the importance of being specific and precise in a client observation?

______________________________________

______________________________________

## SECTION II: APPLYING WHAT YOU KNOW

**Activity F** ***Answer the following questions, which involve the nurse's role in documenting, reporting, and recording client information when providing care.***

The health record facilitates communication among caregivers, provides evidence of accountability, and facilitates health research and education.

1. A nurse is assigned to care for a client with a cardiopulmonary disorder in a healthcare facility. The nurse has to prepare the client's health record.
   a. What information should the nurse document in a health record of the client?
   b. Should the nurse document every single aspect of care given to the client? If yes, then why?

2. A nurse is caring for a client with cancer in a healthcare facility. When preparing the health record, the nurse also has to prepare the assessment documents. In addition, the nurse has to measure the client's ability to perform activities of daily living.
   - a. What information should the nurse include in his assessment document?
   - b. Which assessment form should the nurse work on to measure the client's ability to perform activities of daily living?
3. A nurse is caring for a client with a pulmonary disorder and has to document the client's treatment and responses. For this the nurse will have to use progress records.
   - a. What are the different of data entry systems that can be used in the progress notes?
   - b. What are the different types of progress notes that can be maintained?
4. A nurse caring for a client is required to "report off" to another nurse when her shift is complete. The nurse has to give information about her client to the incoming nurse through change-of-shift reporting. What guidelines should the outgoing nurse follow under change-of-shift reporting?

## SECTION III: GETTING READY FOR NCLEX

**Activity G** *Answer the following questions.*

1. When documenting client information in the electronic health record, a nurse makes an error in documentation. Which of the following steps should the nurse take to correct the error and add the relevant information?
   - a. Correct the error by using "recorded in error."
   - b. Delete the error and replace with relevant information.
   - c. Highlight the error and put it in parentheses.
   - d. Correct the error by using "late entries."
2. The nurse caring for clients in a healthcare facility has to ensure that all the clients are assessed in the same way. Which of the following assessment forms should the nurse use to ensure that her clients are similarly assessed?
   - a. Minimum data set
   - b. Charting by exception
   - c. Medication administration record
   - d. Clinical care path
3. A nurse is caring for a client who has undergone organ transplant surgery. Which of the following steps should the nurse implement to facilitate financial accountability for the care given to the client? (Select all that apply.)
   - a. Meet the standards of care set by the government.
   - b. Verify care given through quality assurance programs.
   - c. Record all treatments given to the client.
   - d. Record use of any special equipment for the client.
   - e. Record all examinations administered when caring for the client.
4. A nurse is caring for a client who is taking longer than expected to achieve the desired outcome. The nurse understands that, because of the client's specific health problem, it is necessary to perform the best nursing interventions to help the client achieve his goal. Which of the following steps should the nurse be aware of that will help determine the best intervention for the client?
   - a. Conduct research on the client's health record.
   - b. Closely monitor the client's vital signs.
   - c. Increase interactions with the client.
   - d. Gather client-related information from his family.

5. A client who is being discharged from a healthcare facility is required to regularly visit a community-based care center for further care. Which of the following factors should the nurse include in his discharge plan to ensure continuity of care by other caregivers?
   a. Importance of the client's maintaining a flow sheet of vital signs
   b. Importance of the client's maintaining a progress note
   c. Teaching plans for the client to follow
   d. Short-term goals to be achieved by the client
6. A nurse is caring for a client with hypertension. The client's family observes the nurse diligently maintaining the health record and are curious to know the importance of this record for the client. Which of the following should the nurse tell the family about the importance of a health record for the client?
   a. It verifies care through quality assurance programs.
   b. It helps in employment and disability applications.
   c. It helps in providing safe and effective care.
   d. It helps in meeting standards of care set by the government.
7. An LPN is addressing a group of unlicensed assistive personnel (UAPs) on the importance of a health record. Which of the following statements correctly reflect the importance of maintaining a health record? (Select all that apply.)
   a. It maintains effective communication among all caregivers.
   b. It specifies expected outcomes and treatments at specified times.
   c. It helps in research and educational purposes.
   d. It helps documentation in the medical information system.
   e. It provides written evidence of accountability.
8. A nurse at the end of her shift is required to introduce the nurse coming on duty to the clients before she leaves. Which of the following steps should the outgoing nurse take to ensure personalized client care by the incoming nurse and development of a good rapport between the incoming nurse and the clients?
   a. Schedule and prioritize the incoming nurse's time for each client.
   b. Provide information to the incoming nurse through walking rounds.
   c. Help establish a rapport between the incoming nurse and the client's family.
   d. Brief the incoming nurse thoroughly on each client's health records.
9. A nurse caring for a client in a healthcare facility is required to prepare the client's health record and to document his observations. Which of the following steps should the nurse implement to ensure that the observations are documented in a clear and concise manner?
   a. Avoid using any abbreviations.
   b. Record the date and time for each day.
   c. Get the physician's signature for every observation.
   d. Sign the health record with the first initial and last name.
10. Which of the following factors need to be documented in the client's manual health record? (Select all that apply.)
   a. Treatment plans for the client
   b. Weekly progress made by the client
   c. Client's vital signs that are monitored
   d. Assessment data of the client
   e. Pharmacy orders for the client

CHAPTER 38

# The Healthcare Facility Environment

## SECTION I: TESTING WHAT YOU KNOW

**Activity A** *Match the support services in Column A with their functions in Column B.*

| Column A | Column B |
|---|---|
| ____ 1. Consulting nurse service | a. Cleans and sterilizes equipment and instruments for use throughout the facility |
| ____ 2. Case management department | b. Provides telephone advice to callers who need assistance |
| ____ 3. Volunteer services | c. Provides service coordination, health assessment, education, and discharge planning |
| ____ 4. Central service supply | d. Brings clients to the nursing unit from the admitting department and transports clients for discharge or special tests |

**Activity B** *Mark each statement as either "T" (True) or "F" (False). Correct any false statements.*

1. T F The morgue is under a pathologist's direction and is the place where dead bodies are kept until identified and released to a funeral home or family.
2. T F The pediatric unit is responsible for the care of mothers and newborns.
3. T F The electroencephalography department records results of the brain wave test, which determines electrical activity within a client's brain.
4. T F The occupational therapy department directs its efforts toward preventing physical disability.
5. T F The emergency department gives care to persons whose conditions require immediate attention.

**Activity C** *Fill in the blanks.*

1. Pathologists also perform ____________ which are examinations conducted after death.
2. The ____________ care unit provides care for clients who require a moderate amount of skilled nursing care.
3. The ____________ care unit cares for clients with serious heart disorders.
4. Some large teaching hospitals also include a ____________ laboratory, where studies and experiments on animals are conducted to understand, cure, or prevent human disease.
5. The ____________ is an instrument used to examine inside the ears, nose, and throat.
6. ____________ enables healthcare providers to communicate with clients in different locations using a telephone and a computer.

**Activity D** *Consider the following figure.*

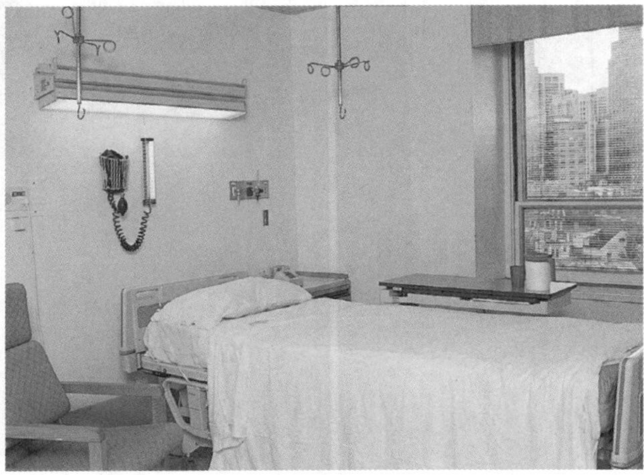

1. What does the figure represent?

______________________________

______________________________

2. What components are represented in the figure?

______________________________

______________________________

**Activity E** *Briefly answer the following:*

1. Which procedure does the radiology department conduct?

______________________________

______________________________

2. What are the functions of the occupational therapy department?

______________________________

______________________________

3. What care does a clinical decision unit provide?

______________________________

______________________________

4. What are the responsibilities of the staff working in an operating room and the post-anesthesia care unit?

______________________________

______________________________

## SECTION II: APPLYING WHAT YOU KNOW

**Activity F** *Answer the following questions, which relate to a nurse's understanding of hospital services.*

Hospitals offer a variety of services and are staffed with people experienced in many different areas. A nurse should have a general understanding of these departments and services and be able to explain them to clients when providing care.

1. A nurse is caring for a client in the physical therapy department of a healthcare facility.
   a. What is the role of the physical therapy department in providing healthcare?
   b. Who are the employees in the physical therapy department?
2. A client admitted to a local healthcare facility requires clinical diagnostic testing.
   a. What specimens does a pathologist include for clinical diagnostic testing?
   b. What are the different diagnostic departments?
3. A client involved in a motor vehicle accident is admitted to an intensive care unit (ICU) in a local healthcare facility. ICU is one of the specialized client care departments. What are the other specialized client care departments that assist in providing client care in healthcare facilities?

## SECTION III: GETTING READY FOR NCLEX

**Activity G** *Answer the following questions.*

1. A client is admitted to the mental health unit of a healthcare facility. Which of the following conditions must the client be experiencing?
   a. Psychiatric disorders
   b. Migraine
   c. Meningitis
   d. Substance abuse

2. A nurse is assigned to care for a client with a cardiopulmonary disorder in an emergency department (ED). What skills should the nurse have to provide effective care to this client? (Select all that apply.)
   a. Able to manage traumatic injuries
   b. Able to provide a moderate amount of skilled nursing care
   c. Able to provide cardiopulmonary resuscitation
   d. Able to provide cardiac care to the client
   e. Able to care for clients in critical conditions
3. A nurse is responsible for maintaining an ideal room temperature to make the client comfortable. What is the ideal room temperature that must be ensured to maintain balance between heat lost and heat produced?
   a. Temperature between 55° and 60° Fahrenheit
   b. Temperature between 68° and 72° Fahrenheit
   c. Temperature between 80° and 85° Fahrenheit
   d. Temperature between 50° and 55° Fahrenheit
4. What measures should the nurse take to ensure that the client's room is odor free to enhance client comfort?
   a. Always keep the windows of the room open.
   b. Use mild cologne, perfume, or an aftershave lotion.
   c. Remove bedpans and urinals immediately after use.
   d. Spray freshener in the room from time to time.
5. What nursing interventions should the nurse perform when issuing early morning care to the client?
   a. Give the client a bath or assist with bathing.
   b. Assist the client to ambulate and move around.
   c. Change the linens according to facility policy.
   d. Adjust the table for the breakfast tray.
6. What advantages of housekeeping should the nurse remember when attending to a client? (Select all that apply.)
   a. Good housekeeping makes the client recover faster.
   b. Good housekeeping helps to carry out nursing care efficiently.
   c. Good housekeeping helps prevent accidents and infections.
   d. Good housekeeping helps make the client feel secure.
   e. Good housekeeping ensures customized rooms for clients.
7. What type of care is issued by the palliative care unit?
   a. The palliative care unit cares for dying individuals.
   b. The palliative care unit cares for clients after discharge.
   c. The palliative care unit offers psychosocial support and rehabilitative services.
   d. The palliative care unit offers physical medicine and rehabilitation.
8. What is the role of the occupational therapy department in providing healthcare?
   a. The occupational therapy department assists clients with cardiac or respiratory disorders.
   b. The occupational therapy department assists clients in regaining function.
   c. The occupational therapy department directs its efforts toward preventing physical disability.
   d. The occupational therapy department helps clients rehabilitate.
9. A nurse is caring for a client with a severe respiratory disorder. The nurse observes that the client's family is distressed about the expense involved in the client's care and also seems to be unsure about the living arrangements that they should provide to the client after discharge. The nurse should refer the client's family to which of the following services in order to help them overcome their distress?
   a. Telecommunications
   b. Social services
   c. Chaplaincy services
   d. Volunteer services

**10.** A nurse is taking care of a patient in the occupational therapy department of a health care facility. What are the functions of the occupational therapy department? (Select all that apply.)

**a.** Help clients move toward rehabilitation with emphasis on gross motor muscle activity.

**b.** Help clients move toward rehabilitation with emphasis on fine motor muscle activity.

**c.** Help clients to regain use of affected areas through individualized programs of exercise and activity.

**d.** Help clients with activities of daily living.

CHAPTER 39

# Emergency Preparedness

## SECTION I: TESTING WHAT YOU KNOW

**Activity A** ***Match the hazardous substances in Column A with their examples in Column B.***

| Column A | Column B |
|---|---|
| ____ 1. Flammables | a. Clorosorb |
| ____ 2. Skin or eye irritants | b. Formalin |
| ____ 3. Poisons | c. Alcohol, oxygen |
| ____ 4. Carcinogens | d. Hibiclens |

**Activity B** ***Match the types of fire extinguishers in Column A with their uses in Column B.***

| Column A | Column B |
|---|---|
| ____ 1. Type C | a. Fire due to flammable liquids |
| ____ 2. Type A | b. Electrical fires |
| ____ 3. Type B | c. Fire due to wood, paper, cloth |

**Activity C** ***Mark each statement as either "T" (True) or "F" (False). Correct any false statements.***

1. T F Clients on "critical" status do not wish to have anyone know that they are in the facility.
2. T F A personal emergency preparedness plan describes the actions to take in the event of a disaster.
3. T F Simple triage and rapid treatment (START) is taught to first responders in the community who are trained in advanced first aid.
4. T F The nurse should alert the client and family to the particular dangers of smoking when oxygen is in use.
5. T F RACE provides assistance and support in many environments both inside and outside healthcare facilities.

**Activity D** ***Fill in the blanks.***

1. The ____________ system is a means of notifying staff by telephone that a disaster has occurred and that their assistance is needed immediately.
2. A disaster plan identifies the location of the ____________ center, the purpose of which is to provide overall direction of the facility's activities.
3. The ____________ safety data sheet provides information about a substance's potential dangers and describes the product, its ingredients, its physical properties, fire or explosion hazards, and reactivity.

4. ___________ disaster may be caused by a fire, an explosion, terrorist activity, radiation, a chemical spill, or a storm within the area the healthcare facility serves.

5. ___________ is the process of sorting and classifying injured persons to determine priority of needs.

**Activity E** *Consider the following figure.*

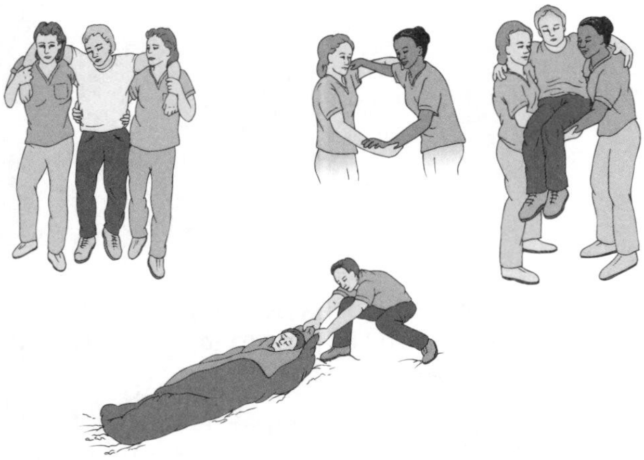

1. Identify the different methods of emergency evacuation.

___________________________________________

___________________________________________

2. How is an immobile client rescued during an emergency evacuation?

___________________________________________

___________________________________________

**Activity F** *Briefly answer the following.*

1. What are the responsibilities of the safety committee?

___________________________________________

___________________________________________

2. What safety measures should a healthcare facility provide for client safety?

___________________________________________

___________________________________________

3. What preventive measures should the nurse teach the client and the family members about dealing with electrical apparatus?

___________________________________________

___________________________________________

4. What does the employees right-to-know law state?

___________________________________________

___________________________________________

5. What does a disaster plan include?

___________________________________________

___________________________________________

6. What helps the nurse to assess a client's risk for falling?

___________________________________________

___________________________________________

## SECTION II: APPLYING WHAT YOU KNOW

**Activity G** ***Answer the following questions, which involve a nurse's understanding of the operations of disaster plans.***

The healthcare facility's disaster plan describes the duties and responsibilities of individuals within the organization in case of a disaster.

1. A number of clients who have suffered burns in an apartment fire are admitted to a local healthcare facility. The disaster medical assistance team (DMAT) is assisting the staff of the healthcare facility.
   a. What are the functions of a DMAT?
   b. Which members of the healthcare facility are included in the DMAT?
2. A healthcare facility requires an emergency evacuation from fire.
   a. What equipment should the nurse relocate after evacuating the clients?
   b. What are the functions of local emergency preparedness agencies?

## SECTION III: GETTING READY FOR NCLEX

**Activity H** *Answer the following questions.*

1. A nurse is caring for a left-handed client. What should the nurse consider when assisting the client out of bed or ambulating?
   a. Provide the client with crutches.
   b. Provide the client with a wheelchair.
   c. Keep in mind that client is also "left-footed."
   d. Provide the client with a walking stick.
2. A nurse is caring for a client who is recovering from surgery. The nurse receives a signal at the central station. Where should the nurse expect to find the client?
   a. Client is in bed
   b. Client is in the bathroom
   c. Client has managed to get out of bed
   d. Client has left the room
3. One of the floors in the healthcare facility is on fire. The nurses are evacuating clients to safer areas. Which of the following interventions should the nurse take in rescuing the clients? (Select all that apply.)
   a. Lead clients who can walk to safer areas.
   b. Carry clients who cannot walk.
   c. Drag immobile clients out of the room on a sheet.
   d. Assist clients in wheelchairs into the elevator.
   e. Close all doors to confine the fire after evacuation.
4. A nurse manager is briefing a newly appointed nurse on the guidelines followed by the healthcare facility for using hazardous substances. Which of the following safety tips should the nurse manager inform the newly appointed nurse about? (Select all that apply.)
   a. Avoid using substances that are not labeled.
   b. Read labels carefully and note emergency information.
   c. Label and store hazardous substances in food containers.
   d. Use protective equipment when handling hazardous substances.
   e. Store aerosol products along with oxygen cylinders.
5. A member of the safety committee is training the nurse on PASS. If a nurse must put out a fire, what would the nurse do first with the fire extinguisher?
   a. Pull the pin
   b. Aim at the base of the fire, near the edge
   c. Squeeze the handles together
   d. Sweep across the base of the fire, with a back and forth motion
6. The client at risk for falling has been identified with a distinctive wrist band. How often does the nurse need to document a fall risk?
   a. 6 hours
   b. 12 hours
   c. 18 hours
   d. 24 hours
7. What is the purpose of a material safety data sheet (MSDS) in a healthcare facility?
   a. It provides information about the physical properties of products.
   b. It maintains a list of the chemical properties of products.
   c. It provides a list of medications and manufacturers.
   d. It describes the method of disposing of hazardous substances.
8. A member of the disaster medical assistance team (DMAT) is explaining the functioning of DMAT during an emergency. What is the role of a DMAT?
   a. It provides financial support during disaster.
   b. It provides safety equipment in an emergency.
   c. It provides relief when there is a shortage of workers.
   d. It provides ambulating services during emergency.

9. A member of the safety committee in a healthcare facility is training the nurses on safety measures at the facility. What guidelines should the trainer provide the nurses?
   a. Assist clients in wheelchairs into elevators to escape fire.
   b. Assist clients who can walk into elevators to escape fire.
   c. Tape the frayed ends of wires on any equipment.
   d. Never turn appliances on when in contact with water.

10. A nurse has been asked to assist in triage in a disaster area. What should the nurse be prepared to do in this situation?
   a. Provide mental support to family members.
   b. Assign victims to proper places for treatment.
   c. Provide first aid to the victims.
   d. Assist people with minor injuries.

CHAPTER 40

# Introduction to Microbiology

## SECTION I: TESTING WHAT YOU KNOW

**Activity A** *Match the types of transmission in Column A with their methods of transmission in Column B.*

| Column A | Column B |
|---|---|
| ____ 1. Vectors | a. Dust particles and spores in the air, droplets from sneezing |
| ____ 2. Bloodborne | b. Bites by infected insects, dogs, cats, rodents |
| ____ 3. Airborne | c. Touching, kissing, shaking hands, sexual intercourse |
| ____ 4. Direct or indirect contact | d. Transfusions, kidney dialysis, injections |

**Activity B** *Match the bacteria in Column A with the categories they belong to in Column B.*

| Column A | Column B |
|---|---|
| ____ 1. Coccus | a. Rod-shaped bacterium |
| ____ 2. Bacillus | b. Spiral-shaped bacterium |
| ____ 3. Spirillum | c. Round or spherical bacterium |

**Activity C** *Mark each statement as either "T" (True) or "F" (False). Correct any false statements.*

1. T F Microorganisms survive only in environments with a pH that is acidic.
2. T F Protozoa are single-celled microorganisms that are visible under an ordinary laboratory microscope.
3. T F Viruses are protein-covered sacs containing the genetic material DNA.
4. T F Rickettsiae are transmitted to people through the bite of an infected insect or tick.
5. T F Contagious diseases are communicable diseases that are transmitted to many individuals quickly and easily.
6. T F The second phase of infection is called the incubation period; it is the period from the onset of initial symptoms to more severe symptoms.
7. T F A pathogen's strength to cause a disease is called its virulence.

**Activity D** *Fill in the blanks.*

1. Microorganisms that cause diseases are called ____________.
2. Microorganisms that require oxygen for growth are called obligate ____________.

3. An infection caused by a fungus is called a ____________.
4. Growth of microorganisms prepared for laboratory study is called a ____________.
5. Some bacteria are capable of locomotion, which is possible because of a cellular organelle called a ____________.
6. A ____________ is a place where a microorganism can survive before moving to a place where it can multiply.
7. ____________ are the toxins manufactured by the microorganism and excreted into the surrounding tissue.

**Activity E** *Consider the following figure.*

1. What does the figure represent?

________________________________________

________________________________________

2. Name and describe the various elements that compose that which is depicted in the figure.

________________________________________

________________________________________

**Activity F** ***When an infection occurs, it usually follows a progressive course. Stages of infection are given below in random order. Write the correct sequence of the phases in the boxes provided.***

1. Convalescence stage
2. Incubation period
3. Full stage of illness
4. Prodromal stage

☐ → ☐ → ☐ → ☐

**Activity G** ***Briefly answer the following questions.***

1. Why do microorganisms require nitrogen?

________________________________________

________________________________________

2. What is the effect of cold temperatures on the growth of microorganisms?

________________________________________

________________________________________

3. Where are cultures usually grown?

________________________________________

________________________________________

4. What is the purpose of a culture and sensitivity (C&S) test?

________________________________________

________________________________________

5. What is the primary cause of malaria?

________________________________________

________________________________________

6. Which tool does a microbiologist use to identify different species of bacteria?

________________________________________

________________________________________

7. Define the term "antibiosis."

________________________________________

________________________________________

## SECTION II: APPLYING WHAT YOU KNOW

**Activity H** ***Answer the following questions, which involve a nurse's understanding of microbiology.***

Microorganisms grow when the number of them at an individual site increases. As bacteria reproduce, they form groups of many millions of individual cells, collectively called colonies.

1. A nurse in a local healthcare facility is caring for a client with a bacterial infection.
   a. Which environmental factors related to the growth of microorganisms should the nurse be aware of when caring for a client infected by a microorganism?
   b. What interventions should the nurse perform to prevent the spread of an infection from one client to another by destroying the microorganism or retarding its growth?
2. A nurse in a local healthcare facility is caring for a client infected by obligate anaerobes. What interventions should the nurse perform to prevent organisms from entering a host?

## SECTION III: GETTING READY FOR NCLEX

**Activity I** ***Answer the following questions.***

1. A client with a high fever visits a healthcare facility. The physician suspects that the client's condition is caused by infection by a microorganism. Which test will be performed to identify the pathogenic microorganism?
   a. Blood test
   b. Culture and sensitivity test
   c. Urine test
   d. Gram's staining
2. A nurse is caring for a client with symptoms that indicate a bacterial infection. What instruction should the nurse offer the client to help prevent the development of drug-resistant bacteria?
   a. Do not share the antibiotics with others.
   b. Take the antibiotics only with warm water.
   c. Stop taking antibiotics if symptoms disappear.
   d. Do not take antibiotics for mild bacterial infections.
3. A nurse informs the client that it is important to complete the antibiotic therapy prescribed by the healthcare provider. Which of the following should the nurse inform the client is the reason for completing the antibiotic therapy prescribed, even if the client feels better after a few days of the therapy?
   a. To prevent nosocomial infections
   b. To prevent transmission of infection to others
   c. To prevent generation of drug-resistant bacteria
   d. To prevent an epidemic of the infection
4. A nurse is caring for a hospitalized client who is susceptible to infections because of a compromised immune system. What interventions should the nurse perform to help reduce the client's susceptibility to infection? (Select all that apply.)
   a. Suggest that the client reduce his or her fluid intake.
   b. Help the client to reduce anxiety.
   c. Isolate the client from the general ward.
   d. Provide adequate rest and skin care.
   e. Provide proper nutritional support.
5. A client who has undergone treatment for food poisoning is being discharged from the healthcare facility. What instruction should the nurse offer the client to kill pathogenic microorganisms in order to prevent any further occurrences?
   a. Refrigerate all edibles.
   b. Heat food in a microwave oven.
   c. Use a steam sterilization technique.
   d. Wash edibles with warm water.

6. A nurse is caring for a client who has had surgery. The nurse knows that the client is at a risk of becoming a reservoir for microorganisms. What measure should the nurse take to destroy the microorganisms or retard their growth in order to break the chain of infection at the reservoir level?
   a. Change dressings promptly every hour.
   b. Avoid using soap when bathing the client.
   c. Sterilize instruments used in the operating room.
   d. Avoid using labeled biohazard bags for disposal.

7. A nurse is caring for a client with an abscess. The nurse should be aware that the major route of transmission of this illness is which of the following?
   a. Contaminated food
   b. Contact with infected client
   c. Contaminated articles
   d. Contaminated hands of healthcare worker

8. A nurse is caring for a postsurgical client using catheters. The client also has impaired mobility. What interventions should the nurse perform to prevent the entry of microorganisms into the client's body? (Select all that apply.)
   a. Provide clean, dry, wrinkle-free linen.
   b. Keep breaks in the skin covered.
   c. Avoid applying moisturizers to skin.
   d. Avoid repositioning the client frequently.
   e. Use sterile technique when using catheters.

9. A nurse is conducting a seminar on the microorganisms that cause trichomonas infection. Which mode of transmission should the nurse highlight for the spread of *Trichomonas vaginalis* infection?
   a. Sexual intercourse
   b. Physical contact
   c. Contaminated water
   d. Insect bite

10. A nurse is caring for a client who is on contact precautions for a bacterial infection. Which environmental factors should the nurse be aware of when caring for a client infected by a microorganism? (Select all that apply.)
   a. Oxygen
   b. Nutrients
   c. Cold temperature
   d. Dry table surface
   e. Light

CHAPTER 41

# Medical Asepsis

## SECTION I: TESTING WHAT YOU KNOW

**Activity A** *Match the links in the chain of infection in Column A with the actions taken to break these links in Column B.*

| Column A | Column B |
|---|---|
| ____ 1. Causative agent | a. Nursing care helps to eliminate areas in which pathogens might grow and multiply. |
| ____ 2. Reservoir for growth of pathogens | b. Nursing care helps to prevent pathogens from being allowed to enter a client's system. |
| ____ 3. Vehicle of transmission | c. Nursing care helps to reduce the number and/or virulence of pathogens. |
| ____ 4. Portal of entry | d. Nursing care eliminates the transmission of pathogens between people. |

**Activity B** *Mark each statement as either "T" (True) or "F" (False). Correct any false statements.*

1. T F Chemicals that decrease the number of pathogens in an area are called antimicrobial agents.
2. T F Chemical asepsis refers to the practice of reducing the number of microorganisms.
3. T F A nurse should use a gown or protective apron to keep her clothing clean when the potential exists for body substances to splash.
4. T F Aseptic techniques include the use of personal protective equipment (PPE): gloves, eye protection, gowns, and masks.
5. T F Masks are disposed of to reduce the risk of cross-contamination.

**Activity C** *Fill in the blanks.*

1. ____________ refers to practices that minimize or eliminate organisms that can cause infection and disease.
2. Chemicals that decrease the number of pathogens in an area are called ____________ agents.
3. A generalized bacterial infection in the blood is termed a ____________.
4. ____________ is the single most important measure to prevent the spread of disease.
5. Masks protect both clients and healthcare personnel from upper ____________ infections and communicable diseases.

**Activity D** *Consider the following figure.*

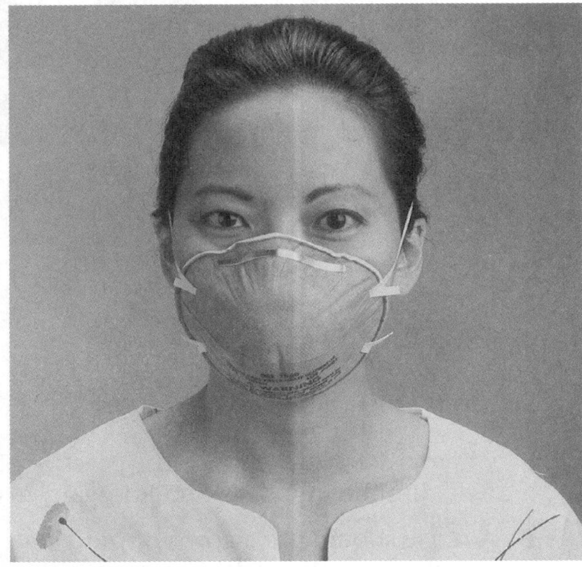

1. What protective equipment should the nurse use while caring for clients with active pulmonary tuberculosis?

_______________________________________________

_______________________________________________

2. List the different forms in which the masks are available.

_______________________________________________

_______________________________________________

**Activity E** *Given below, in random order, are the steps of the nursing procedure for removing and disposing of gloves. Write the correct sequence in the boxes provided.*

1. Drop gloves into the appropriate waste receptacle.
2. Roll the two gloves together, with the side that was nearest the hands on the outside.
3. Grasp the outside of one glove, near the cuff, with the thumb and forefinger of the other hand. Pull the glove off.
4. Wash the hands again.
5. Hook the bare thumb or finger inside the other glove and pull it off, turning it inside out and over the already-removed glove.

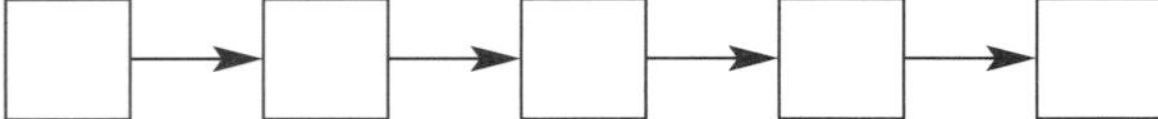

**Activity F** *Briefly answer the following questions.*

1. What are the three levels of latex sensitivity?

_______________________________________________

_______________________________________________

2. What is terminal disinfection?

_______________________________________________

_______________________________________________

3. Which items of personal protective equipment (PPE) should a nurse use?

_______________________________________________

_______________________________________________

4. What are the different components of medical asepsis?

_______________________________________________

_______________________________________________

5. Which are the most common nosocomial infections?

_______________________________________________

_______________________________________________

## SECTION II: APPLYING WHAT YOU KNOW

**Activity G** *Answer the following questions, which involve the nurse's role in the management of clients with infections.*

A nurse's role in treating clients with nosocomial infections involves assisting the clients with any infections. Careful nursing care can eliminate the transmission of pathogens between people.

1. A nurse is required to assist a client with a severe hand injury. It is suspected that the client may have some skin infections.
   a. What are the functions of the Infection Control Committee?
   b. Which factors contribute to lowering the client's resistance?

2. A nurse is taking care of a client with skin infections admitted to a healthcare facility.
   a. How can the nurse protect herself from infection risks?
   b. Why should the nurse use gloves while caring for a client?

## SECTION III: GETTING READY FOR NCLEX

**Activity H** *Answer the following questions.*

1. A client who has undergone treatment for a foot infection is being discharged. Which of the following should a nurse include in a teaching plan to prevent the spread of infection? (Select all that apply.)
   a. Importance of adequate fluid, food intake, and exercise
   b. Aseptic techniques for self-care activities
   c. Methods for handling and disposing of contaminated material
   d. Methods of washing daily wear
   e. Referral to journals that provide sanitization procedures
2. Which handwashing technique should the nurse adopt when performing invasive procedures?
   a. Wash hands with soap or detergent.
   b. Use hand antisepsis.
   c. Use surgical hand scrub.
   d. Avoid washing hands with warm water.
3. A nurse is caring for a client who is infected with *Neisseria* species endogenous microorganisms. For which of the following infections should the nurse monitor the client?
   a. Moniliasis
   b. Diarrhea
   c. Meningitis
   d. Impetigo
4. A nurse is caring for a client with an infection. What precautions should the nurse take after leaving the client's room? (Select all that apply.)
   a. Scrub the hands at least twice thoroughly, with attention to nails.
   b. Use a wet towel to turn off faucets.
   c. Avoid touching any part of the sink or the faucets.
   d. Discard the paper towels appropriately after drying hands.
   e. Apply hand sanitizer to keep the hands free from odor.
5. A nurse at a healthcare facility is accustomed to using latex gloves when caring for clients. For which of the following clients should the nurse be careful when using latex gloves?
   a. Clients with a history of spina bifida
   b. Clients with a history of skin reactions
   c. Clients receiving chemotherapy
   d. Clients receiving radiation therapy
6. What kind of eye protection should the nurse wear in an operating room for her safety?
   a. Chemical splash goggles
   b. Goggles with side and forehead shields
   c. Full-face shields
   d. Disposable goggles
7. A nurse is caring for a client with an infection at a healthcare facility. Which of the following measures should the nurse follow to prevent the transmission of pathogens between people?
   a. Carefully dispose of soiled dressings.
   b. Suggest that the client takes a bath twice a day.
   c. Sterilize the curtains of the client's room.
   d. Carefully dispose of the client's daily wear.
8. A nurse is explaining the different procedures used to break the chain of infection to a nursing student. In which of the following links in the chain of infection should a nurse provide special attention to the respiratory and gastrointestinal tracts?
   a. Portal of exit
   b. Vehicle of transmission
   c. Portal of entry
   d. Susceptible host

9. While caring for a client in an operating room, the nurse notices that one of his gloves is punctured. What should a nurse do in such a situation?
   a. Remove the gloves and then finish the procedure.
   b. Wear another pair of gloves over the ripped pair.
   c. Continue and then wash hands after completion.
   d. Discard the gloves, wash hands, and wear a new pair.

10. A nurse is caring for a client with tuberculosis. What intervention should the nurse take to protect herself from the risk of infection?
   a. Use appropriate antibiotics.
   b. Get regular checkups done.
   c. Obtain appropriate immunizations.
   d. Avoid parenteral administration of the drug to the client.

CHAPTER 42

# Infection Control

## SECTION I: TESTING WHAT YOU KNOW

**Activity A** *Match the transmission types in Column A with their characteristics in Column B.*

**Column A**

____ 1. Contact transmission

____ 2. Airborne transmission

____ 3. Droplet transmission

**Column B**

a. Transmission occurs when droplets containing microorganisms are propelled through the air from an infected person and deposited on the host's eyes, nose, or mouth.

b. Transmission occurs as a result of direct contact between a susceptible host's body surface and an infected or colonized person.

c. Transmission occurs when tiny microorganisms from evaporated droplets remain suspended or are carried in the air.

**Activity B** *Match the precaution types in Column A with their purposes in Column B.*

**Column A**

____ 1. Standard precautions

____ 2. Special precautions

____ 3. Transmission-based precautions

**Column B**

a. Used for the violent client who spits or bites

b. Used for clients with suspected or diagnosed infections

c. Designed to reduce the risk of transmission of microorganisms from both known and unknown sources of infection

**Activity C** *Mark each statement as either "T" (True) or "F" (False). Correct any false statements.*

1. T F Infection is best controlled by prevention and breaking the links in the chain of infection.

2. T F Disease-specific isolation is also known as neutropenic isolation.

3. T F Hospital Infection Control Practices Advisory Committee requires every healthcare facility it accredits to have an infection control plan.

4. T F Special air handling and ventilation are required to prevent airborne transmission.

5. T F One duty of an infection control committee is to carry out terminal disinfection.

**Activity D** *Fill in the blanks.*

1. Special filtered ___________ masks are often required when caring for a client with known or suspected tuberculosis.
2. ___________ occurs when a microorganism is present in a client but the client shows no clinical signs or symptoms of infection.
3. ___________ isolation attempts to prevent harmful microorganisms from coming into contact with the client.
4. ___________ techniques are designed to prevent microorganisms from leaving a client's room.
5. ___________ transmission is the most frequent mode of disease transmission in healthcare facilities.

**Activity E** *Consider the following figure.*

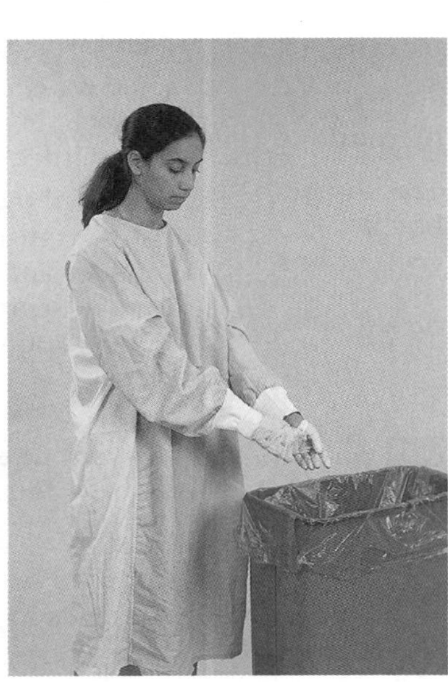

1. Which PPE should be used in case of anticipation of contact with infectious matter?

___________________________________________

___________________________________________

2. Which items should be removed first when using PPE?

___________________________________________

___________________________________________

**Activity F** *Briefly answer the following questions.*

1. What is the BBP standard?

___________________________________________

___________________________________________

2. What are the two primary types of isolation systems?

___________________________________________

___________________________________________

3. How does indirect contact transmission occur?

___________________________________________

___________________________________________

4. What are transmission-based precautions designed for?

___________________________________________

___________________________________________

5. Which infections result from droplet transmission?

___________________________________________

___________________________________________

## SECTION II: APPLYING WHAT YOU KNOW

**Activity G** *Answer the following questions, which involve the nurse's role in infection control.*

The best method of infection control is prevention, which is successful when the chain of infection is successfully broken. A nurse's role in caring for a client in isolation requires special precautions.

1. A client with a respiratory disorder requires isolation in a healthcare facility.
   a. What points should the nurse remember while setting up the client's room for isolation?
   b. What type of specific isolation should be given to this client?

2. A nurse is setting up a client's room for isolation. The client's family wants to know the reasons behind the isolation of the client.
   a. What reason should the nurse give to the client and family while setting up the client's room for isolation?
   b. What should the nurse tell the client and family in order to prepare them for the client's hospital stay in isolation?
3. The physician has ordered a nurse to administer medication to a client in isolation. What precautions should the nurse take when administering medications to the client in isolation?

## SECTION III: GETTING READY FOR NCLEX

**Activity H** *Answer the following questions.*

1. A nurse caring for a client needs to take droplet precautions when transporting the client to an area outside the client's room. Which of the following precautions should the nurse take?
   a. Ask the client to wear a mask.
   b. Drape the wheelchair with a clean sheet.
   c. Drape the client with a bath blanket.
   d. Disinfect the wheelchair or stretcher after use.
2. A healthcare facility is expected to adopt infection control methods. What should the plan to control infection include? (Select all that apply.)
   a. An infection control committee
   b. Procedures for irradiation
   c. Surveillance of nosocomial infections
   d. Procedures for acid treatment
   e. Procedures for environmental sanitation
3. A nurse is caring for a client with tuberculosis. What kind of a personal protective cover should the nurse use while in the vicinity of the client?
   a. Double layer of gloves
   b. Gown
   c. High-filtration particulate respirator
   d. Protective eyewear
4. A nurse is caring for a client with scabies. What precaution should the nurse take when caring for this client? (Select all that apply.)
   a. Wear gloves when entering the room and remove them before leaving.
   b. Change gloves after contact with a client's infective material.
   c. Wash hands with an antimicrobial agent or waterless antiseptic agent.
   d. Wear a mask when working within 3 feet of the client.
   e. Make the client wear a mask during transportation.
5. A nurse caring for a client with typhoid collects a urine specimen from the client in his room. What procedure should the nurse follow when sending the urine specimen to the laboratory?
   a. Place the specimen in "double bagging."
   b. Carefully scrub the urine container outside the room.
   c. Expose the specimen to sunlight if possible.
   d. Use disposable medication cups.
6. Which of the following procedures should the nurse follow when caring for a client in protective isolation?
   a. Recap or break needles immediately after use.
   b. Administer enema to the client periodically.
   c. Ensure handwashing for those coming into contact with the client.
   d. Give fresh fruit and fresh vegetables to the client.
7. Which of the following types of clients are most likely to be placed in protective isolation? (Select all that apply.)
   a. Clients undergoing bone marrow transplantation
   b. Clients undergoing chemotherapy for cancer
   c. Clients with agammaglobulinemia
   d. Clients with diabetes
   e. Clients with cardiovascular diseases

8. What information should the nurse give the client and family while setting up a client's room for isolation?
   a. Teach the client the isolation procedures.
   b. Teach the client OSHA regulations.
   c. Educate the client about the BBP standards.
   d. Explain the reasons for isolation precautions.
9. A nurse is caring for a client with a stab wound in the back. What should be the appropriate nursing intervention when caring for this client?
   a. Place the client on contact precautions.
   b. Place the client on airborne precautions.
   c. Place the client on droplet precautions.
   d. Place the client in an open and airy room.
10. Healthcare facilities have stringent procedures in place for preventing infection. What is the main purpose of designing standard precautions for infection control?
    a. To reduce the risk of transmission of microorganisms
    b. To ensure the cleanliness of the healthcare facility premises
    c. To instill a sense of safety in the client and relatives
    d. To speed the recovery of clients and increase their sense of well-being

CHAPTER 43

# Emergency Care and First Aid

## SECTION I: TESTING WHAT YOU KNOW

**Activity A** *Match the conditions occurring due to motor vehicle accidents or a fall in Column A with their meanings in Column B.*

| Column A | Column B |
|---|---|
| ____ 1. Fracture | a. Displacement of a bone from a joint |
| ____ 2. Sprain | b. Broken bone |
| ____ 3. Strain | c. Twisting of a joint with rupture of ligaments |
| ____ 4. Dislocation | d. Twisting or stretching that damages a muscle or tendon |

**Activity B** *Match the types of shock in Column A with their causes in Column B.*

| Column A | Column B |
|---|---|
| ____ 1. Cardiogenic shock | a. A severe, life-threatening reaction to a substance to which the client is sensitive or allergic |
| ____ 2. Anaphylactic shock | b. Result of overdose of insulin, a skipped meal, or strenuous exercise in a client with insulin-dependent diabetes mellitus (IDDM) |
| ____ 3. Hypoglycemic shock | c. Failure of the heart to accomplish its pumping function |

**Activity C** *Mark each statement as either "T" (True) or "F" (False). Correct any false statements.*

1. T F A splint is a device applied to immobilize a fracture or sprain.
2. T F The primary assessment performed during an emergency involves taking and recording the victim's vital signs and continues with a head-to-toe assessment.
3. T F Clinical death occurs when a person's breathing and heartbeat stop.
4. T F Scalp lacerations cause profuse bleeding, making even the smallest wound appear very serious.
5. T F Classic heat stroke develops from an increased internal heat load due to muscular exertion, along with high external temperature and humidity.

6. T F A tooth that is knocked out is an example of an intrusion injury.

7. T F Caustic substances are those which burn or destroy flesh.

**Activity D** *Fill in the blanks.*

1. ____________ is the process of sorting and classifying to determine priority of needs; it involves determining life-threatening situations and assisting those clients first.
2. ____________ refers to a wound or injury that is caused by an outside force.
3. ____________ death refers to permanent damage of brain cells due to lack of oxygen.
4. The automated external ____________ is considered the definitive initial treatment of clients in cardiac arrest.
5. A tension pneumothorax that remains uncorrected will worsen and results in a ____________ shift.
6. ____________ is the freezing of body tissues that results from exposure to cold temperatures.
7. ____________ occurs when the body loses heat faster than it can burn food to replace it.

**Activity E** *Consider the following figure.*

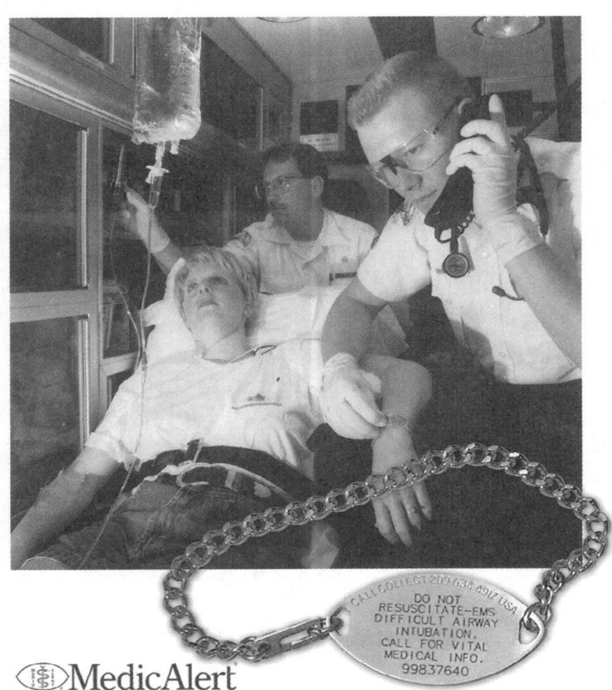


1. What should a paramedic always search for on an injured person when providing first aid?

______________________________________

______________________________________

2. What actions should the paramedic perform in emergency conditions and injuries?

______________________________________

______________________________________

**Activity F** *Assisting a client who has a nosebleed not associated with a fractured skull or severe hypertension requires certain steps be followed. Those steps are given below in random order. Write the correct sequence in the boxes provided.*

1. Place cold compresses on the person's nose and face.
2. Have the person sit down and lean forward slightly if no other injuries prohibit this position.
3. If bleeding continues, place small, clean pieces of gauze in one or both nostrils.
4. Apply pressure to the nostrils or to the bridge of the nose with your thumb and forefinger for 5 to 10 minutes without releasing the pressure.
5. Seek medical assistance if bleeding is uncontrollable.
6. Apply pressure above the person's upper lip if he or she is conscious.

☐ → ☐ → ☐ → ☐ → ☐ → ☐

**Activity G** *Briefly answer the following questions.*

1. What are the causes of flail chest?

______________________________________

______________________________________

2. What are the causes of sudden death?

______________________________________

______________________________________

3. What do Advanced Cardiac Life Support (ACLS) techniques include?

______________________________________

______________________________________

4. What are the common causes of chest injuries?

_______________

_______________

5. When does a tension pneumothorax occur?

_______________

_______________

6. Which danger signs of head injury should the nurse look for in a client?

_______________

_______________

## SECTION II: APPLYING WHAT YOU KNOW

**Activity H** *Answer the following questions, which involve the nurse's role in emergency care.*

Basic emergency care principles provide the foundation to act appropriately when accidents occur. The stress level is usually high during an emergency, and, in such a situation, a nurse should follow a predetermined, orderly plan of action and method of assessment.

1. A nurse witnesses a motor vehicle accident (MVA).
   a. What should the nurse check for before rushing to assist the victim?
   b. How should the nurse identify the problems during an emergency?
2. A nurse is assessing a client in a local health-care facility. The client is in a state of shock due to trauma following a motor vehicle accident.
   a. What is the cause of shock in the client involved in a motor vehicle accident?
   b. What is compensatory circulation?
3. A nurse is providing first aid care to a client who has been involved in an accident. The nurse checks the client for a medical identification or MedicAlert tag.
   a. What does the MedicAlert tag signify?
   b. What is the nurse's responsibility if he or she finds on the client a card indicating that the person wishes to donate tissues or organs after death?

## SECTION III: GETTING READY FOR NCLEX

**Activity I** *Answer the following questions.*

1. Which of the following actions should the emergency personnel perform when reporting an MVA? (Select all that apply.)
   a. Note the vehicle's condition.
   b. Mark the area of accident.
   c. Note areas of intrusion such as the driver's side.
   d. Inquire about the cause of the accident.
   e. Check for any gasoline spill.
2. A nurse is caring for a client with a nosebleed and a possible skull fracture. What basic steps should the nurse take to treat the nosebleed?
   a. Use a clean handkerchief or cloth to wipe the bleeding.
   b. Do not attempt to stop the bleeding.
   c. Place the person on a flat surface to help blood circulation.
   d. Cleanse the nose with warm, soapy water.
3. Which of the following procedures should the nurse follow to monitor the pupillary responses of a client during an emergency?
   a. ABCDE procedure
   b. PERRLA+C procedure
   c. APVU procedure
   d. BCLS procedure
4. A nurse is assigned the responsibility of caring for a client in a home-care setting who has severe anxiety. What should be the nurse's role for such a client? (Select all that apply.)
   a. Encourage the client to engage in voluntary activity.
   b. Avoid making any assumptions or judgments.
   c. Encourage the client to remain calm.
   d. Encourage the client to talk about the cause of anxiety.
   e. Ask the client questions that elicit "yes or no" answers.

5. A nurse is caring for a client with botulism. What steps can the nurse suggest to the client's relatives to prevent further poisoning from botulism?
   a. Do not eat leafy and green salads.
   b. Do not eat items that are canned at home.
   c. Avoid eating fruits and berries.
   d. Do not use food from cans with bulging tops.
6. A client with excessive bleeding has been brought to a healthcare facility. How should the nurse stop the client's bleeding?
   a. Have the client sit down and lean forward.
   b. Place the client on a flat surface and slightly elevate the feet.
   c. Have the client lie on the side not affected by the wound.
   d. Use a tourniquet to stop client's bleeding.
7. A nurse is assigned the responsibility of caring for a client who has been exposed to hazardous chemicals. Which of the following additional precautions should the nurse undertake for this client?
   a. Use soapy water on affected area.
   b. Apply salve over the affected area.
   c. Remove client's clothing and rinse off chemicals.
   d. Cover the area with a dry, non-stick, sterile dressing.
8. What nursing interventions should the nurse perform for a client who has frostbite? (Select all that apply.)
   a. Separate frozen fingers and toes with cotton wedges.
   b. Loosen any tight clothing worn by the client.
   c. Instruct the client to avoid walking if the foot is frostbitten.
   d. Use bandages, ointments, or salves on the frostbitten parts.
   e. Rub the frostbitten parts of the client with snow.
9. What nursing interventions should the nurse perform for a client who has a fractured leg?
   a. Raise the client's injured leg.
   b. Replace the ends of the bones in the fracture.
   c. Apply a roller bandage on the fracture.
   d. Apply ice on the injury site.
10. Which of the following compensatory actions should the nurse perform for a client who has gone into shock as a result of a serious illness?
    a. Maintain the client's airway.
    b. Stabilize the client's cervical spine.
    c. Move the client to a well-ventilated, cool room.
    d. Look for signs of change in the client's level of consciousness.

CHAPTER 44

# Therapeutic Communication Skills

## SECTION I: TESTING WHAT YOU KNOW

**Activity A** ***Match the components of communication in Column A with their descriptions in Column B.***

| Column A | Column B |
|---|---|
| ____ **1.** Sender | **a.** A means of transmitting the idea |
| ____ **2.** Message | **b.** A person who interprets the message |
| ____ **3.** Medium | **c.** An originator or source of the idea |
| ____ **4.** Receiver | **d.** Response to the message through feedback |
| ____ **5.** Interaction | **e.** The idea |

**Activity B** ***Match the terms associated with communication in Column A with their descriptions in Column B.***

| Column A | Column B |
|---|---|
| ____ **1.** Therapeutic communication | **a.** Feeling of harmony |
| ____ **2.** Verbal communication | **b.** Giving, receiving, and interpreting information through any of the five senses by two or more interacting people |
| ____ **3.** Body language | **c.** Sharing information through the written or spoken word |
| ____ **4.** Communication | **d.** Clients talk about and resolve their feelings and problems |
| ____ **5.** Rapport | **e.** Sharing information without using words or language |

**Activity C** ***Mark each statement as either "T" (True) or "F" (False). Correct any false statements.***

**1.** T F The most effective communication occurs when words and actions convey the same message.

**2.** T F Silence is a valuable communication tool.

**3.** T F When two people speak different languages, there is no interaction between the two of them.

**4.** T F A nursing assistant can take verbal orders from the physician.

**5.** T F A smile is part of the universal human language.

**Activity D** *Fill in the blanks.*

1. ____________ space is an area around an individual reserved for only close friends or intimates.
2. ____________ communication is that which stops the communication process or threatens the client.
3. Aphasia often results from a ____________ disorder or injury or a psychiatric disorder.
4. Successful therapeutic communication encourages client coping and ____________ toward self-care.
5. A/An ____________ is a goal-directed conversation in which one person seeks information from the other.

**Activity E** *Consider the following figure.*

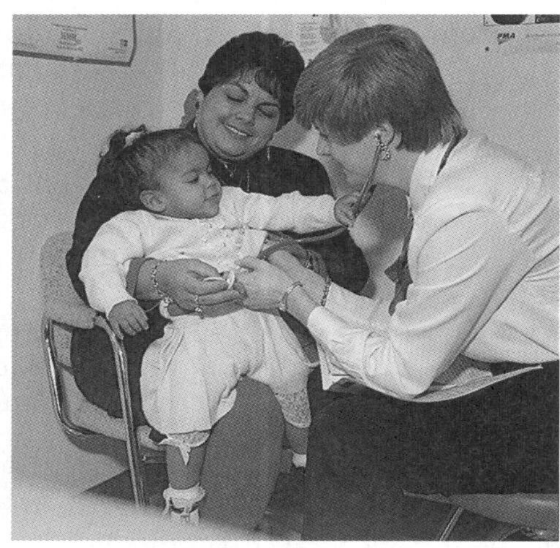

1. What effective communication skills should the nurse use when caring for a child?

______________________________________________

______________________________________________

**Activity F** *Briefly answer the following questions.*

1. What are the verbal barriers to communication?

______________________________________________

______________________________________________

2. List the nonverbal forms of communication.

______________________________________________

______________________________________________

3. How does a firm touch differ from a light touch?

______________________________________________

______________________________________________

4. What are the different forms of verbal communication by the nurse?

______________________________________________

______________________________________________

5. What is proxemics?

______________________________________________

______________________________________________

6. List the factors that affect communication.

______________________________________________

______________________________________________

## SECTION II: APPLYING WHAT YOU KNOW

**Activity G** *Answer the following questions, which involve the nurse's role in communicating with clients.*

The foundation of relationships is effective communication. The art of therapeutic communication does not come naturally; it must be learned and practiced. The nurse must be able to develop a rapport with the client and communicate genuineness and empathy, even when fears or concerns cannot be fully expressed verbally.

1. A nurse is caring for a client who has aphasia due to a stroke. How can the nurse communicate with this client?
2. A nurse is caring for an elderly client. The client seems to be very reserved and disinterested in communicating with the nurse. How can the nurse obtain necessary information from the client that will be helpful in the treatment?

## SECTION III: GETTING READY FOR NCLEX

**Activity H** *Answer the following questions.*

1. A nurse is assessing a client at the healthcare facility. Which therapeutic communication technique helps to communicate to the client that the nurse has understood the client's problem?
   a. Clarification
   b. Reflection
   c. Summarization
   d. Paraphrasing
2. A client has been admitted to the healthcare facility under an alias. What care should the nurse take with respect to this client?
   a. Address the client by his or her actual name only when alone.
   b. Use the client's actual name for records and address the client by his or her alias.
   c. Use the client's alias on the facility's records only.
   d. Address the client by his or her alias at all times.
3. A nurse is preparing a young client for surgery. The nurse understands that the client is worried and is afraid of the surgery. Which of the following nonverbal expressions helps the nurse to understand the client's feelings?
   a. Wringing hands
   b. Slouched appearance
   c. Twitching feet
   d. Bouncing feet
4. Which of the following precautions should the nurse take to ensure the correctness of a telephone message to a healthcare facility? (Select all that apply.)
   a. Write down the message.
   b. Paraphrase the message.
   c. Verify the message.
   d. Remember the message.
   e. Repeat the message.
5. A nurse is caring for a client who does not understand the language spoken by the nurse. Which of the following would be an appropriate method of developing effective communication with the client?
   a. Avoid any verbal interaction with the client.
   b. Request the assistance of an interpreter.
   c. Ask a family member to translate.
   d. Use sign language to communicate.
6. A nurse is caring for a postoperative client who is unconscious. Which of the following should the nurse do when caring for this client?
   a. Avoid introducing himself to the client.
   b. Maintain silence when caring for the client.
   c. Explain to the client the procedure to be performed.
   d. Explain the client's condition to the assisting nurse.
7. What appropriate intervention should the nurse take when caring for a visually impaired client?
   a. Enter the client's room silently without disturbance.
   b. Repeat instructions to ensure that the client has understood.
   c. Introduce herself before entering or leaving the client's room.
   d. Touch the client quietly to make her presence felt.
8. A nurse is conducting a preadmission assessment for a client. Which of the following ensures effectiveness of the interview? (Select all that apply.)
   a. Nurse asks relevant questions.
   b. Nurse does most of the talking.
   c. Nurse asks open-ended questions.
   d. Client responds accurately.
   e. Client is accompanied by a friend.

9. A client is fearful of being admitted to the healthcare facility. What should the nurse do to gain the confidence of this client? (Select all that apply.)
   a. Inform the client of the need for admission.
   b. Explain the treatment process.
   c. Maintain a nonjudgmental attitude.
   d. Remain calm when interacting with client.
   e. Ignore the client's fears.

10. When concluding a preliminary assessment of the client, which of the following ensures that the nurse has clearly understood all relevant information provided by the client?
   a. Echo the client's words.
   b. Record all information on tape.
   c. Document all the information.
   d. Paraphrase the information.

CHAPTER 45

# Admission, Transfer, and Discharge

## SECTION I: TESTING WHAT YOU KNOW

**Activity A** *Match the levels of anxiety in Column A with their symptoms in Column B.*

| Column A | Column B |
|---|---|
| ____ 1. +1 Anxiety | a. Dread |
| ____ 2. +2 Anxiety | b. Increased pulse rate |
| ____ 3. +3 Anxiety | c. Apprehension |
| ____ 4. Panic | d. Paranoia |

**Activity B** *Match the scales in Column A with the type of clients whose weights are measured in Column B.*

| Column A | Column B |
|---|---|
| ____ 1. Balance scales | a. Clients who are immobile |
| ____ 2. Chair scales | b. Clients who can step on the scales |
| ____ 3. Litter scale | c. Clients who are unable to stand |

**Activity C** *Mark each statement as either "T" (True) or "F" (False). Correct any false statements.*

1. T F A master board with all clients' names and room numbers should be placed at the nursing station so that passers-by can read the names.
2. T F Fluctuating weight may indicate when the client is or is not retaining fluids.
3. T F If a person's lower-level needs are not being met, he or she will have difficulty concentrating and learning.
4. T F Nursing data collection and assessment begin after admission to the facility.
5. T F The hospital laundry facility is responsible for laundering the client's own clothing.

**Activity D** *Fill in the blank.*

1. Each continuous period of time a client spends in a facility is considered one ____________.
2. A client's bed should be put in ____________ position, regardless of whether the client can get in and out of bed without assistance.
3. Temperature, pulse, ____________ and blood pressure are called vital signs because they must be present for a person's life to continue.
4. ____________ deprives a person of personality, spirit, privacy, and other human qualities.
5. If the height of a client who cannot stand is measured when he is in bed, it is recorded as ____________ height.

**Activity E** *Consider the following figure.*

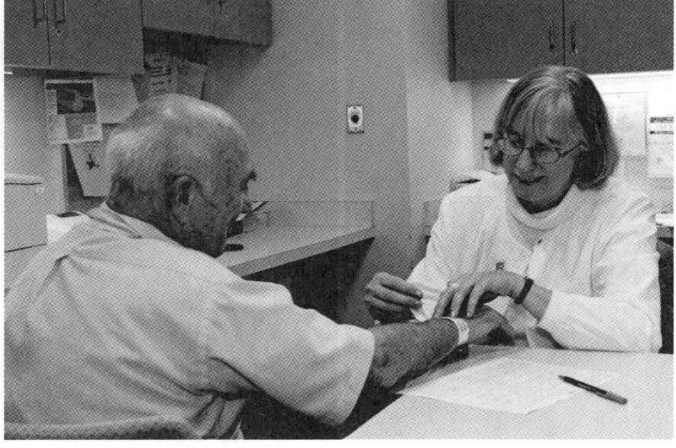

1. What does the figure show?

______________________________

______________________________

2. What is it used for?

______________________________

______________________________

3. What information does the object in the figure contain?

______________________________

______________________________

**Activity F** *Briefly answer the following questions.*

1. What are the responsibilities of the admitting department?

______________________________

______________________________

2. What are the responsibilities of the nurse once the client arrives at the nursing unit?

______________________________

______________________________

3. What are the financial concerns of a client admitted to a healthcare facility?

______________________________

______________________________

4. How can the nurse assist in orienting the client to the room?

______________________________

______________________________

5. What is the purpose of an advance directive?

______________________________

______________________________

6. What are the reasons a client may be transferred to another unit?

______________________________

______________________________

## SECTION II: APPLYING WHAT YOU KNOW

**Activity G** *Answer the following questions, which involve the nurse's role in admitting clients.*

Effective care can be provided if the nurse is aware of the client's needs, attitudes, and emotions. By maintaining safety and drawing on communication and interviewing skills, nurses help clients express and work through their feelings about admission to the healthcare facility.

1. A nurse is caring for an elderly client who needs assistance in dressing and undressing. How can the nurse help the client who is embarrassed and uneasy during the procedure?
2. A client with Alzheimer's disease has just been admitted to the Alzheimer's unit of the healthcare facility. What care should the nurse take with respect to the client's personal belongings?

## SECTION III: GETTING READY FOR NCLEX

**Activity H** *Answer the following questions.*

1. A nurse is assigned to care for a client who is to be admitted to the healthcare facility. What care should the nurse take with respect to the client's bed? (Select all that apply.)
   a. Explain the bed controls to the client and family.
   b. Adjust the height of the bed according to the client's height.
   c. Adjust the entire bed to a lower position.
   d. Adjust the foot of the bed for the client's comfort.
   e. Adjust the head of the bed so that it is always flat.
2. A nurse is caring for an elderly client with urine incontinence. How can the nurse care for the client while maintaining the client's privacy?
   a. Explain that street clothes are not convenient to perform tests and procedures.
   b. Ask the client not to leave the room without prior permission.
   c. Ask the client to change into hospital clothes as per hospital rules.
   d. Explain that gowns help to identify the unit to which the client belongs.
3. A client has been admitted to the healthcare facility for the first time. The client is anxious about being alone in an unfamiliar environment, especially when he is ill. What should the nurse do to alleviate anxiety and fear in the client?
   a. Ask a family member to accompany the client at all times.
   b. Explain how the signal light in the bathroom can help the client.
   c. Tell the client to wait until the nurse comes by during rounds.
   d. Assume that the client is aware of the use of the "nurse call" signal.
4. A 5-year-old child with a high fever is admitted to the healthcare facility. The child is scared of being in a new place with strangers and is throwing tantrums, making it difficult to care for her. How can the nurse help this child?
   a. Ask a colleague to help in feeding the child.
   b. Prevent the parents from fussing over the child.
   c. Provide the child with toys and books.
   d. Ask a colleague to help in dressing the child.
5. Which of the following instructions should the nurse provide the client who has been admitted to a healthcare facility regarding his eyeglasses?
   a. Place them on the bedside table or drawer and inform him where they have been placed.
   b. Hand them over to the client's family for safekeeping.
   c. Keep them in the facility's safe along with other valuables.
   d. Tell the client that the facility is not liable for his possessions.
6. An LPN is assigned to care for a client at the healthcare facility. Which of the following is the role of the LPN?
   a. Notify the physician of the client's arrival.
   b. Check the physician's orders for the client's diet.
   c. Confirm that the client's diet order has been placed.
   d. Assess the vital signs of the client.
7. During the admission interview, the nurse measures and records the initial height and weight of the client. Why is it necessary to compare the client's weight with the height?
   a. To determine the effectiveness of feedings
   b. To determine whether the client is overweight
   c. To calculate the medication dosage
   d. To identify the possibility of fluid retention
8. Which of the following clients would need to be transferred to another unit?
   a. A client who has just delivered a baby
   b. A client who is capable of going home to self-care
   c. A client who returns after leaving the facility without information
   d. A client who might leave the facility against medical advice

9. A client has been admitted to the healthcare facility for the first time. Which of the following is the responsibility of the nurse once the client arrives at the nursing unit?
   a. Attaching an identification band with the client's name and agency identification
   b. Arranging for diagnostic tests
   c. Preparing the client for the admission examination
   d. Ensuring the client signs documents giving consent for treatment

10. A nurse has been told that the assigned client has to be transferred to another unit. What are reasons a client may be transferred to another unit? (Select all that apply.)
   a. The patient requires a more active environment for recovery.
   b. Assignment to a certain unit is permanent.
   c. The client is disturbing others and needs a private room.
   d. The client's condition is more acute than originally determined.
   e. The client needs to be moved to postsurgical care unit after surgery.

CHAPTER 46

# Vital Signs

## SECTION I: TESTING WHAT YOU KNOW

**Activity A** ***Match the methods to measure body temperature in Column A with the appropriate average normal temperature range for afebrile adults in Column B.***

**Column A**

____ **1.** Oral

____ **2.** Rectal

____ **3.** Axillary

**Column B**

**a.** 36.6°–38.0° degrees Celsius (97.9°–100.4° Fahrenheit)

**b.** 34.7°–37.3° Celsius (94.5°–99.1° Fahrenheit)

**c.** 35.5°–37.5° Celsius (95.9°–99.5° Fahrenheit)

**Activity B** ***Match the types of fever in Column A with the related description in Column B.***

**Column A**

____ **1.** Intermittent fever

____ **2.** Remittent fever

____ **3.** Crisis

____ **4.** Lysis

____ **5.** Relapsing fever

**Column B**

**a.** A temperature that rises several degrees above normal and returns to normal or near normal.

**b.** A sudden drop from fever to normal temperature.

**c.** Fever that returns to normal for at least a day, and then occurs again.

**d.** A temperature that alternates between a fever and a normal or subnormal reading.

**e.** The gradual return of an elevated temperature to normal.

**Activity C** ***Mark each statement as either "T" (True) or "F" (False). Correct any false statements.***

**1.** T F If a person is angry or excited, the adrenal glands become very active and he or she feels warm.

**2.** T F Body temperature is usually highest in the morning.

**3.** T F Hyperthermia indicates impending death.

**4.** T F The rectal temperature is the least accurate measurement method for assessing body temperature.

**5.** T F The pulse of a newborn ranges from 120 to 140 beats per minute.

**6.** T F Cheyne-Stokes respirations are serious and usually precede death in cases of cerebral hemorrhage, uremia, or heart disease.

**7.** T F If blood volume is normal but the elasticity or caliber of the arteries is reduced, the blood pressure lowers.

**8.** T F Any blood pressure that is much higher than normal for the person's age is a sign of shock.

**Activity D** ***Fill in the blanks.***

**1.** Normal body temperature using oral measurement remains at approximately ______ Fahrenheit.

**2.** The ____________ which is the brain's heat-regulating center, controls body temperature by controlling blood flow.

3. A condition in which the pulse rate is consistently above normal (100 beats per minute) is called ___________.

4. When the pulse occasionally skips a beat, this irregularity is described as a/an ___________ pulse.

5. ___________ breathing occurs when air passes through secretions present in the air passages.

6. The ___________ pulse is located posterior to the knee.

**Activity E** *Consider the following figure.*

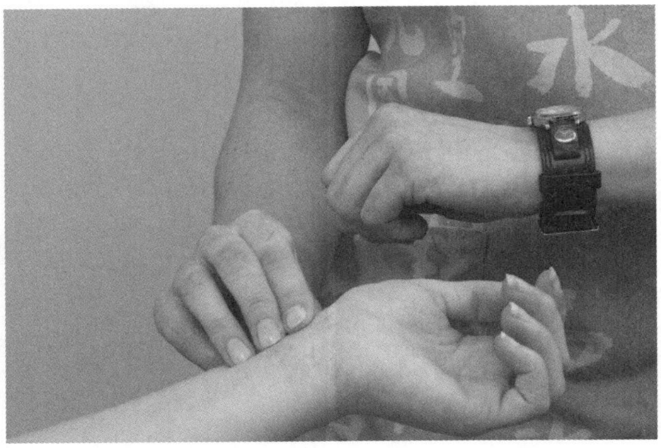

1. Identify the pulse being assessed by the nurse.

___________________________________

___________________________________

2. List the steps involved in measuring this pulse. Provide an appropriate rationale for each step involved in the measurement of this pulse.

___________________________________

___________________________________

**Activity F** ***Given below are characteristics of the phases of Korotkoff's sounds, in random order. Write the correct sequence in the boxes provided below.***

1. Turbulence
2. Final silence
3. Initial silence

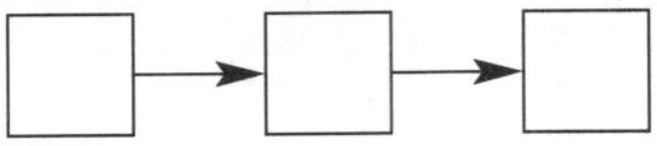

☐ → ☐ → ☐

**Activity G** ***Briefly answer the following questions.***

1. What is the benefit of recording a client's vital signs?

___________________________________

___________________________________

2. Why are electronic thermometers rarely used in isolation units?

___________________________________

___________________________________

3. What does an abnormally rapid pulse rate indicate?

___________________________________

___________________________________

4. When is the pulse referred to as "full" or "bounding"?

___________________________________

___________________________________

5. What are the characteristic signs of breathing difficulty?

___________________________________

___________________________________

6. What are two factors that determine the degree of blood pressure?

___________________________________

___________________________________

7. Why is it possible to estimate only the *systolic* pressure through palpation?

___________________________________

___________________________________

## SECTION II: APPLYING WHAT YOU KNOW

**Activity H** *Answer the following questions, which involve the nurse's role in taking vital signs.*

Body temperature, pulse, respiration, and blood pressure are basic client assessments. These measurements are indicators of functions necessary to sustain life. A nurse takes the vital signs of the client as ordered or may use judgment to determine whether a client requires more frequent assessment of vital signs.

1. A nurse is required to assess the tympanic temperature of a 19-year-old client.
   a. What are the steps involved when assessing the tympanic temperature? Provide a rationale for each step.
   b. Should the nurse also inform the client about the alternative equipment used to measure body temperature? If yes, then list the alternative equipment used to measure the body temperature, stating the advantages of each.
2. A nurse is preparing to measure the pulse of a 45-year old client. It is suspected that the client's heart is not effectively pumping blood.
   a. Which is the appropriate pulse the nurse should assess for?
   b. List the steps involved in measuring this pulse.
   c. In what situation should the nurse report the assessment to the physician?
3. A nurse is taking care of a mastectomy client with an intravenous line and is required to measure the client's blood pressure.
   a. What are the steps involved when measuring the blood pressure of this client?
   b. What points should a nurse keep in mind when using an alternative site for measuring this client's blood pressure?
4. When assessing the vital signs of a client, the nurse observes that the client's respirations are slow and shallow at first, gradually grow faster and deeper, and then taper off until they stop entirely.
   a. Identify the type of respiration.
   b. List the steps involved in counting respirations, and provide a rationale for each step.
   c. What is the appropriate intervention required when observing this client's respirations?
   d. What could be the possible indication of this respiration?

## SECTION III: GETTING READY FOR NCLEX

**Activity I** *Answer the following questions.*

1. When monitoring a client, a nurse observes that the client's body temperature alternates between a fever and a normal or subnormal reading. This observation indicates which of the following types of fever?
   a. Intermittent fever
   b. Remittent fever
   c. Relapsing fever
   d. Lysis
2. The nurse has received a report from unlicensed assistive personnel in relation to the morning vital signs. Which statement would indicate that the oral temperature method is contraindicated in this client?
   a. "The client is exhibiting persistent coughing."
   b. "The client has passed three stools since morning."
   c. "The client was on oxygen when I took the reading."
   d. "The client has recently undergone rectal surgery."

3. Which of the following signs of a subnormal temperature should a nurse monitor for when assessing the body temperature of a client? (Select all that apply.)
   a. Flushed face
   b. Clammy skin
   c. Unusually bright eyes
   d. Restlessness
   e. Cold, pale skin

4. The nurse is taking care of a newborn. When preparing to assess the vital signs, the nurse knows that which of the following is the most preferred method for measuring the temperature of a newborn?
   a. Oral temperature
   b. Axillary temperature
   c. Rectal temperature
   d. Tympanic temperature

5. A nurse is caring for a group of clients in the community clinic and is required to assess their vital signs regularly. Which of the following clients should the nurse closely monitor for Cheyne-Stokes respiration? (Select all that apply.)
   a. Clients with congestive heart failure
   b. Clients with electrolyte disturbances
   c. Clients with drug overdose
   d. Clients with increased intracranial pressure
   e. Clients with neurologic disturbances
   f. Clients with renal failure

6. A nurse is required to take the vital signs of an adult client. Which of the following is the most accurate assessment of the pulse rate?
   a. Manual palpation
   b. Doppler ultrasound
   c. Auscultation and counting the apical pulse
   d. Sphygmomanometer

7. In which of the following situations should a nurse measure the client's apical pulse? (Select all that apply.)
   a. Concern about heart's rhythm or rate
   b. When the heart appears to have stopped beating
   c. To determine the need for cardiopulmonary resuscitation
   d. By physician's order
   e. When the heart is not effectively pumping blood

8. Which of the following sites should a nurse use to assess the status of circulation to the lower leg?
   a. Popliteal pulse
   b. Pedal pulse
   c. Carotid pulse
   d. Apical-radial pulse

9. When assessing the respiration of an elderly client, the nurse observes bubbling noises. Which of the following is the possible cause of this sound?
   a. The air passageway is partially blocked.
   b. Obstruction has occurred near the glottis.
   c. The air passage is filled with mucus.
   d. Spasms and edema of the bronchi have occurred.

10. Given below are the steps for measuring the radial pulse, in random order. Arrange the steps in the correct order.
   a. Place the tips of the first, second, and third fingers over the client's radial artery on the inside of the wrist on the thumb side.
   b. Using a watch, count the pulse beats for 30 seconds and multiply by 2 to get the rate per minute.
   c. Record the rate (BPM) on paper or on the flow sheet.
   d. Position the client's forearm comfortably with the wrist extended and the palm down.
   e. Press gently against the client's radial artery, to the point at which pulsations can be felt distinctly.
   f. Report any irregular findings to the appropriate person.

CHAPTER 47

# Data Collection in Client Care

## SECTION I: TESTING WHAT YOU KNOW

**Activity A** *Match the examination techniques in Column A with their descriptions in Column B.*

**Column A**

____ 1. Observation

____ 2. Inspection

____ 3. Palpation

____ 4. Auscultation

____ 5. Percussion

**Column B**

a. Tapping or striking fingers against the body

b. Listening for sounds from within the body using a stethoscope or an ultrasound blood-flow detector

c. Watching for general characteristics or factors that do not require closer scrutiny or the use of measurement aids

d. Feeling body tissues or parts with hands or fingers

e. Careful, close, and detailed visual examination of a body part

**Activity B** *Match the various diagnostic procedures in Column A with their explanations in Column B.*

**Column A**

____ 1. Endoscopy

____ 2. Biopsy

____ 3. Lumbar puncture

____ 4. X-ray examinations

____ 5. Treadmill stress test

**Column B**

a. Helps determine fractures and other pathology

b. Helps determine a client's digestive or respiratory structure and function

c. Helps determine the presence of cancer or other disorders

d. Helps evaluate a client's cardiovascular status

e. Helps determine the status of the client's nervous system

**Activity C** *Mark each statement as either "T" (True) or "F" (False). Correct any false statements.*

1. T F Evidence of disease that can be seen or measured, such as a rash or swelling, is called a symptom.

2. T F Infection is the invasion of cells, tissues, or organs by pathogens.

3. T F A purulent exudate is a clear drainage from a wound.

4. T F Examination of the rectum using an endoscope is called sigmoidoscopy.

5. T F Disease is a definite pathologic process.

**Activity D** *Fill in the blanks.*

1. The formation of pus is called ___________.
2. A canal or passage leading to a/an ___________ is called a wound sinus.
3. The ___________ diagnosis focuses on the person and his or her needs in response to the disease, rather than on the disease itself.
4. A/An ___________ disease develops suddenly and runs its course in days or weeks.
5. ___________ is the inflammation of the gallbladder.

**Activity E** *Consider the following figure.*

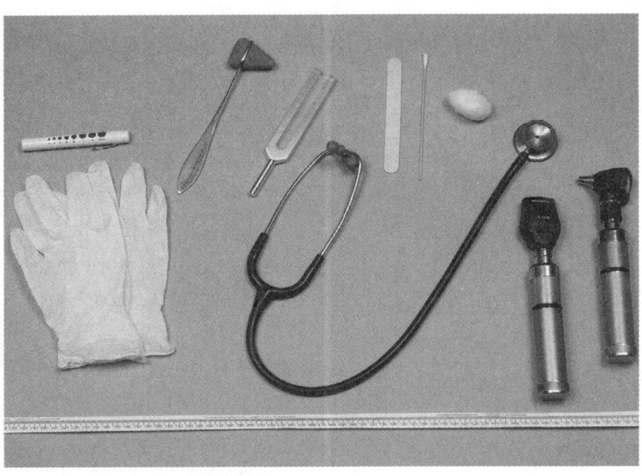

1. Identify the objects in the image.

___________________________________________

___________________________________________

2. What are they used for?

___________________________________________

___________________________________________

**Activity F** *Briefly answer the following questions.*

1. Who determines the medical diagnosis in a healthcare facility?

___________________________________________

___________________________________________

2. What does the nursing diagnosis focus on?

___________________________________________

___________________________________________

3. What is complementary and alternative medicine (CAM)?

___________________________________________

___________________________________________

4. What are the different stages of complications that may occur in a client?

___________________________________________

___________________________________________

5. What is the importance of laboratory tests?

___________________________________________

___________________________________________

## SECTION II: APPLYING WHAT YOU KNOW

**Activity G** *Answer the following questions, which involve the nurse's role in data collection.*

Physical examination and data collection through various tests and procedures help in formulating the medical and nursing diagnoses. A nurse must understand all the methods of data collection and may be required to prepare and assist clients for various tests or procedures.

1. A nurse is caring for a client who is to undergo to a diagnostic test. What are the nursing responsibilities before a diagnostic test?
2. A nurse is caring for a client who is to undergo a radiology treatment. What precaution should the nurse take when assisting the client for radiology?
3. A nurse is to measure the knee-jerk reflexes of an adult client. What should the nurse do to obtain knee-jerk reflexes?

## SECTION III: GETTING READY FOR NCLEX

**Activity H** *Answer the following questions.*

1. A nurse is preparing a pregnant client for a physical examination. What format of physical examination will be used for this client?
   a. Head-to-toe examination
   b. Body system examination
   c. Focused physical examination
   d. Toe-to-head examination
2. A nurse is interviewing a client with eczema. Which of the following should the nurse record as a sign of the disease?
   a. Pain
   b. Nausea
   c. Itching
   d. Rash
3. A nurse is caring for a client who has swelling on his leg after a fall. The nurse informs the client that swelling is a sign of inflammation, which is one of the ways that the body responds to the injury. Which of the following is a cause of inflammation? (Select all that apply.)
   a. Invasion of cells by pathogens
   b. Destruction of tissues in the area
   c. Rush of white blood cells into the area
   d. Loss of blood after an injury
   e. Reduction in the red blood cell count
4. A nurse is caring for a client with a wound. There is a clear discharge from the wound. How should the nurse document this finding?
   a. Purulent
   b. Mucoid
   c. Serum
   d. Necrosis
5. A nurse is caring for a client who is to undergo a colonoscopy. The nurse explains to the client that an endoscope is used for the procedure. What are the uses of an endoscope? (Select all that apply.)
   a. Obtain magnetic resonance image
   b. Isolate pathogens
   c. Examine the internal structures
   d. Perform a biopsy
   e. Remove polyps
6. A nurse is preparing a client who is to undergo a biopsy at the healthcare facility. When is a biopsy performed?
   a. When determining the structure of the organ
   b. When analyzing arterial blood gases
   c. When determining the function of the organ
   d. When determining the presence of cancer
7. A nurse is assessing the function of a client's cranial nerves. Which of the following actions should the nurse ask the client to perform?
   a. Move the hands up and down.
   b. Stand with eyes closed.
   c. Open and close the fist.
   d. Hold an object firmly.
8. A client is to undergo a chest radiograph. What should the nurse do before the radiograph?
   a. Ensure that the client's chart is up-to-date.
   b. Develop a nursing care plan.
   c. Collect data for a nursing care plan.
   d. Evaluate the outcome of nursing care.
9. Which of the following techniques involves tapping or striking of fingers on the client's body?
   a. Auscultation
   b. Palpation
   c. Percussion
   d. Observation
10. A nurse is caring for a client who complains of constipation and gas pains. How should the nurse examine the client?
    a. Palpate, inspect, and auscultate
    b. Inspect, palpate, and auscultate
    c. Auscultate, palpate, and inspect
    d. Inspect, auscultate, and palpate

CHAPTER 48

# Body Mechanics and Positioning

## SECTION I: TESTING WHAT YOU KNOW

**Activity A** *Match the client positions in Column A with their descriptions in Column B.*

**Column A**

____ **1.** Supine dorsal recumbent position

____ **2.** Prone position

____ **3.** Sims' position

____ **4.** Fowler's position

____ **5.** Dorsal lithotomy position

**Column B**

**a.** Side-lying (usually left side), upper knee flexed sharply, bottom arm behind body

**b.** Back-lying, with head raised and knees elevated slightly

**c.** Lying on the abdomen, head to side with arms above the head or beside the body

**d.** Back-lying, with legs separated, knees acutely flexed, and feet in stirrups

**e.** Back-lying, legs extended with arms up or down

**Activity B** *Match the crutch-walking gaits in Column A with their descriptions in Column B.*

**Column A**

____ **1.** Two-point gait

____ **2.** Three-point gait

____ **3.** Four-point gait

____ **4.** Tripod gait

**Column B**

**a.** The client places one crutch forward and then advances the contralateral foot; he then brings the second crutch forward, and the other foot follows.

**b.** The client stands on the strong leg, moves both crutches forward the same distance, rests his weight on his palms, and swings forward slightly ahead of the crutches.

**c.** The client puts his body weight on one leg and on the contralateral crutch.

**d.** The client moves the weak leg and both crutches forward together, balancing his weight on the unaffected leg.

**Activity C** ***Mark each statement as either "T" (True) or "F" (False). Correct any false statements.***

1. T F A person with hemiplegia is paralyzed from the waist area down.
2. T F A person's feet provide the base of support.
3. T F Leaning on crutches in the axilla can cause brachial paralysis.
4. T F A person's center of gravity is located in the abdominal area.
5. T F Joint movement is never forced when doing range-of-motion exercises.

**Activity D** ***Fill in the blanks.***

1. ___________ exercises are performed by tightening and releasing certain muscle groups.
2. ___________ refers to allowing the client to sit on the edge of the bed with the legs down and the feet supported on a footstool or on the floor.
3. A ___________ is a four-legged tubular device with hand grips.
4. A ___________ is a slender, hand-held, curved stick that provides support for walking.
5. The client doing individual, self-directed exercises is performing ___________ range of motion.

**Activity E** ***Briefly answer the following questions.***

1. What kinds of clients would use a Lofstrand crutch?

___________________________________________

___________________________________________

2. What are the advantages of this type of crutch?

___________________________________________

___________________________________________

3. What are the disadvantages of this device?

___________________________________________

___________________________________________

**Activity F** ***Briefly answer the following questions.***

1. Which are the three basic types of canes?

___________________________________________

___________________________________________

2. What is body mechanics?

___________________________________________

___________________________________________

3. How can a person achieve proper body alignment?

___________________________________________

___________________________________________

4. What disorders can be caused by immobility?

___________________________________________

___________________________________________

5. What is the logroll turn?

___________________________________________

___________________________________________

## SECTION II: APPLYING WHAT YOU KNOW

**Activity G** ***Answer the following questions, which involve the nurse's role in positioning clients.***

Nurses need to care for clients who may have restricted or no mobility. It is not physical strength but efficient use of body mechanics that determines how effectively and safely a nurse is able to move clients. Nurses must understand and practice proper body mechanics and often need to teach clients the use of proper body mechanics for safe walking and movement.

1. A nurse is caring for a client with a respiratory disorder. The client is uncomfortable in the supine position.
   a. Into what position should the nurse assist the client?
   b. How can the nurse assist the client into the required position?

2. A nurse is caring for a client with restricted movement of his hands. What measures should the nurse take to ensure that the client does not develop contractures?

3. A nurse is caring for a client who has undergone arthroscopic repair of a knee.
   a. What device is used to provide continuous motion to the specific joint?
   b. How should the nurse explain this to the client?

## SECTION III: GETTING READY FOR NCLEX

**Activity H** *Answer the following questions.*

1. A nurse is to assist a client who has been lying in bed to the bathroom. Which of the following interventions should the nurse perform before taking him to the bathroom?
   a. Assist the client to the Sims' position.
   b. Assist the client to sit at the edge of the bed.
   c. Assist the client to support his feet on the floor.
   d. Assist the client to a supine position.

2. A nurse is required to move an immobile client frequently to prevent skin breakdown. Which of the following should the nurse keep in mind when using a lifting sheet to turn the client with the help of a colleague?
   a. Position the client's arms on her chest.
   b. Lift the neck region of the client first.
   c. Position the client's arms along her side.
   d. Lift the legs and thighs of the client first.

3. A nurse is to prepare a client for a colonoscopy. How should the nurse position the client for the assessment?
   a. Sims' position
   b. Dorsal recumbent position
   c. Orthopneic position
   d. Lithotomy position

4. A nurse is caring for an elderly client who has been confined to bed with rheumatoid arthritis. Which of the following interventions should the nurse perform to prevent skin breakdown?
   a. Raise and lower the head of the bed at frequent intervals.
   b. Adjust the pillows on the bed as often as required.
   c. Assist the client with range-of-motion exercises.
   d. Change the client's body position regularly.

5. A nurse is caring for a violent client in the psychiatry division of a healthcare facility. The physician has ordered the application of leather safety devices to the client. Which of the following interventions should the nurse perform in this situation? (Select all that apply.)
   a. Apply device on emergency order from the charge nurse.
   b. Interview client after device is removed to determine his or her feelings.
   c. Notify client's family immediately on application of device.
   d. Visit the client 1 hour after application of device.
   e. Maintain one-to-one nursing observation for the violent client.

6. A nurse is to assist a client with pulmonary disorders to the radiography unit on a stretcher. Which of the following interventions should the nurse perform when helping the client move from the bed to the wheeled stretcher? (Select all that apply.)
   a. Place the stretcher parallel to the bed.
   b. Cover the client with a blanket over the bedclothes.
   c. Lock the wheels of the bed and the stretcher.
   d. Ensure that the level of the bed is higher than that of the stretcher.
   e. Hold the stretcher tightly against the bed during the move.

7. A nurse is teaching a client with arthritis in both legs to use crutches for walking. Which of the following instructions should the nurse provide the client?
   a. Walk with a two-point gait.
   b. Walk with a three-point gait.
   c. Walk with a four-point gait.
   d. Walk with a tripod gait.

8. A nurse is teaching a client with a fracture to walk with the help of crutches. Which of the following should the nurse tell the client about descending stairs with no handrails?
   a. The affected leg and the crutches should move together.
   b. The crutches and the strong leg should move first.
   c. The affected leg should follow the crutches.
   d. Both crutches should be held on the affected side.

9. A nurse is to assist a client with a fractured left leg from the bed to a wheelchair. How should the nurse perform this task?
   a. Place the chair on the left side of the client.
   b. Raise the head of the bed to a semi-sitting position.
   c. Adjust the chair and bed to the same height.
   d. Move the client from bed to chair quickly.

10. A nurse caring for a client who is confined to bed is required to turn the client on her side. How should the nurse assist the immobile client to turn on her side?
   a. Lower the side rails to be able to turn the client easily.
   b. Position the client to the center of the bed.
   c. Turn the client to her side and support her lower arm on a pillow.
   d. Turn the client to her side and place a pillow between her legs.

CHAPTER 49

# Beds and Bed Making

## SECTION I: TESTING WHAT YOU KNOW

**Activity A** *Match the types of beds in Column A with their descriptions in Column B.*

**Columns A**

____ **1.** Closed bed

____ **2.** Open bed

____ **3.** Occupied bed

____ **4.** Unoccupied bed

____ **5.** Postoperative bed

**Column B**

**a.** A bed that is empty at the time it is made and is the easiest bed to make

**b.** A bed that is made with a weak or immobile client in it

**c.** A bed that is prepared for a client returning from a procedure that requires transfer into bed from a stretcher or wheelchair

**d.** A bed which has its top covers pulled up to the head of the bed over the bottom covers

**e.** A bed which has its top covers fanfolded to the foot of the bed so the client can get in easily

**Activity B** *Match the attachments or accessories for beds in Column A with the type of clients who would need to use them in Column B.*

**Column A**

____ **1.** Bed cradle

____ **2.** Side rails

____ **3.** Footboard

**Column B**

**a.** Used for clients who are in danger of falling out of bed

**b.** Used for immobile clients who are confined to bed for a long period of time

**c.** Used for clients who have fractures, extensive burns, and open or painful wounds

**Activity C** *Mark each statement as either "T" (True) or "F" (False). Correct any false statements.*

**1.** T F The nurse should leave the bed in a low position after having completed caring for the client.

**2.** T F When making a bed, the nurse should put the soiled linen on the floor.

**3.** T F Egg crate mattresses provide client comfort and prevent skin breakdown.

**4.** T F Proper body mechanics are an essential part of bed making.

**5.** T F The trapeze is used by the paraplegic client to pull up to a sitting position.

**Activity D** *Fill in the blanks.*

1. Hospital beds are equipped with a means for attaching a ____________ that holds bags for intravenous (IV) or blood therapy.
2. Clients with ____________ disorders often require head-to-toe linen changes.
3. A ____________ bed, which adjusts to different positions, is most commonly used in health-care facilities.
4. A client may be placed in ____________ to keep a body part such as a leg in proper alignment.
5. The ____________ mattress or pad supports the body or body part so as to avoid creating pressure points.

**Activity E** *Consider the following figure.*

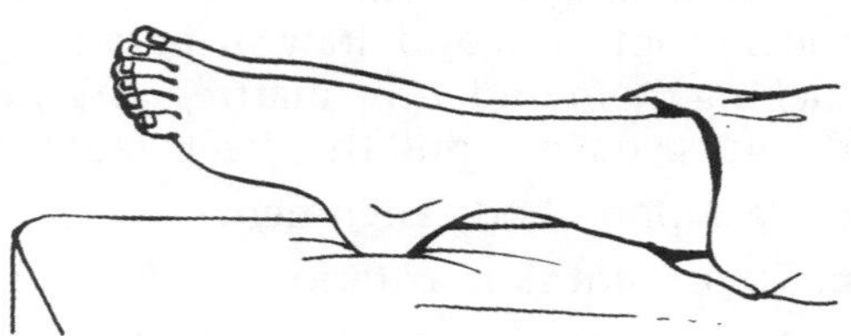

1. Identify the condition shown in the figure.

______________________________________

______________________________________

2. What causes this condition?

______________________________________

______________________________________

3. What care should be taken to prevent this condition?

______________________________________

______________________________________

**Activity F** ***It is important to provide clients with a neat, wrinkle-free bed. Making mitered corners gives a neat appearance and keeps the sheet secured under the mattress. Given below, in random order, are steps used to make mitered sheet corners. Write the correct sequence in the boxes provided below.***

1. Drop the triangle over the side of the bed.
2. Pick up the selvage edge nearest the foot of the bed.
3. Tuck the hanging edge under the mattress.
4. Fold down a triangle on the bed.
5. Tuck the hanging part of the sheet under the mattress.

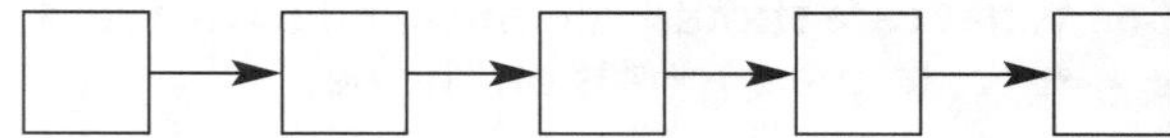

**Activity G** ***Briefly answer the following questions.***

1. Why is it necessary to provide a bed to the client?

______________________________________

______________________________________

2. What are the characteristics of an ideal bed?

______________________________________

______________________________________

3. What are the necessary supplies that should be included in bed making?

______________________________________

______________________________________

4. What is the purpose of bed making?

______________________________________

______________________________________

5. What are the schedules for changing beds?

______________________________________

______________________________________

## SECTION II: APPLYING WHAT YOU KNOW

**Activity H** *Answer the following questions, which involve the nurse's role in bed making.*

Every client needs a smooth, clean bed for comfort. Sometimes the nurse may need to make beds for clients who are immobile or who are to be transferred from one unit of the healthcare facility to another.

1. A nurse is caring for a client with an unset fracture. Changing the bed may prove harmful for this client.
   - **a.** How can the nurse ensure that the client is comfortable in bed even if it is not changed?
   - **b.** What care should the nurse take with respect to the controls on the bed?
2. A nurse is caring for a client who is weak and cannot get out of bed. The nurse is required to make an occupied bed.
   - **a.** How is making an occupied bed different from making an unoccupied bed?
   - **b.** How can the nurse ensure proper body mechanics when making beds?

## SECTION III: GETTING READY FOR NCLEX

**Activity I** *Answer the following questions.*

1. A nurse is caring for a semiconscious client in a bed with a bed cradle attached. How does the bed cradle help the client?
   - **a.** It protects the client from accidental falls.
   - **b.** It rocks the bed from side to side.
   - **c.** It prevents linen from touching the client.
   - **d.** It reduces pressure on one side of the body.
2. A client who is injured in an accident has the side rails of the bed raised. How is the side rail helpful for the client? (Select all that apply.)
   - **a.** It holds the nurse call signal.
   - **b.** It prevents the client from falling.
   - **c.** It provides cushioned comfort.
   - **d.** It helps the client to change position.
   - **e.** It supports the body in correct alignment.
3. A nurse is caring for a client with paraplegia, who has a horizontal bar hanging on chains attached to a large overhead frame fastened to the bed. What is this attachment called?
   - **a.** Bed cradle
   - **b.** Bed board
   - **c.** Traction
   - **d.** Trapeze
4. A nurse is making an open bed for a client. Which of the following should the nurse keep in mind when changing the linens?
   - **a.** Place soiled linens on the side table.
   - **b.** Keep the side rails on the far end of the bed up.
   - **c.** Slide the mattress toward the foot of the bed.
   - **d.** Adjust the bed to a low position after it is made.
5. When making a bed, the nurse should pull the bottom sheet and draw sheet taut before tucking them under the mattress. Why does the nurse have to pull the sheets taut?
   - **a.** To support body alignment
   - **b.** To prevent skin irritation
   - **c.** To prevent the mattress from sliding
   - **d.** To provide comfort and hygiene
6. A nurse is preparing a bed for a client who is returning from surgery. Which of the following should the nurse do if the linen used by the client is not soiled?
   - **a.** Pull the sheets and tuck them under the mattress.
   - **b.** Fanfold the top linen to the side next to the stretcher.
   - **c.** Use only clean linen and do not place pillows.
   - **d.** Remake the bed with the used linen and place pillows.
7. A nurse is caring for a client who had a paralytic stroke. Which of the following would be beneficial for this client?
   - **a.** Flotation mattress
   - **b.** Egg crate mattress
   - **c.** Flotation pad
   - **d.** Circ-O-Lectric bed

**8.** A nurse is caring for a client with a bleeding wound. What should the nurse keep in mind about the schedule for making the bed?

**a.** Early in the morning

**b.** After bed bath only

**c.** Whenever linen is soiled

**d.** Just before bedtime

**9.** The physician has suggested the use of an air-fluidized bed for a client with paralysis. Which of the following is the purpose of an air-fluidized bed?

**a.** It rocks the client from side to side.

**b.** It reduces the effects of pressure against the skin.

**c.** It keeps the body in straight alignment.

**d.** It provides alignment to a part of the body.

**10.** A nurse is caring for a client with foot drop. The client moves about the bed a great deal. Which of the following would be most beneficial to this client?

**a.** Padded footboard

**b.** High top shoes

**c.** Bed cradle

**d.** Bed board

CHAPTER 50

# Personal Hygiene

## SECTION I: TESTING WHAT YOU KNOW

**Activity A** ***Match the conditions related to personal hygiene in Column A with their definitions in Column B.***

**Column A**

____ 1. Halitosis

____ 2. Pyorrhea

____ 3. Sordes

____ 4. Pediculosis

**Column B**

a. Infestation by lice

b. Brownish deposits on tongue

c. Inflammation of tooth sockets

d. Bad breath

**Activity B** ***Match the various backrub techniques in Column A with their procedures in Column B.***

**Column A**

____ 1. Pétrissage

____ 2. Effleurage

____ 3. Tapotement

____ 4. Friction

**Column B**

a. Light tapping with the edge of the hands farthest from the thumb

b. Rubbing around the bony prominences at the end of the spine and along each shoulder blade

c. Picking up and squeezing muscle groups or single muscles

d. Stroking in the direction of venous circulation in a circular pattern

**Activity C** ***Mark each statement as either "T" (True) or "F" (False). Correct any false statements.***

1. T F A nurse should encourage clients to brush their teeth by placing the bristles at a 90-degree angle to the teeth.

2. T F Flossing removes debris that could cause tooth decay and offensive breath odor.

3. T F Thickened and raised nails can be a sign of a bacterial infection.

4. T F Some oral conditions cause infection or pain in other body parts.

5. T F Scabies is a common contagious condition caused by pediculosis capitis.

**Activity D** ***Fill in the blanks.***

1. ___________ are the eggs of lice, which look like solid specks found on hairy body parts.

2. A product called a Shampoo ___________ is very handy for clients who cannot get out of bed for a shampoo.

3. A hand massage is an example of ___________ touch, providing a connection between client and nurse.

4. Tears are produced by the ___________ glands, which are situated at the top and outer portion of each eye.

5. The ___________ bath is a special type of bath used for a client after rectal surgery and sometimes after childbirth.

**Activity E** *Consider the following figures.*

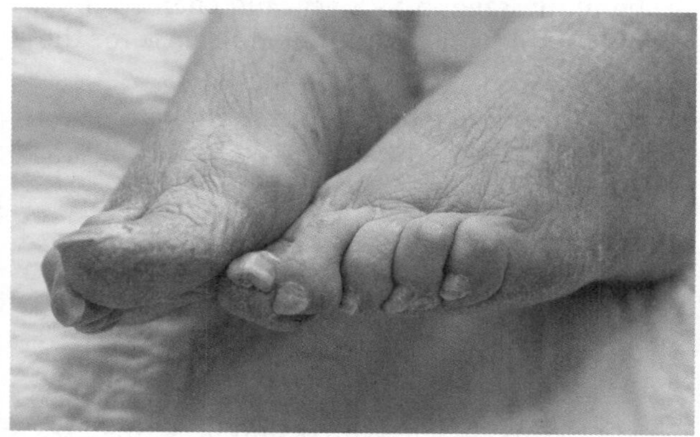

1. Identify the toenail abnormalities shown in the figure.

______________________________

______________________________

2. Explain the need for toenail care.

______________________________

______________________________

3. What are the steps in toenail care?

______________________________

______________________________

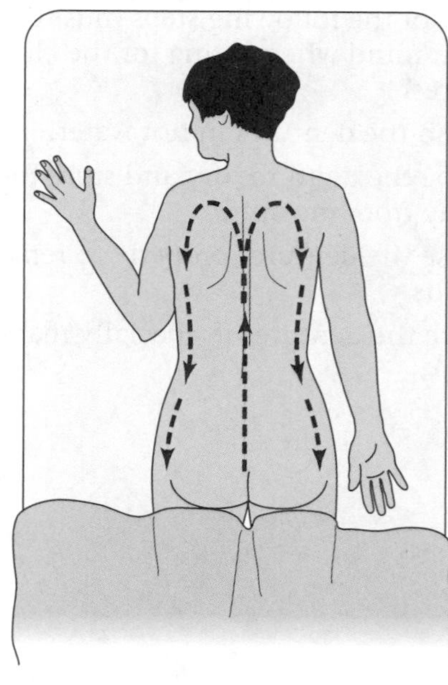

4. Identify the pattern of backrub shown in the figure.

______________________________

______________________________

5. Why is a backrub given?

______________________________

______________________________

6. How is the procedure performed?

______________________________

______________________________

**Activity F** ***The nurse needs to be careful with care of the nails if the client is diabetic or hemophilic. The steps in caring for fingernails are listed below in random order. Write the correct sequence in the boxes provided.***

1. Shape the fingernails with an emery board.
2. Clip hangnails with manicure scissors or cuticle snippers.
3. Trim the client's fingernails straight across with nail clippers.
4. Soak the client's fingers in a basin of warm water and mild soap.

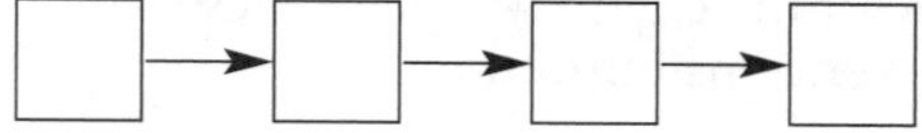

**Activity G** *Briefly answer the following questions.*

1. How should a nurse at a healthcare center manage a client's dentures?

______________________________

______________________________

2. When do clients require special mouth care?

______________________________

______________________________

3. What nursing care is necessary when caring for a client with a blocked lacrimal gland duct?

______________________________

______________________________

4. What are the benefits of hand massage?

______________________________

______________________________

5. Why is warm water used for a foot soak?

______________________________

______________________________

## SECTION II: APPLYING WHAT YOU KNOW

**Activity H** ***Answer the following questions, which involve the nurse's role in management of personal hygiene and skin care.***

A nurse's role in managing the client's personal hygiene and skin care includes assisting the client in bathing.

1. A 65-year-old client with a respiratory disorder is admitted to a healthcare center. The attending nurse is asked to assist the client in taking a tub bath. What are the appropriate nursing interventions required when assisting the client?
2. A nurse is caring for a 50-year-old client who is unresponsive. What are the nursing interventions involved when maintaining the oral hygiene of the client? Why are these interventions important?
3. A nurse is required to give a backrub to a 30-year-old client who has been admitted to a healthcare center after a stroke.
   a. Why is a backrub necessary for this client?
   b. What preparations are required before giving a backrub to the client?
   c. What are the various nursing considerations involved when giving a backrub to the client?

## SECTION III: GETTING READY FOR NCLEX

**Activity I** ***Answer the following questions.***

1. A nurse in a healthcare center needs to give a hand massage to a 45-year-old client. Which of the following would the nurse use for the procedure?
   a. Gently shake the client's hand before starting the procedure.
   b. Avoid rotating and bending each finger back and forth.
   c. Do not massage the webbed area between the client's thumb and first finger.
   d. Massage the fingers from the tip to the hand.
2. A nurse in a healthcare facility is caring for an 11-year-old client with a chronic fever. Which of the following instructions should the nurse suggest to the client for maintaining oral care and hygiene?
   a. Hold the floss gently between the index finger and thumb when using it.
   b. Place the bristles at a 30-degree angle to the tooth when brushing.
   c. Brush the inner and outer surface of the teeth with a horizontal motion.
   d. Use floss by moving it up and down on each side of the tooth.
3. A client wearing dentures is required to remove them before undergoing a colonoscopy. Which of the following steps must the nurse keep in mind when caring for the client's dentures?
   a. Wash the dentures in hot water.
   b. Wipe the dentures dry and store them away from moisture.
   c. Rinse the dentures properly to remove deposits.
   d. Store the dentures in specially marked cups.

**4.** A nurse is caring for a client who is unresponsive. Which of the following nursing interventions related to the client's personal hygiene should the nurse perform when caring for the client?

**a.** Restrict oral care to once every day.

**b.** Turn the client's head frequently.

**c.** Keep the client undisturbed in the same position.

**d.** Give frequent tub baths.

**5.** A 40-year-old diabetic client with a previous history of heart attack is admitted to a healthcare facility to undergo a surgery early the next day. Which of the following must the nurse ensure when caring for the client?

**a.** Ensure removal of any nail polish or artificial nails on the client's fingers.

**b.** Ensure that the client's toenails are clean and clipped if they are long.

**c.** Provide daily baths to the client whether the skin is oily or dry.

**d.** Provide a towel bath to the client by vigorously rubbing the skin.

**6.** A 25-year-old client who has delivered a baby requires special perineal care. Which of the following nursing interventions should the nurse perform when providing special perineal care?

**a.** Wash the client's genitals first and then the thighs and groin area.

**b.** Begin cleaning the perineal area from the center to the outside.

**c.** Use a single portion of the washcloth for cleaning the entire perineal area.

**d.** Wash the client's perineal area from the pubic to the anal area.

**7.** When performing a perineal wash for a 56-year-old client, the nurse notices tiny oval, grayish insects moving around the client's genital region. The nurse suspects which of the following conditions in the client?

**a.** Pediculosis capitis

**b.** Sordes

**c.** Crab lice infestation

**d.** Scabies

**8.** A nurse is asked to give a towel bath to a 60-year-old unresponsive client. Which of the following should the nurse keep in mind when performing the procedure?

**a.** Friction over the client's body is achieved by gentle rubbing with the nurse's hands.

**b.** A dry or damp towel is used to rub the client's body during the procedure.

**c.** Friction during the procedure causes the blood vessels in the client's body to constrict.

**d.** Firm pressure during the procedure promotes improved circulation in the skin.

**9.** A nurse is assisting an 80-year-old client to take a shower. Which of the following nursing procedures would be preferable for this client?

**a.** Encourage the client to take the shower immediately after food.

**b.** Ensure that the shower room has no rails to prevent injury.

**c.** Provide a stool or shower chair.

**d.** Allow the client to take the shower by himself.

**10.** A nurse in a healthcare center is assisting a 25-year-old client with her personal hygiene. Which of the following nursing interventions should the nurse perform when providing care to the client's toenails?

**a.** Place the client's feet in a basin of cold water and soak them.

**b.** Cut (with a physician's order) and file very thick and hard nails.

**c.** Shape the corners of the nails by rounding them.

**d.** Clean under the client's nails with a metal file.

CHAPTER 51

# Elimination

## SECTION I: TESTING WHAT YOU KNOW

**Activity A** *Match the patterns of urinary elimination in Column A with their descriptions in Column B.*

**Column A**

____ 1. Nocturia

____ 2. Polyuria

____ 3. Oliguria

____ 4. Urinary retention

**Column B**

a. Increase in the expected amount of urine a person excretes over a period of time; may be a symptom of diabetes mellitus or certain types of kidney disease

b. Decrease in the expected amount of urine a person excretes; possible indication of a kidney disorder or urinary tract obstruction

c. Frequent voiding during the night, usually accompanied by urinary frequency; may not indicate a structural or organic problem

d. Inability to empty the bladder of urine because of inability to feel the urge to void or to relax the urethral muscles; a temporary condition may follow abdominal surgery

**Activity B** *Match the types of enemas in Column A with their descriptions in Column B.*

**Column A**

____ 1. Carminative enema

____ 2. Emollient enema

____ 3. Cleansing enema

____ 4. Medicated enema

**Column B**

a. This enema consists of a small amount of olive or cottonseed oil, given to protect or soothe the mucous membrane of the colon.

b. This enema introduces enough fluid into the colon to soften feces, stimulate peristalsis, and produce a bowel movement that empties the rectum and lower colon.

c. In this enema, a drug is inserted into the rectum in combination with a small amount of oil or saline to reduce its irritating effect and to lessen the client's desire to expel it.

d. This enema is given to stimulate peristalsis so that flatus (gas) is expelled from the intestine.

**Activity C** ***Mark each statement as either "T" (True) or "F" (False). Correct any false statements.***

1. T F Gray- or clay-colored stools usually indicate constipation.
2. T F Projectile vomiting can be a sign of a serious condition such as a brain tumor or brain trauma.
3. T F Normally, feces are yellowish-brown due to the presence of microorganisms.
4. T F Incontinence is defined as the retention of urine in the bladder.
5. T F Normal kidneys produce about 1 milliliter of urine per every kilogram of body weight each hour.

**Activity D** ***Fill in the blanks.***

1. Involuntary voiding of urine in bed is called ___________.
2. ___________ is an inflammation of the bladder.
3. ___________ is the expulsion of loose, watery, unformed stools.
4. The type of enema used to introduce contrast solution into the bowel for a radiographic procedure is called a ___________.
5. Normal urine has a specific gravity, when compared with water, of 1.010 to ___________.

**Activity E** ***Consider the following figure.***

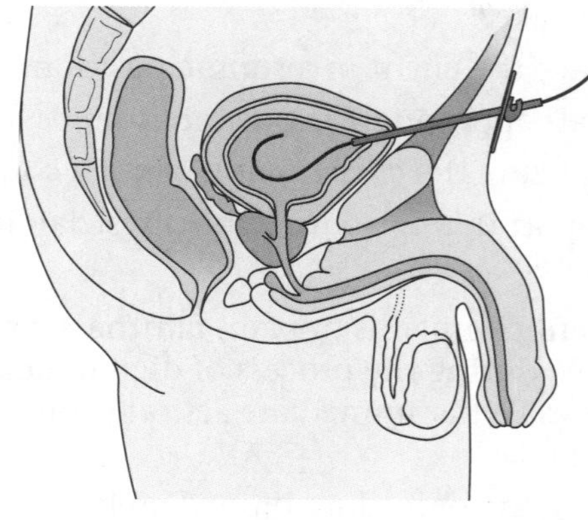

1. Identify the procedure being done.

___________________________________

___________________________________

2. How is this procedure done?

___________________________________

___________________________________

3. Can urine also be voided naturally after the procedure is done?

___________________________________

___________________________________

**Activity F** ***The goal of bladder retraining is to help the client regain the sensation of voiding by allowing the bladder to refill, which causes the bladder muscles to stretch and signal the brain. The steps for bladder training with closed urinary drainage are given below in random order. Write the correct sequence in the boxes provided.***

1. Open the clamp and allow the bladder to drain by gravity into the drainage bag. Repeat the procedure.
2. Explain the procedure and position the client in supine position.
3. Record the procedure on the client's record, including urinary output. Clamp the catheter tubing for 1 to 2 hours.
4. Put on disposable gloves and clamp the catheter tubing for 1 to 2 hours.

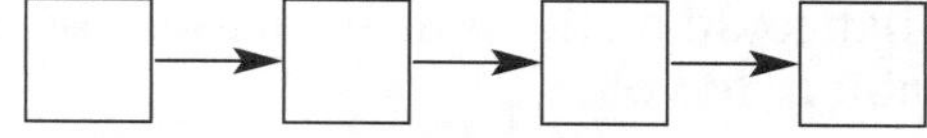

**Activity G** ***Briefly answer the following questions.***

1. What is renal colic?

___________________________________

___________________________________

2. What do long, thin, pencil-like stools indicate?

___________________________________

___________________________________

3. What is the mechanism of production of bowel sounds?

______________________________________________

______________________________________________

4. When is digital removal of feces contraindicated?

______________________________________________

______________________________________________

5. Vomiting is dangerous and needs to be prevented in what situations?

______________________________________________

______________________________________________

## SECTION II: APPLYING WHAT YOU KNOW

**Activity H** ***Answer the following questions, which involve the nurse's role in managing clients' elimination.***

Assessing the client's products of elimination (urine and feces), observing his or her bladder and bowel function, and assisting the client who is facing a problem with these functions are fundamental nursing responsibilities.

1. After a hysterectomy, a 35-year-old female client is unable to void urine.
   a. List the nursing measures to relieve this condition.
   b. What could be the possible reason for this inability to void?
   c. In what situation should the nurse report her assessment to the physician?
2. A client is unable to pass stools after administration of a barium enema. A rectal examination reveals a hard or putty-like mass.
   a. Identify the condition.
   b. Suggest the nursing measure to relieve this condition.
   c. List the steps for this procedure.

## SECTION III: GETTING READY FOR NCLEX

**Activity I** ***Answer the following questions.***

1. A client tells the nurse that he has alternate-day bowel movements and is otherwise symptom free. What action should the nurse take?
   a. Give abdominal pressure.
   b. Report to the physician at once.
   c. Perform a digital evacuation.
   d. Reassure him that it is not a concern.
2. A nurse is preparing a client for an enema. Which of the following should the nurse administer to protect or soothe the mucous membrane of the colon?
   a. Oil retention enema
   b. Emollient enema
   c. Anthelminthic enema
   d. Cleansing enema
3. A client is complaining of urgency, frequency, dysuria, chills, abdominal discomfort, and pain. What action should the nurse take?
   a. Encourage the client to perform Kegel exercises.
   b. Send a urine specimen for culture, and report to the physician.
   c. Begin catheterization immediately.
   d. Strain the urine specimen for urinary calculi.
4. A 25-year-old client with complaints of frequent headaches has an episode of projectile vomiting. What immediate action should the nurse take?
   a. Place the client in a supine position.
   b. Start appropriate intravenous fluids.
   c. Reassure the client that it is not a concern.
   d. Report this episode to the physician immediately.
5. A client complains of pain, faintness, and nausea during the process of digital removal of feces. What immediate action should the nurse take?
   a. Stop the procedure immediately.
   b. Reassure and continue.
   c. Give an enema immediately.
   d. Auscultate for bowel sounds.

**6.** During bladder retraining, a client develops a few random episodes of incontinence. What action should the nurse take?

**a.** Notify the physician.

**b.** Limit fluid intake.

**c.** Catheterize immediately.

**d.** Reassure the client.

**7.** A 30-year-old client complains of abdominal discomfort. What is the first step to be taken by the nurse?

**a.** Provide a bedpan.

**b.** Give a cleansing enema.

**c.** Auscultate for bowel sounds.

**d.** Notify the physician.

**8.** A client with a retention catheter in situ complains that the catheter has come off. What actions should the nurse take if the catheter has fallen off? (Select all that apply.)

**a.** Report this immediately to the physician.

**b.** Reinsert the same retention catheter.

**c.** Discontinue if the client is now able to void.

**d.** Insert a new, sterile retention catheter.

**e.** Obtain a physician's order and reinsert the catheter.

**9.** Given below are the steps for listening to bowel sounds, in random order. Arrange the steps in the correct orders.

**1.** Auscultate all areas of the abdomen.

**2.** Document the findings on the client's chart.

**3.** Place the diaphragm of the stethoscope against the abdomen.

**4.** Warm the stethoscope in your hands.

**5.** Position the client in supine position.

**6.** Listen for peristalsis, which makes a gurgling sound.

**7.** Expose the abdomen, keeping other areas covered.

**a.** 7, 6, 1, 2, 4, 3, 5

**b.** 5, 7, 4, 3, 1, 6, 2

**c.** 7, 5, 4, 3, 6, 1, 2

**d.** 5, 1, 6, 4, 3, 2, 7

**10.** When monitoring a 70-year-old male client, a nurse observes that the client is voiding more often than usual without an increase in total urine volume. What term best describes this condition?

**a.** Incontinence

**b.** Urinary frequency

**c.** Enuresis

**d.** Urgency

CHAPTER 52

# Specimen Collection

## SECTION I: TESTING WHAT YOU KNOW

**Activity A** ***Match the steps for stool specimen collection and examination in Column A with their rationales in Column B.***

**Column A**

____ 1. Label the container.

____ 2. Use a tongue blade to transfer a portion of the feces to the container.

____ 3. Take a portion of feces from three different areas of the specimen.

____ 4. Stools should be examined when fresh.

**Column B**

a. Examinations for parasites, ova, and organisms must be made when the stool is warm

b. Helps the laboratory to correctly identify the specimen

c. Specimen is grossly contaminated

d. Enhances the accuracy of the results

**Activity B** ***Match the steps involved in collecting a urine specimen from a retention catheter in Column A with their rationales in Column B.***

**Column A**

____ 1. Clamp the drainage tubing.

____ 2. Unclamp the retention catheter.

____ 3. Cleanse the aspiration port with antiseptic.

____ 4. Draw urine using a sterile needle and syringe.

**Column B**

a. Prevents contamination of the bladder

b. Guarantees collection of a fresh specimen

c. Prevents urinary stasis by allowing free flow

d. Prevents microorganisms from entering the catheter

**Activity C** ***Mark each statement as either "T" (True) or "F" (False). Correct any false statements.***

1. T F Consuming adequate amounts of fluids makes it easier for the client to cough up sputum.

2. T F A sputum specimen should be collected over 24 hours and stored in the refrigerator before the test is conducted.

3. T F To distend the veins before venipuncture at the antecubital space, a tourniquet is tied around the forearm.

4. T F Routine specimen collection is usually scheduled for early in the morning.

5. T F Fluid intake includes all fluids consumed only through the gastrointestinal tract.

**Activity D** ***Fill in the blanks.***

1. Venipuncture is often done on the inside surface of the forearm near the elbow, called the ____________ space.

2. During 24-hour fractional urine specimen collection, each new time slot begins with a/an ____________ bladder.

3. The urine-collecting bag should not be higher than the level of the ____________.

4. The Hematest or Hemoccult brand method is used to test for occult __________ in the stool.

5. Breathing __________ air makes it easier for the client to expectorate.

**Activity E** *Consider the following figure.*

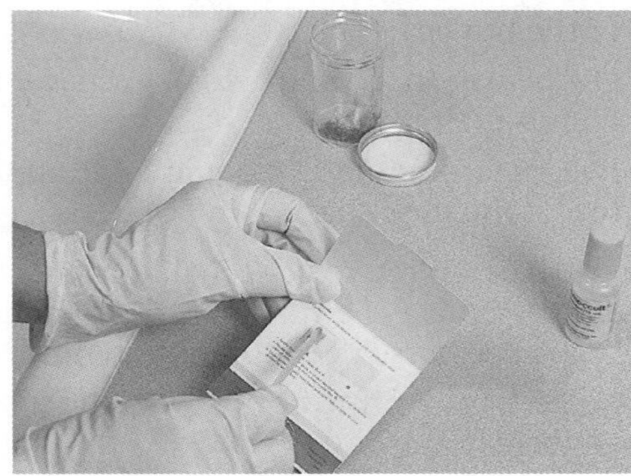

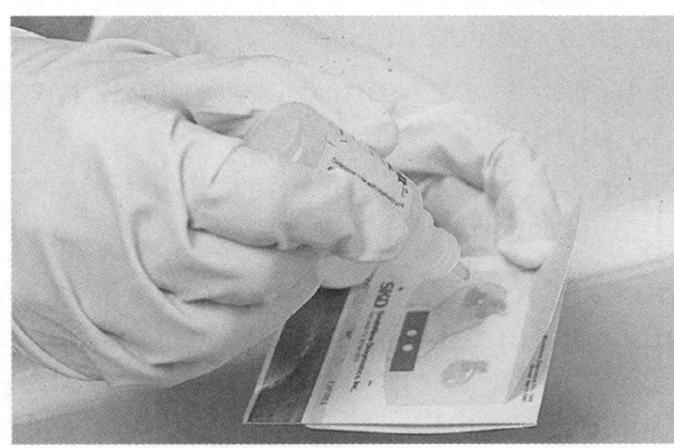

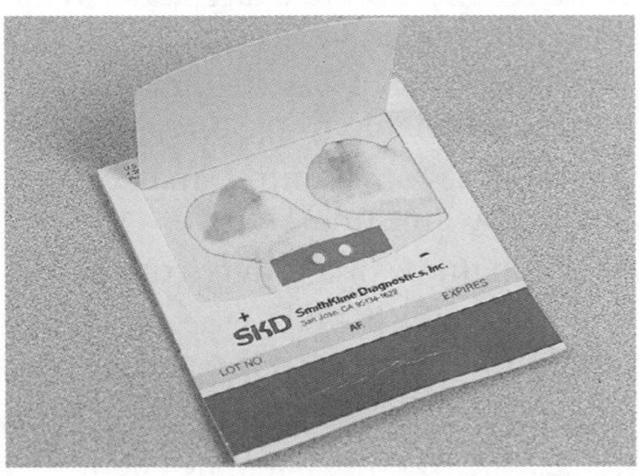


1. What test does the figure depict?

______________________________

______________________________

2. What is the purpose of the test?

______________________________

______________________________

3. How does a nurse perform this test?

______________________________

______________________________

**Activity F** ***The steps in collection of a urine specimen from a retention catheter are given below in random order. Write the correct sequence in the boxes provided.***

1. Unclamp the catheter to allow free urinary flow.
2. Draw urine from the aspiration port into a syringe.
3. Explain the procedure to the client.
4. Clamp the drainage tubing.

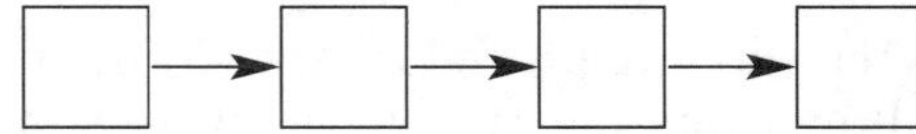

**Activity G** ***Briefly answer the following questions.***

1. What is understood by the term "specific gravity of urine"?

______________________________

______________________________

2. What is the purpose of obtaining a midstream urine specimen?

______________________________

______________________________

3. What are the two most common tests done on stool specimens? What do they detect?

______________________________

______________________________

4. What is the most common indication for collection of a sputum specimen?

______________________________

______________________________

## SECTION II: APPLYING WHAT YOU KNOW

**Activity H** *Answer the following questions, which involve the nurse's role in specimen collection.*

A nurse's role in helping healthcare providers learn about the health status of a client involves assisting in the collection of urine, stool, and sputum specimens. The nurse also helps the primary caregiver or the laboratory professional in collecting blood specimens by venipuncture.

1. A nurse has been ordered to measure the urinary output of a client with suspected nephritis.
   a. What supplies and equipment does the nurse need to keep ready for the procedure?
   b. What nursing procedure should the nurse follow when measuring the urinary output?
2. A client has been admitted into the gastroenterology department of a healthcare agency. A nurse is required to collect a stool specimen and send it to the laboratory for examination. Before sending it, the nurse is required to conduct a Hemoccult test at the bedside.
   a. What supplies and equipment may be required to collect the stool specimen?
   b. What nursing procedure does the nurse need to follow when collecting a stool specimen?
   c. What nursing alerts should the nurse keep in mind when conducting a Hemoccult test?

## SECTION III: GETTING READY FOR NCLEX

**Activity I** *Answer the following questions.*

1. As part of data collection, a nurse is required to maintain an intake and output (I&O) record for each client. Which of the following should the nurse keep in mind when maintaining the I&O record?
   a. Measure in units of deciliters (dL).
   b. Record total food and fluid intake of the client.
   c. Keep records in the records room of the healthcare facility.
   d. It provides a guide for decision-making about fluid administration.
2. A nurse has been asked to measure the volume and specific gravity of the urine of a client. Which of the following standard precautions does the nurse need to adhere to?
   a. The beaker should be filled to about half its capacity.
   b. The hydrometer should just touch the side of the beaker.
   c. The beaker should be held at eye level to obtain the reading.
   d. The reading should be obtained from the top of the meniscus.
3. A nurse is required to collect a 24-hour urine specimen from a client. Which of the following does the nurse need to keep in mind?
   a. Collection of urine begins with the first voiding of the day.
   b. The sample must be sent to the laboratory as it is collected.
   c. Exposure to air might decompose the urine to ammonia.
   d. Urine from each voiding is kept in a separate container.
4. A nurse is required to collect a stool specimen from a client for a Hemoccult test. After realizing that the client has been taking high doses of vitamin C, the nurse advances the specimen collection to a later date. What is the possible reason for this?
   a. Stool color may be altered, making the test results unreliable.
   b. Excess doses of vitamin C may cause bleeding in the intestine.
   c. Stool might be of a watery consistency and unsuitable for the test.
   d. Vitamin C reacts with the reagents to give a false-positive result.
5. A nurse is instructing a female client on how to obtain a clean-catch urine specimen. What instruction is most important in such a case?
   a. Clean the urethral area from front to back.
   b. Void the first stream of urine into the container.
   c. Wash the hands only after specimen collection.
   d. Label the container after specimen collection.

**6.** A stool specimen has to be collected from a client with normal bowel movements. The client has been asked to let the nurse know when there is an urge to have a bowel movement. What is the reason for this?

**a.** Client will need to be assisted to the bathroom.

**b.** Client may not be able to move bowels on command.

**c.** Nurse may need to report to the primary care provider.

**d.** Nurse needs to give a purgative before collecting stool.

**7.** As part of the Standard Precautions for specimen collection, all specimens need to be placed in biohazard bags. Why is this done?

**a.** To prevent risk of infection to the staff

**b.** To prevent contamination of the specimen

**c.** To prevent exposure to air

**d.** To facilitate immediate transportation

**8.** A nurse is required to collect a sputum specimen from a client. Which of the following should the nurse keep in mind?

**a.** The specimen should be collected just before bedtime.

**b.** The client should expectorate directly into the container.

**c.** The specimen should be stored in the refrigerator.

**d.** The client should label the container before handing it over.

**9.** A nurse is instructing a client on the steps needed to collect a clean-catch urine specimen. The required steps are given below in random order. Arrange the steps in the correct order.

**a.** Hold the urine for some time.

**b.** Void the urine directly into the container.

**c.** Void a small amount of urine into the toilet.

**d.** Cleanse the urethral area with a wipe.

**10.** A nurse is instructing a 45-year-old male client about how to collect a midstream urine specimen. In what direction should he be instructed to cleanse the urethral area?

**a.** Back to front direction

**b.** Front to back direction

**c.** Circular motion going inward

**d.** Circular motion going outward

CHAPTER 53

# Bandages and Binders

## SECTION I: TESTING WHAT YOU KNOW

**Activity A** *Match the bandage type in Column A with its use in Column B.*

| Column A | Column B |
|---|---|
| ____ 1. Elastic roller bandage | a. To support a specific body part and to hold a dressing in place |
| ____ 2. Antiembolism stockings | b. To enable frequent dressing changes |
| ____ 3. T-binders | c. To support a dressing and to exert pressure over a bleeding point |
| ____ 4. Montgomery strap | d. To ensure adequate return circulation to the heart and to prevent blood clots |

**Activity B** *Match the conditions in Column A with the type of bandage used for them in Column B.*

| Column A | Column B |
|---|---|
| ____ 1. Thromboembolitic disease | a. Tape |
| ____ 2. To hold rectal or perineal dressings in place | b. Kerlix gauze |
| ____ 3. To hold dressings in place or apply pressure | c. T-binder |
| ____ 4. Sprained ankle or fractured ribs | d. Antiembolism stockings |

**Activity C** *Mark each statement as either "T" (True) or "F" (False). Correct any false statements.*

1. T F Elasticized bandages are often used to provide muscle or joint support and to increase circulation.
2. T F Elastic roller bandages are often used to control bleeding by applying direct pressure over the bleeding point.
3. T F Antiembolism stockings are applied after the client gets out of the bed following surgery.
4. T F An arm sling is a type of binder that supports the dislocated arm in place.
5. T F To avoid discomfort to the client, a tape should always be removed in the direction opposite to that of the hair growth.
6. T F The dressing is held in place by the adhesive end of the Montgomery strap.

**Activity D** *Fill in the blanks.*

1. When applying antiembolism stockings, the color, motion, and sensation of the client's extremity are checked every ____________ hours.
2. Before applying an antiembolism stocking, it is ensured that the client has been lying down for at least ____________ minutes.
3. Binders are used to provide ____________ to specific body parts.
4. Abdominal binders are used after abdominal surgery and after ____________.

5. Tight application of bandages and binders usually results in ____________ type of edema over the extremities.

**Activity E** *Consider the following figure.*

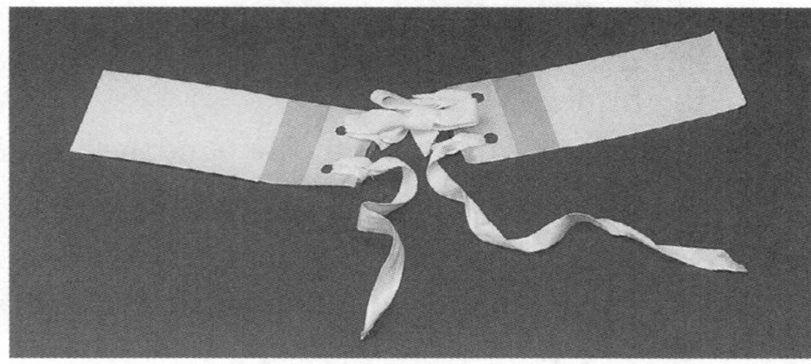

1. Identify the object shown in the figure. What are its advantages?

_______________________________________

_______________________________________

2. How is it applied?

_______________________________________

_______________________________________

**Activity F** *The steps that occur during the application of an antiembolism stocking are given below in random order. Write the correct sequence in the boxes provided.*

1. Applying the antiembolism stocking
2. Taking measurement of the legs for proper size
3. Explaining the procedure to the client
4. Checking for the integrity of the stocking

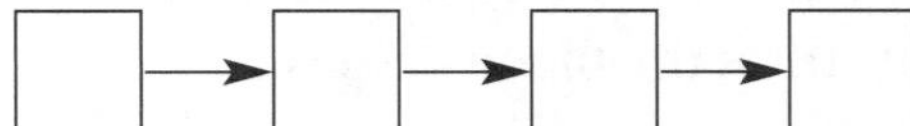

**Activity G** *Briefly answer the following questions.*

1. What are bandages and binders? Where are they used?

_______________________________________

_______________________________________

2. What are the various types of bandages and binders?

_______________________________________

_______________________________________

3. What are the precautions to be taken while applying and removing tapes?

_______________________________________

_______________________________________

4. How is an abdominal binder applied?

_______________________________________

_______________________________________

## SECTION II: APPLYING WHAT YOU KNOW

**Activity H** *Answer the following questions, which involve the nurse's role in postoperative care.*

A nurse's management of injuries and postoperative care depends on the application and management of bandages.

1. A nurse is required to apply a bandage to a client who has injured his leg in an accident.
   a. What type of bandage is preferred for the client?
   b. What are the signs and symptoms that are evaluated by the nurse to indicate whether there is any circulatory disturbance in the client?
2. A nurse is required to apply an antiembolism stocking to a client who has undergone surgery.
   a. What benefits do antiembolism stockings offer over the cotton elastic bandages?
   b. What are the precautions to be taken while using the antiembolism stocking?
3. A nurse is caring for a postoperative client who is using a sequential compression device. What is the purpose of using a sequential compression device?

## SECTION III: GETTING READY FOR NCLEX

**Activity I** *Answer the following questions.*

1. A client had tapes applied to hold her dressing in place. The nurse applied acetone to the skin at the edges of the tape. Why did the nurse need to do so?
   a. To hold the tape in place.
   b. To provide antisepsis for the wound.
   c. To relieve the itching sensation.
   d. To loosen up the adhesion.
2. A client complains of itching when his hand is wrapped with a bandage. What should the nurse immediately assess for?
   a. Rise in body temperature
   b. Fall in blood pressure
   c. Presence of bleeding
   d. Macular eruptions on the skin
3. When assessing a client whose leg is wrapped in a bandage, the nurse notices that her toes are colder than the rest of her body. What immediate step should the nurse take in such a case?
   a. Apply a hot compress to the client's toes.
   b. Ask the client to soak her foot in lukewarm water.
   c. Apply alternating hot and cold compresses.
   d. Alert the team leader to this condition at once.
4. Which of the following should the attending nurse keep in mind when applying a bandage to a client's extremity?
   a. Overlap each layer about half the width of the strip.
   b. Wrap the bandage firmly and tightly.
   c. Anchor the top of the bandage with pins.
   d. Release the bandage once every 2 hours.
5. A nurse is caring for a 35-year-old client who has been hospitalized with an injury to his leg. What specific measures should the nurse take after application of a bandage to the client's leg?
   a. Monitor the circulation and nerve function of the extremity.
   b. Ensure that the client is continuously moving his legs.
   c. Apply hot compresses to the bandage area.
   d. Record the client's blood pressure and temperature.
6. Which type of bandage or binder should the nurse use for the client who requires alternating pressure to the legs?
   a. All-cotton elastic roller bandage
   b. Intermittent sequential compression device
   c. Antiembolism stockings
   d. Montgomery strap
7. A 15-year-old client is brought to the hospital with a sprained ankle. Which of the following binders should the attending nurse choose?
   a. Montgomery strap
   b. Abdominal binder
   c. 3M Micropore tape
   d. T-binder
8. An elastic bandage is applied to a client's lower limb. How does this bandage help to increase return circulation to the heart?
   a. It causes contraction of calf muscles.
   b. It puts gentle pressure on the tissue.
   c. It constricts the blood vessels.
   d. It increases the local temperature.

**9.** A nurse is caring for a client with a Montgomery strap. What is the purpose of the Montgomery strap?

**a.** To support a specific body part and to hold a dressing in place.

**b.** To enable frequent dressing changes and to not have to remove the tape from the client's skin with each change.

**c.** To support a dressing and to exert pressure over a bleeding point.

**d.** To ensure adequate return circulation to the heart and to prevent blood clots.

**10.** A client has a broken right arm after falling off a skateboard. What signs and symptoms would indicate that the client has a circulatory disturbance? (Select all that apply.)

**a.** Pain with movement of fingers

**b.** Pale, white fingers

**c.** Complaints of numbness and tingling in hand

**d.** No edema or swelling in hand

**e.** Temperature of hand is the same as general temperature of client's body

CHAPTER 54

# Heat and Cold Applications

## SECTION I: TESTING WHAT YOU KNOW

**Activity A** ***Match the equipment used for heat therapies in Column A with their descriptions in Column B.***

| Column A | Column B |
|---|---|
| ____ 1. Aquathermia pad | a. A bed cradle that has a lamp, light bulb, or special heater inside it |
| ____ 2. Heat cradle | b. Covered network of wires that emits heat when electricity passes through it |
| ____ 3. Hypothermia blanket | c. Waterproof pad through which flows temperature-controlled distilled water |
| ____ 4. Electric heating pad | d. A plastic mattress pad through which very cold water flows continuously |

**Activity B** ***Mark each statement as either "T" (True) or "F" (False). Correct any false statements.***

1. T F Cold applications help to reduce edema.
2. T F Alcohol is used in tepid sponge baths because it cools quickly.
3. T F Cold application is more effective than heat for sprains or other soft tissue injuries.
4. T F Moist heat applications warm the skin more quickly than do dry heat applications.
5. T F Skin maceration may develop when dry heat is applied directly to the skin for long periods.

**Activity C** ***Fill in the blanks.***

1. Application of ____________ to an abscess or infected appendix may cause rupture of the area.
2. A warm soak may be combined with a whirlpool bath, usually in the ____________ therapy department.
3. Cold causes ____________ which decreases the amount of blood flow to an area, slowing the body's metabolism and its demand for oxygen.
4. A child who requires a cold ____________ treatment may be placed in a croupette.
5. ____________ from heat application over a large area of the body may cause hypotension.

**Activity D** *Consider the following figure.*

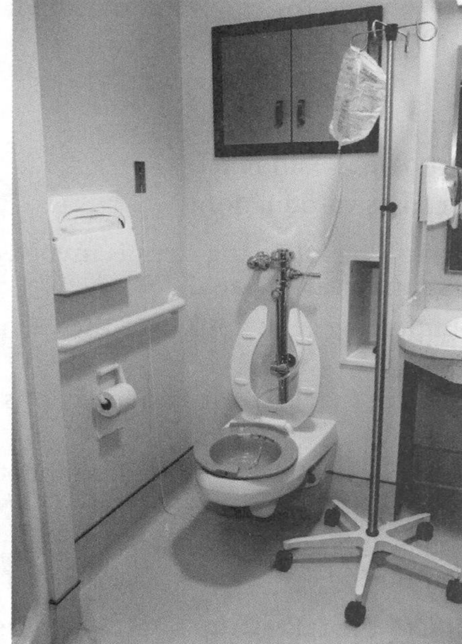

1. Identify the equipment shown in the figure.

______________________________

______________________________

2. Explain how the equipment works.

______________________________

______________________________

3. What is the purpose of the equipment?

______________________________

______________________________

**Activity E** ***The steps used to administer a tub soak to an arm with a wound are given below in random order. Write the correct sequence in the boxes provided.***

1. Apply a sterile dressing to the wound.
2. Wear gloves and remove the dressing from the client's wound.
3. Cover the client with a protective sheet, and prepare the water in the tub (37.8° to 40.6°C).
4. Gradually lower the client's arm into the water, resting the elbow on the padded edge of the tub.
5. Remove the client's arm from the bath after 15 to 20 min or as ordered, and dry the client's skin.
6. Test the water's temperature frequently; add hot water carefully as needed, and stir the water.

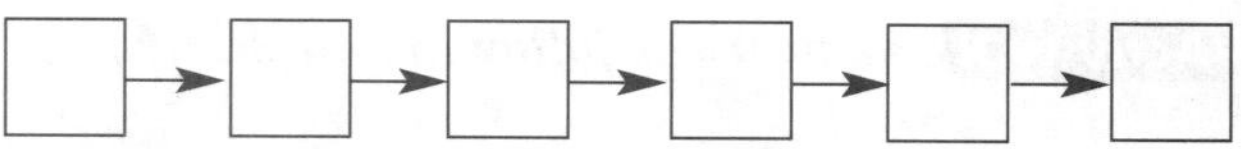

**Activity F** ***Briefly answer the following questions.***

1. What is the purpose of infrared treatment?

______________________________

______________________________

2. How is ultraviolet ray treatment helpful?

______________________________

______________________________

3. For what type of clients is the use of electric heating pads unsafe?

______________________________

______________________________

4. What are refreezable ice packs?

______________________________

______________________________

## SECTION II: APPLYING WHAT YOU KNOW

**Activity G** ***Answer the following questions, which involve the nurse's role in applying heat or cold.***

Heat or cold applications are beneficial for certain health conditions. A nurse should administer these therapies safely and effectively to prevent complications that can occur due to extreme heat or cold.

1. Cold humidity has been ordered for a client with a tracheostomy.
   a. How should the nurse provide humidified oxygen to this client?
   b. Why should oxygen administered to all clients with breathing difficulties be humidified?
2. A nurse is caring for a client with a very high temperature. The client has been prescribed the use of a hypothermia blanket. What precautions should the nurse take when caring for this client?

## SECTION III: GETTING READY FOR NCLEX

**Activity H** *Answer the following questions.*

1. Which of the following steps should the nurse follow for disassembling the aquathermia pad?
   a. Unplug the unit and discard the aquathermia pad.
   b. Empty the water out of the pump and unplug unit.
   c. Disconnect the tubes, empty the water, and unplug the unit.
   d. Return the pump unit and pad to the equipment department.
2. A nurse is educating a client who has been asked to take moist heat applications at home. Which of the following conditions may occur if there is prolonged exposure to moisture?
   a. Vasoconstriction
   b. Numbness
   c. Skin maceration
   d. Slow circulation
3. Which of the following should the nurse do when applying warm compresses to a client's eyes?
   a. Use warm water for the compress.
   b. Send reusable equipment for sterilization.
   c. Wash the compress if the eye is draining.
   d. Use the same equipment for both eyes.
4. A nurse is assigned to assist a client with a foot soak. Which of the following should the nurse know are reasons for giving a warm soak? (Select all that apply.)
   a. It loosens scabs and crusts.
   b. It cleans draining wounds.
   c. It controls hemorrhage.
   d. It applies medications.
   e. It blocks pain receptors.
5. Which of the following should the nurse ensure when assisting the client with a sitz bath?
   a. Set the temperature to 45° Celsius.
   b. Set the reservoir level with the basin.
   c. Ask client to wear only a hospital gown.
   d. Provide a stool to support the legs.
6. A client has been asked to apply an ice pack after a tooth extraction. Which of the following should the nurse tell the client is the benefit of an ice pack?
   a. It increases blood flow.
   b. It increases drainage.
   c. It provides pain relief.
   d. It causes vasodilation.
7. Which of the following steps is involved in ultrasound heat therapy?
   a. Lubricating gel is applied to the client's skin.
   b. Rays are used to treat skin infections and wounds.
   c. A special heater is mounted on the inside of a bed cradle.
   d. The heat lamp is regulated to prevent injury during exposure.
8. Which of the following should the nurse consider when providing a tepid sponge bath to a client?
   a. Set the temperature of the water between 20° and 25°C.
   b. Place dry, warm cloths on the client's axillae and groin.
   c. Stop sponging as the client's temperature approaches normal.
   d. Sponge each limb and the back for at least 10 minutes.
9. A nurse is required to apply ice bags with capsules for a client with a muscle injury. Which of the following should the nurse consider during the treatment?
   a. Monitor the client's temperature continuously.
   b. Observe the client for shivering or chilling.
   c. Know that ice bags take longer to cool.
   d. Ask client to report sensations of burning pain.
10. In which of the following conditions does the nurse know that a sitz bath is contraindicated?
    a. After active bleeding
    b. After rectal surgery
    c. After childbirth
    d. After perineal surgery

CHAPTER 55

# Client Comfort and Pain Management

## SECTION I: TESTING WHAT YOU KNOW

**Activity A** *Match the types of pain in Column A with their descriptions in Column B.*

| Column A | Column B |
|---|---|
| ____ 1. Acute pain | a. Discomfort that continues for 6 months or longer, often interfering with a person's normal functioning |
| ____ 2. Cancer pain | b. Discomfort that usually is intermittent and typically lasts for 6 months or less |
| ____ 3. Chronic pain | c. Discomfort that results from some sort of malignancy |

**Activity B** *Match the phases of nociception in Column A with their descriptions in Column B.*

| Column A | Column B |
|---|---|
| ____ 1. Transduction | a. The impulses travel from their original site to the brain. |
| ____ 2. Transmission | b. The body activates needed inhibitory responses to the effects of pain. |
| ____ 3. Perception | c. The nervous system changes painful stimuli in the nerve endings to impulses. |
| ____ 4. Modulation | d. The brain recognizes, defines, and responds to pain. |

**Activity C** *Mark each statement as either "T" (True) or "F" (False). Correct any false statements.*

1. T F A person with continued chronic pain should be physically inactive to obtain pain relief.
2. T F Lack of or excessive appetite could be a symptom of depression.
3. T F Intake of certain foods, such as caffeine, salt, and sugar, increases endorphin production.
4. T F Pain is to be evaluated each time the other vital signs are measured.
5. T F The Wong Faces Scale was developed primarily for preverbal children, usually those younger than 3 years of age.
6. T F Application of heat and cold is a nonpharmacologic technique that has been proven to relieve pain.

**Activity D** *Fill in the blanks.*

1. ___________ pain originates in one body part but is perceived in another part of the body.
2. ___________ nursing is often involved with the management of cancer pain.
3. The feeling of suffering or agony caused by stimulation of specialized nerve endings is called ___________.
4. Individuals with the ___________ type of pain typically report constant burning, tingling sensations, and/or shooting pain.

5. The central nervous system produces __________ a naturally occurring substance that relieves pain.

**Activity E** *Consider the following figures.*

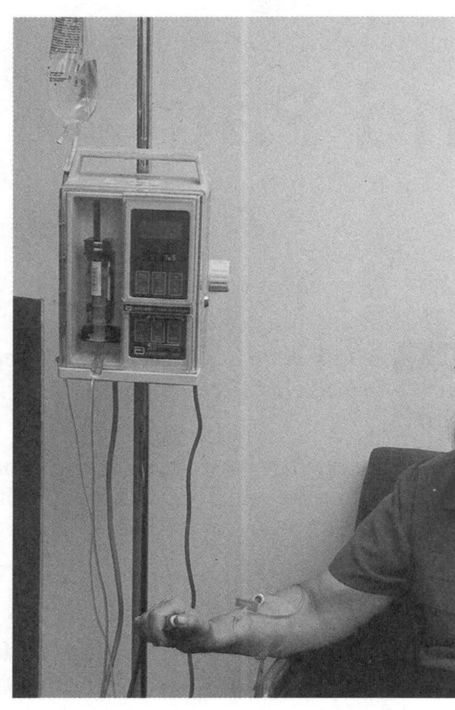

1. Identify the equipment in the figure.

2. How is the equipment useful to a client?

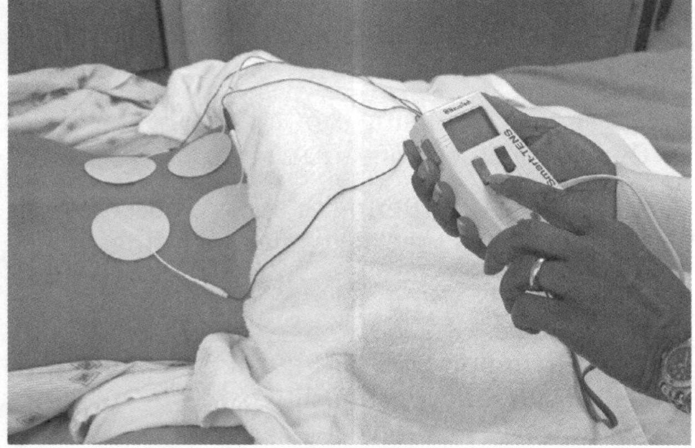

3. Identify the equipment in the figure.

4. What is the purpose of the equipment?

**Activity F** *Briefly answer the following questions.*

1. What is nociception?

2. What are the common causes of acute pain?

3. What is meant by a person's pain threshold?

4. What does a person's pain tolerance denote?

## SECTION II: APPLYING WHAT YOU KNOW

**Activity G** *Answer the following questions, which involve the nurse's role in pain management.*

Providing pain relief and comfort through administration of medication and various other interventions is an important nursing responsibility and challenge.

1. A nurse is caring for a client with chronic pain. The nurse suggests that the client and family should join a support group.
   a. How can joining a support group help the client?
   b. How do family members benefit from participation in a support group?

2. A nurse is caring for a client with cancer. The physician has suggested the use of guided imagery for the client.
   a. What should the nurse tell the client about guided imagery?
   b. How does the guided imagery technique help the client in pain management?

## SECTION III: GETTING READY FOR NCLEX

**Activity H** *Answer the following questions.*

1. Which of the following should the nurse suggest to a client to manage stress? (Select all that apply.)
   a. Well-balanced diet
   b. Adequate fluids
   c. Recreation
   d. Acupuncture
   e. Hypnosis
2. A client with chronic pain has been ordered a regimen of exercise. Which of the following should the nurse tell the client regarding exercise?
   a. Maintain the same level of activity every day.
   b. Exercise to the point of severe pain.
   c. Push just beyond the tolerance level.
   d. Repeat the same set of exercises each day.
3. A nurse is caring for a client with a terminal illness. Which of the following is a physical comfort measure that the nurse can provide the client?
   a. Assist the client in intense exercise.
   b. Provide a gentle massage.
   c. Provide restful music.
   d. Arrange for a semilighted room.
4. A client with chronic pain has been prescribed medication. Which of the following instructions should the nurse give the client regarding the use of medication?
   a. Take medication on a regular schedule.
   b. Take medication if pain crosses the tolerance level.
   c. Take medication before the pain starts.
   d. Reduce the intake of medication gradually.
5. A client with chronic pain is being cared for by a nurse at the healthcare facility. Which of the following should the nurse identify as symptoms of depression associated with the chronic pain? (Select all that apply.)
   a. Sleeping for long hours
   b. Withdrawing from social activities
   c. Displaying lack of interest in surroundings
   d. Expressing feelings of pain and fear
   e. Feeling extremely exhausted
6. A nurse is gathering data regarding the character of pain experienced by the client. Which of the following questions helps the nurse to determine the duration of the pain?
   a. "Where does the pain start?"
   b. "Is the pain internal or external?"
   c. "Is the pain always in the same place?"
   d. "Is the pain constant, occasional, or recurring?"
7. A client who is being cared for by a nurse at the healthcare facility is ordered to receive an adjuvant drug. Which of the following is a function of adjuvant drugs?
   a. They treat moderate to severe pain.
   b. They assist in muscle relaxation.
   c. They treat mild to moderate pain.
   d. They increase temperature and circulation.
8. The physician has recommended the use of deep relaxation techniques for a client with long-term intractable pain. When educating the client on the recommended technique, the nurse identifies which of the following as a benefit of deep relaxation technique that will help manage the client's pain?
   a. It helps the client develop concentration.
   b. It helps the client express feelings about pain.
   c. It helps the client loosen up taut muscles.
   d. It helps the client visualize destruction of pain.

9. A nurse is caring for a client who is in pain. Which of the following are cognitive–behavioral techniques to help in pain management? (Select all that apply.)
   a. Herbal remedies
   b. Games and television
   c. Deep relaxation techniques
   d. Physical activity and recreation
   e. Essences of flowers

10. A client who is to undergo surgery for lower back pain is stressed out and complains of lack of sleep. Which of the following should the nurse tell the client with reference to relaxation and sleep?
   a. Take naps during the day.
   b. Exercise until pain is severe.
   c. Stay in bed for a long time.
   d. Exercise alone at own pace.

CHAPTER 56

# Preoperative and Postoperative Care

## SECTION I: TESTING WHAT YOU KNOW

**Activity A** *Match the postoperative complications in Column A with their nursing interventions in Column B.*

| Column A | Column B |
|---|---|
| ____ 1. Urinary retention | a. Assist in splinting the incision |
| ____ 2. Atelectasis | b. Place client's hand in warm water |
| ____ 3. Postoperative pneumonia | c. Move the client from side to side |
| ____ 4. Abdominal distention | d. Administer antibiotic medications as ordered |

**Activity B** *Match the types of anesthesia procedures in Column A with their indications in Column B.*

| Column A | Column B |
|---|---|
| ____ 1. General | a. Chronic back pain |
| ____ 2. Local infiltration | b. Surgeries of lower extremities |
| ____ 3. Spinal | c. Hip joint replacement surgery |
| ____ 4. Conduction block | d. Third molar extractions |

**Activity C** *Mark each statement as either "T" (True) or "F" (False). Correct any false statements.*

1. T F Angioplasty after a heart attack is a required or nonelective choice of surgery.
2. T F During the moderate sedation stage of anesthesia, the client responds to pain and is able to follow some commands.
3. T F Specific medications that affect blood coagulation are discontinued at least 7 days before surgery to reduce the risk of excessive bleeding.
4. T F The client should be in a lying position when using an incentive spirometer.
5. T F Occult bleeding after surgery is mainly revealed through signs of shock.

**Activity D** *Fill in the blanks.*

1. ____________ is a postoperative respiratory complication that develops due to the reluctance of the client to cough or breathe deeply because of pain over the incision area.
2. ____________ care is the term used to describe the nursing care in the operating room, post-anesthesia recovery unit, or post-anesthesia care unit.
3. ____________ anesthesia is defined as the degree of anesthesia at which an operation can safely be performed and be tolerated by the client.

4. In clients with abdominal distention due to gas, nutrition begins with a/an ___________ diet to avoid further complications.

5. ___________ is the splitting open or separation of the surgical incision.

**Activity E** *Consider the following figures.*

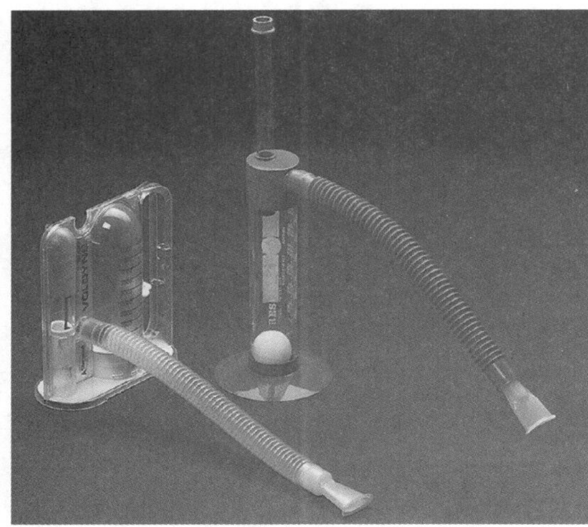

1. Identify the equipment in the figure.

_______________________________________________

_______________________________________________

2. What is the equipment used for?

_______________________________________________

_______________________________________________

3. Describe the two varieties and explain how they work.

_______________________________________________

_______________________________________________

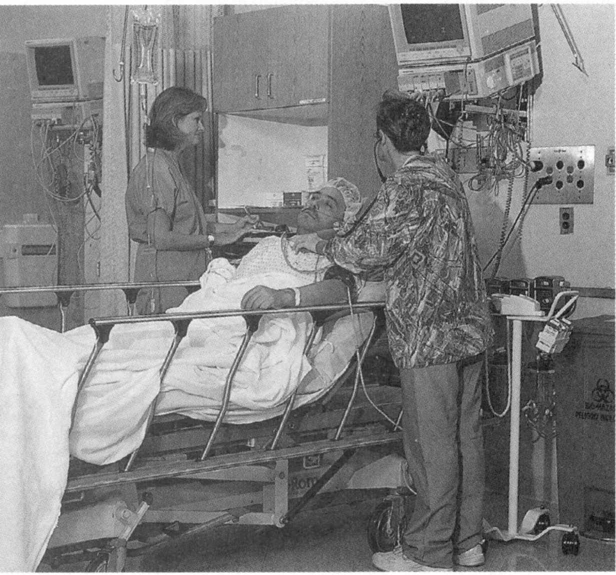

4. Identify the unit of the healthcare facility shown in the figure.

_______________________________________________

_______________________________________________

5. Describe the unit.

_______________________________________________

_______________________________________________

**Activity F** ***The steps that occur during the transport of a client from the post-anesthesia unit to the recovery room are given below in random order. Write the correct sequence in the boxes provided.***

1. Notify the client's family that the client is back in the recovery room.
2. Check the client's vital signs and compare them with previous recordings for any significant discrepancies.
3. Place the bed in its highest position, and keep the head of the bed flat.
4. Arrange for all necessary equipment before the client arrives in the recovery room.

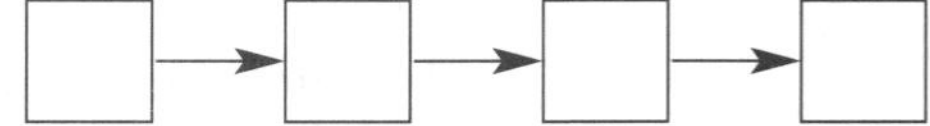

**Activity G** ***Briefly answer the following questions.***

1. How is postoperative hypovolemic shock managed?

______________________________

______________________________

2. Who is a circulating nurse?

______________________________

______________________________

3. What are the advantages of using staples to close a surgical incision?

______________________________

______________________________

4. How are postoperative infections managed?

______________________________

______________________________

5. What are the symptoms and complications of embolism?

______________________________

______________________________

6. What are the signs of a pulmonary embolism?

______________________________

______________________________

## SECTION II: APPLYING WHAT YOU KNOW

**Activity H** ***Answer the following questions, which involve the nurse's role in preoperative and postoperative care.***

A nurse's role in managing preoperative and postoperative care involves assisting the clients by providing necessary instructions and support.

1. A 60-year-old client has a tumor in the intestine. He is admitted at a healthcare facility for surgical removal of the tumor under general anesthesia. The client shows anxiety and fear about the procedure.
   a. What nursing evaluations should the nurse consider before the surgery?
   b. What preoperative instructions must the nurse provide the client to alleviate his fears and anxiety?
2. A 15-year-old client is rushed to a healthcare facility after complaints of severe abdominal pain. On further examination, the client is diagnosed with appendicitis that requires emergency surgery.
   a. What are the various considerations to be noted in the preoperative checklist?
   b. What nursing considerations should be employed when caring for a client who is receiving anesthesia?

## SECTION III: GETTING READY FOR NCLEX

**Activity I** ***Answer the following questions.***

1. An 18-year-old client wants to have minor plastic surgery done on her nose. Which of the following can make the client feel more comfortable while in the operating room?
   a. The procedure is performed under general anesthesia.
   b. The anesthesiologist or nurse anesthetist visits the client before surgery.
   c. The client's vitals are recorded before the surgery is started.
   d. Breathing exercises are taught to the client before the surgery.
2. A nurse is preparing a client for gastric bypass surgery under general anesthesia. The client has been prescribed certain presedation medications before being moved to the operation room. Which of the following must the nurse ensure before giving any presedation medications to the client?
   a. The client has signed the consent to surgery.
   b. The client has had a healthy diet.
   c. The oxygen saturation has been checked.
   d. The client has provided transportation details.
3. An 18-year-old client needs periodontal flap surgery due to a gum disorder. Which of the following type of anesthesia will be used during the surgery?
   a. General anesthesia
   b. Local anesthesia
   c. Spinal anesthesia
   d. Conduction block

4. A client who underwent an abdominal surgery under general anesthesia is transported from the post-anesthesia unit to the recovery unit in a semiconscious state. What nursing procedure must the attending nurse perform after receiving the client from the post-anesthesia care unit?
   a. Position the client with legs slightly raised.
   b. Provide complete privacy to the client and family members.
   c. Check the client's temperature at least once every 8 hours.
   d. Reinforce the client's dressing without changing it.

5. A client is undergoing thoracic surgery under general anesthesia. Which of the following personnel is responsible for assisting the surgeon with suturing the incision?
   a. Circulating nurse
   b. Registered nurse first assistant
   c. Sterile assistant
   d. Vocational nurse

6. A client who underwent surgery 2 days earlier arrives at the healthcare facility with complaints of continuous fever and severe pain over the incision area, along with redness and swelling around it. On further examination, the client's white blood cell count is high. Which of the following symptoms does the client's white blood cell count represent?
   a. Infection
   b. Dehiscence
   c. Evisceration
   d. Embolism

7. After an extensive surgical procedure under general anesthesia, a client complains of severe pain in the calves of her legs. On further examination, the client is diagnosed with thrombophlebitis. Which of the following should the nurse do when caring for such a client?
   a. Raise the head end of the client's bed.
   b. Assist the client in exercising the leg.
   c. Apply cold compression and gently rub the area.
   d. Check for progress with a positive Homans' sign.

8. An elderly client is being prepared to undergo abdominal surgery under general anesthesia. Which of the following nursing measures must the nurse perform when providing preoperative nursing care to the client?
   a. Ensure that the client has recently eaten a nutritious meal.
   b. Ensure that the client has used a cathartic solution before the surgical procedure.
   c. Check the preoperative checklist as soon as the client is moved to the operating room.
   d. Request that family members converse with the client after sedative administration.

9. A 14-year-old client is admitted to the healthcare facility to undergo an appendicectomy. Which of the following should the nurse ensure when assisting in the preoperative nursing care of the client?
   a. Ensure that the client is able to participate in his or her own care as much as possible.
   b. Ensure that needs for water, oxygen, sleep, food, and elimination are met, in that order.
   c. Ensure that the client understands the procedure but does not necessarily verbalize it.
   d. Ensure that the client has had adequate food and fluids before the surgery.

10. A 45-year-old client who is about to undergo a surgical procedure is administered general anesthesia. The client gradually exhibits lack of reflexes, weak and thready pulse, flaccid respiration, lowered blood pressure, and widely dilated pupils. Which of the following stages of general anesthesia should the nurse document this as?
    a. Analgesia and amnesia stage
    b. Dreams and excitement stage
    c. Surgical anesthesia stage
    d. Toxic or danger stage

CHAPTER 57

# Surgical Asepsis

## SECTION I: TESTING WHAT YOU KNOW

**Activity A** *Match the terms related to asepsis in Column A with their descriptions given in Column B.*

| Column A | Column B |
|---|---|
| ____ 1. Dirty | a. Free of many of the most harmful microorganisms |
| ____ 2. Clean | b. Not cleaned or sterilized for removal of microorganisms |
| ____ 3. Sterile | c. Free of all microorganisms and spores |

**Activity B** *Match the objects or surfaces in Column A with the agents used to disinfect or sterilize them in Column B.*

| Column A | Column B |
|---|---|
| ____ 1. Scalpels | a. Povidone-iodine scrub |
| ____ 2. Heart-lung machine | b. Dry heat |
| ____ 3. Countertops | c. Moist heat under pressure |
| ____ 4. Skin | d. Chlorine bleach |

**Activity C** *Mark each statement as either "T" (True) or "F" (False). Correct any false statements.*

1. T F The client should always lie on the left side for side-lying position catheterization.
2. T F After catheterization, the drainage bag must always be higher than the client's bladder.
3. T F A retention catheter can be cut for removal.
4. T F A contaminated object can be clean or dirty.
5. T F Self-catheterization may be performed on a client with chronic neurologic bladder atony.

**Activity D** *Fill in the blanks.*

1. In order to avoid pulling and discomfort, urinary catheter tubing is secured by hypoallergenic tape to a female client's ____________.
2. The ____________ heat used in an autoclave may dull the sharp cutting edges of scalpels and suture removal scissors.
3. The catheter balloon is ____________ when removing a retention catheter.
4. Before catheterization of a male client, the head of the ____________ is cleansed in a circular motion from the meatus outward.
5. A surgical mask acts as a barrier to prevent the transmission of pathogens from the ____________ and the mouth.

**Activity E** *Consider the following figures.*

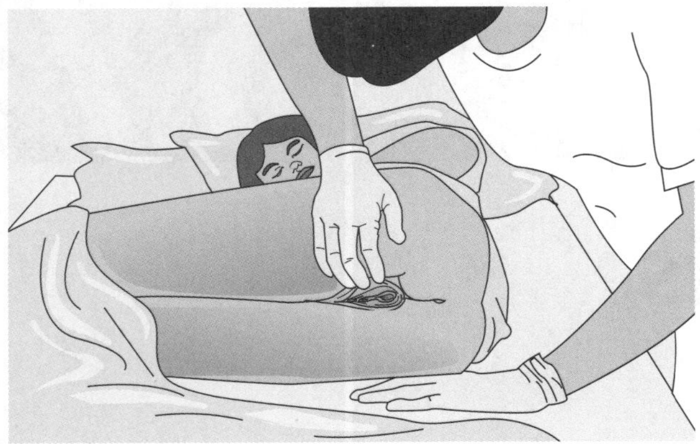

1. Identify the procedure shown in the figure.

_______________________________________

_______________________________________

2. How is this procedure done?

_______________________________________

_______________________________________

3. List the advantages of this procedure.

_______________________________________

_______________________________________

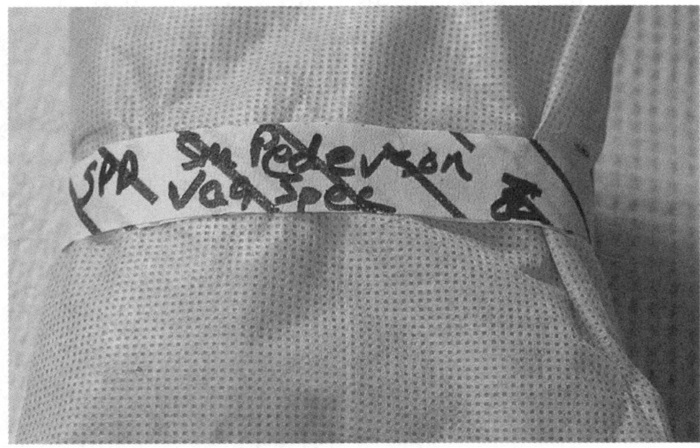


4. Identify the object in the figure.

_______________________________________

_______________________________________

5. What is sterilization?

_______________________________________

_______________________________________

6. How does a nurse identify sterilized items after the sterilization procedure?

_______________________________________

_______________________________________

**Activity F** ***The primary goal of wearing gloves is to keep the nurse's hands and arms free from any contamination. The steps for putting on sterile gloves are given below in random order. Write the correct sequence in the boxes provided.***

1. Grasp the glove for the dominant hand using the nondominant hand, touching only the inside upper surface of the glove's cuff.
2. Open the outer package of the sterile gloves on a clean, dry, flat surface.
3. Insert the fingers of the sterile gloved hand between the cuff and the glove to put on the second glove.
4. Insert the dominant hand into the glove, placing the thumb and fingers in the appropriate openings.

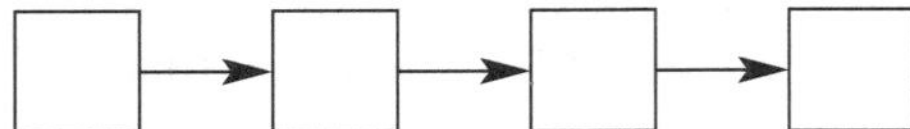

**Activity G** *Briefly answer the following.*

1. What is an autoclave?

_______________________________________

_______________________________________

2. What is the advantage of using chemical disinfectants?

_______________________________________

_______________________________________

3. What is the difference between medical asepsis and surgical asepsis?

_______________________________________

_______________________________________

4. What is the procedure for removing sterile gloves?

_______________________________________

_______________________________________

5. What is the purpose of wearing eye protection in operating rooms?

_______________________________________

_______________________________________

## SECTION II: APPLYING WHAT YOU KNOW

**Activity H** *Answer the following questions, which involve the nurse's role in catheterization.*

Catheterizing male and female clients, monitoring their bladder and kidney function, and assisting clients who have problems with these functions are fundamental nursing responsibilities.

1. A nurse caring for a 60-year-old male client with chronic neurologic bladder atony is required to insert a retention catheter as per physician's order.
   a. What information should the nurse provide to the client before beginning the procedure?
   b. What priority assessment should the nurse make before catheterization? Why is this important?
2. A 70-year-old male client is unable to pass urine due to urinary obstruction caused by a hypertrophied prostate gland. A nurse is required to catheterize the client according to the healthcare provider's order.
   a. What nursing care is given after catheterization of the client?
   b. What information should a nurse give the client after catheterization?

## SECTION III: GETTING READY FOR NCLEX

**Activity I** *Answer the following questions.*

1. A nurse is preparing to inject insulin into a diabetic client. Which of the following techniques is appropriate for the process?
   a. Clean technique
   b. Disinfection
   c. Medical asepsis
   d. Surgical asepsis
2. A nurse is required to care for a newborn. Which of the following should be used to disinfect the nurse's hands before she handles the baby?
   a. Chlorine bleach
   b. Hexachlorophene
   c. Ethylene oxide
   d. Distilled water
3. A 35-year-old female client is catheterized after a hysterectomy, and the urine flow seems undiminished after withdrawal of a normal quantity of urine. What immediate action should the nurse take?
   a. Check for regularity of the client's pulse rate.
   b. Check the position of the catheter.
   c. Remove the catheter and inform the physician.
   d. Remove and reinsert the catheter properly.
4. A nurse has to clean the inanimate objects in the blood collection room. Which of the following should the nurse use for the mechanical cleansing of inanimate objects?
   a. Antiseptic cleanser
   b. Hexachlorophene
   c. Betadine
   d. Ethylene oxide
5. A nurse is preparing to assist the healthcare provider in performing a lumbar puncture, which is a sterile procedure. The nurse has put on sterile gloves and a sterile gown. Where on the surgical gown can the nurse safely place his gloved hands while waiting for the healthcare provider to be ready?
   a. Between the neck and the nipples
   b. Between the nipples and the waist
   c. Between the waist and the hips
   d. Between hips and the knees
6. In the operating room, a nurse touches the strings of the sterile gown worn by another nurse with a sterile gloved hand. What is the next step to be taken by the nurse?
   a. Soak the gloved hand in warm saline water.
   b. Wash the gloved hands with a povidone-iodine scrub.
   c. Discard the gloves and use a fresh pair.
   d. Continue wearing the gloves, because the gown was sterile.

7. A 30-year-old male client is catheterized after major abdominal surgery. For which of the following reasons is the drainage bag placed in a position lower than that of the client's urinary bladder after catheterization?
   a. For proper drainage of urine
   b. For general comfort of the client
   c. For proper positioning of the drainage tube
   d. For preventing any type of infection

8. A nurse is preparing to assist the surgeon in a major operation. What are the guidelines taken into consideration to maintain sterility? (Select all that apply.)
   a. Only clean equipment should be used for any surgical procedure.
   b. Reaching over a sterile field should be avoided, unless sterile clothing is worn.
   c. The mask must be changed for a new sterile mask if it becomes wet.
   d. Sterile packages should be placed on a clean working area.
   e. When the nurse is pouring a sterile solution, the inside of the bottle should not be touched.

9. Given below are a few steps for removal of a retention catheter. What is the correct order for the nurse to remove the retention catheter?
   a. Gently and slowly pull the catheter out.
   b. Deflate the balloon by completely aspirating all the fluid.
   c. Ask the client to inhale and exhale slowly and deeply.
   d. Adjust bed to a comfortable height.

10. A 30-year-old client has received multiple wounds on her arm and face in a motor vehicle accident. The nurse uses Betadine to clean the wounds. What term best describes this process?
    a. Sterilization
    b. Disinfection
    c. Mechanical cleansing
    d. Surgical asepsis

CHAPTER 58

# Special Skin and Wound Care

## SECTION I: TESTING WHAT YOU KNOW

**Activity A** ***Match the types of wounds in Column A with their descriptions in Column B.***

| Column A | Column B |
|---|---|
| ____ 1. Abrasion | a. A wound with clean edges |
| ____ 2. Puncture | b. A wound with torn, ragged edges |
| ____ 3. Laceration | c. Rubbing off of the skin's surface |
| ____ 4. Surgical incision | d. A deep stab wound |

**Activity B** ***Match the common causes of wounds in Column A with their descriptions in Column B.***

| Column A | Column B |
|---|---|
| ____ 1. Pressure | a. Superficial abrasion as a result of the skin rubbing another surface |
| ____ 2. Shear | b. Unintentional mechanical removal of the epidermis |
| ____ 3. Friction | c. Interaction of gravity and friction against the surface of the skin |
| ____ 4. Stripping | d. External force that occludes capillaries, resulting in tissue anoxia and tissue death |

**Activity C** ***Mark each statement as either "T" (True) or "F" (False). Correct any false statements.***

1. T F Retention sutures are removed by the nurse.
2. T F Debridement is the removal of dead or infected tissue.
3. T F Medication should be applied to the skin's edges, but not to the wound itself.
4. T F Dry skin is more subject to breakdown than well-hydrated skin.
5. T F Deep open wounds heal from the outside inward.

**Activity D** ***Fill in the blanks.***

1. The Braden scale rating considers the following factors: ____________ perception, moisture, activity, mobility, nutrition, and friction/shear.
2. Drainage containing a great deal of protein and cellular debris is called ____________.
3. The ____________-assisted closure machine applies controlled localized negative pressure to a wound site.
4. Drainage and wound debris slow the ____________ process.
5. A surgical incision is a/an ____________ wound.

**Activity E** *Consider the following figure.*

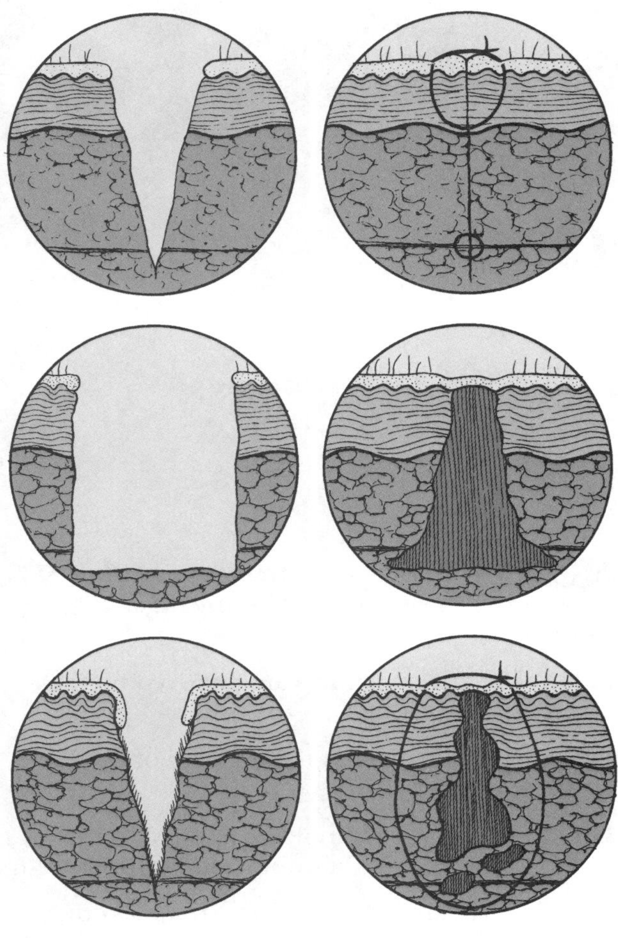

1. Identify what is shown in the figure.

2. Describe what is meant by primary intention healing.

3. List three methods of wound healing.

**Activity F** ***The purpose of wound dressing is to protect wounds from contamination, to collect exudate, and to protect against any damage during healing. The steps that need to be taken during the changing of a dry sterile dressing are given below in random order. Write the correct sequence in the boxes provided.***

1. Cleanse the wound and the area around the wound, and then dry the wound.
2. Put on clean gloves and remove the used dressing using sterile saline.
3. Apply medications as ordered and a dry sterile dressing over the wound area.
4. Observe the condition of the wound, drainage, and surrounding tissues.

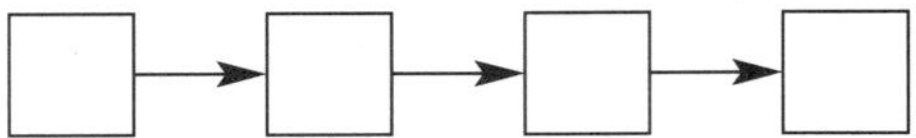

**Activity G** *Briefly answer the following questions.*

1. What is drainage? How does a nurse manage drainage?

2. How are perianal wounds due to urinary or fecal incontinence prevented?

3. When is wound packing done?

4. What is a vacuum-assisted closure machine?

5. What is a Norton scale?

## SECTION II: APPLYING WHAT YOU KNOW

**Activity H** *Answer the following questions, which involve the nurse's role in the management of wound care.*

A nurse's role in wound care involves inspecting the client's skin for any signs of pressure or skin breakdown and, if it occurs, reporting it and treating it as ordered. The nurse also observes and documents descriptions of wounds.

1. A nurse is assessing the infected surgical incision of a client who has undergone a herniotomy at the healthcare facility.
   a. What should be included in the description of the wound?
   b. What procedure should the nurse perform for this client before dressing the wound?
   c. What dressing should the nurse apply for this client?
2. A client has come to the healthcare facility for suture removal.
   a. When are sutures usually removed?
   b. What should the nurse use to remove sutures?
   c. What is the procedure for suture removal?

## SECTION III: GETTING READY FOR NCLEX

**Activity I** *Answer the following questions.*

1. A client admitted to a healthcare facility develops a pressure ulcer in his gluteal region. Which of the following nursing measures would have prevented the occurrence of this pressure ulcer?
   a. Application of antifungal powder
   b. Application of transparent dressing
   c. Frequent change of position
   d. Application of a wet cloth
2. A large, infected wound of a client is temporarily kept open till debridement is performed. Wound healing will most likely occur through which of the following?
   a. Third-intention healing
   b. Cutaneous stimulation
   c. Thermal application
   d. First-intention healing
3. A nurse is required to apply a dressing to the incision area, healing by primary intention, of a client who has undergone an appendectomy. Which of the following dressings should the nurse apply to this client?
   a. Wet-to-dry dressing
   b. Dry sterile dressing
   c. Wet-to-wet dressing
   d. Hydrocolloid dressing
4. A nurse observes a reddened area that does not return to a normal hue after pressure is removed on the lower back of a postoperative client. Which of the following actions should the nurse take?
   a. Massage that area
   b. Decrease dietary protein
   c. Apply porous tape
   d. Report to the physician
5. A client's abdominal wound is draining clear, thin, and watery discharge. Which of the following terms will the nurse use to describe the drainage?
   a. Serous
   b. Sanguineous
   c. Serosanguineous
   d. Purulent
6. A client has developed a painful shallow pressure ulcer. Which of the following stages will the nurse document the ulcer to be in?
   a. Stage 1
   b. Stage 2
   c. Stage 3
   d. Stage 4
7. A 25-year-old client who is paralyzed from below the hips is put on a special mattress to prevent skin breakdown. Which of the following factors contributes to skin breakdown?
   a. Younger age
   b. High calorie intake
   c. Low level of activity
   d. Fluid intake of 2 L/day

8. A client develops discoloration on her left big toe due to arterial insufficiency. Which of the following measures are used to prevent development of a wound in the area of discoloration? (Select all that apply.)
   a. Adequately remoisturize.
   b. Apply Steri-strips.
   c. Elevate feet and legs.
   d. Avoid compression.
   e. Apply powder.

9. A nurse is emptying the drainage container of a client with a closed drainage system. Which of the following are closed drainage systems? (Select all that apply.)
   a. EnzySurge
   b. Jackson-Pratt
   c. Hemovac
   d. Penrose
   e. Davol

10. A nurse needs to handle a closed drainage system. What is the correct order for the steps in working with a closed drainage system?
   a. Check for leaks in the closed drainage system.
   b. Empty the drainage receptacle if it is full.
   c. Measure and record the amount of drainage.
   d. Wear gloves when working with wound drainage.

CHAPTER 59

# End-of-Life Care

## SECTION I: TESTING WHAT YOU KNOW

**Activity A** *Match the stages of dying in Column A with the expressions of clients in Column B.*

| Column A | Column B |
|---|---|
| ____ 1. Denial | a. "I promise to be a better person if only . . ." |
| ____ 2. Anger | b. "I don't care anymore." |
| ____ 3. Bargaining | c. "Why is this happening to me?" |
| ____ 4. Depression | d. "This isn't happening to me!" |

**Activity B** *Match the symptoms of a dying client in Column A with the medications used to treat or prevent them in Column B.*

| Column A | Column B |
|---|---|
| ____ 1. Nausea | a. Docusate |
| ____ 2. Constipation | b. Atropine |
| ____ 3. Pain | c. Metoclopramide |
| ____ 4. Secretions | d. Opioids |

**Activity C** *Mark each statement as either "T" (True) or "F" (False). Correct any false statements.*

1. T F Vision is the last sense to fail in a dying client.
2. T F Milk is usually contraindicated in the final stages of life.
3. T F Biological death is defined as the irreversible cessation of heart and lung function.
4. T F The client's pain may ease or disappear just before death.
5. T F Crying and being sad in front of the client are often discouraged.

**Activity D** *Fill in the blanks.*

1. Irreversible cessation of total brain function is termed brain death or ____________ death.
2. Careful positioning of the dying client is vital to maintain a patient ____________.
3. ____________ care emphasizes nursing care and medical treatments that relieve or reduce symptoms of a disease or illness.
4. ____________ death occurs when both respiration and heartbeat stop.
5. ____________ breathing often occurs if a person experiences acidosis.

**Activity E** *Consider the following figures.*

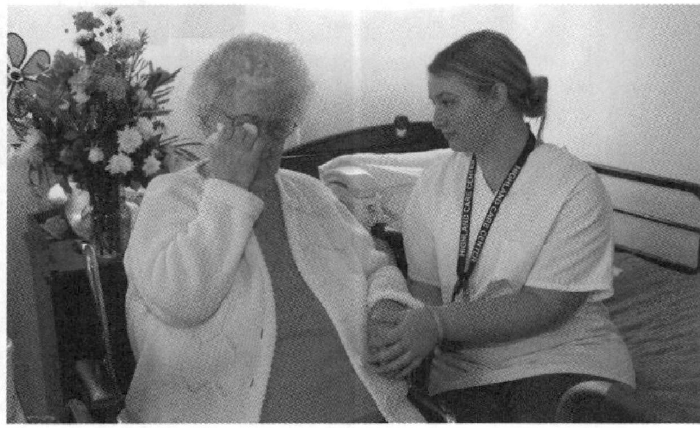

1. Identify what is shown in the figure.

2. What is the importance of performing this procedure?

3. What are the various other needs of the dying client?

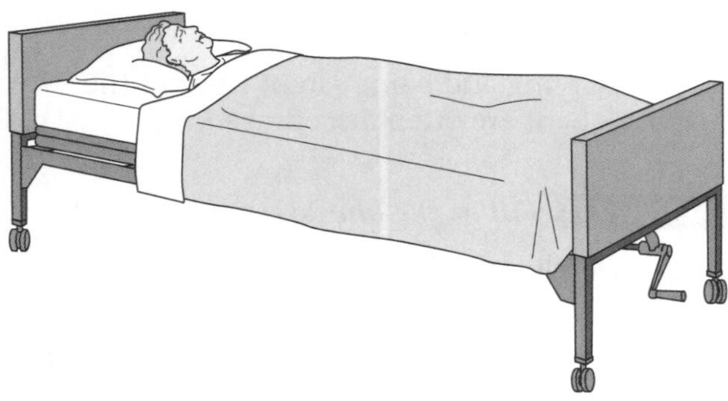

4. Identify the procedure in the figure.

5. What is the need for performing this procedure?

6. How is the procedure done?

**Activity F** ***The nurse needs to recognize the signs of approaching death to provide the required care and also to support the client and the client's family members. The steps that occur during the last stage of life and indicate approaching death are given below in random order. Write the correct sequence in the boxes provided.***

1. The client's sense of hearing is slowly lost.
2. The client experiences sweating.
3. The client's extremities feel colder to the touch.
4. The client's sense of touch is gradually diminished.

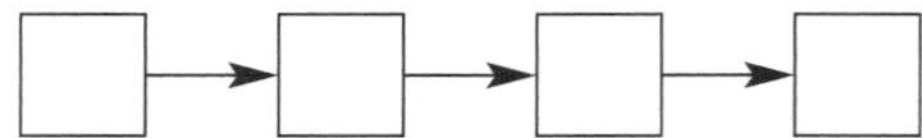

**Activity G** ***Briefly answer the following questions.***

1. What is an advance directive?

2. What is the procedure for a client who chooses to die at home?

3. What is the cause of the loud respiratory sounds in a dying client? How is it managed?

4. What is the legal procedure for organ donation after the death of a client?

5. What is the importance of self-esteem in a dying client? How does the nurse help with regard to self-esteem?

## SECTION II: APPLYING WHAT YOU KNOW

**Activity H** *Answer the following questions, which involve the nurse's role in management of the dying client.*

A nurse's role in managing a dying client involves assisting the client with end-of-life care and support.

1. An 89-year-old client with lung cancer is being cared for at a healthcare facility. The attending nurse notices that the client's condition is gradually deteriorating with each hour.
   a. What are the various signs of approaching death noticed by the nurse in this client?
   b. What are the various signs the nurse could expect to find at the point of death?
2. A 90-year-old client diagnosed with intestinal carcinoma is being cared for at a healthcare facility. The client's relatives are experiencing emotional trauma and difficulty coping with the situation.
   a. What nursing measures must the nurse ensure for implementation of care and support to the dying client and his family members?
   b. What measures must the nurse take to prepare and plan for the client and his relatives to cope with the situation?

## SECTION III: GETTING READY FOR NCLEX

**Activity I** *Answer the following questions.*

1. A 60 year-old-client with human immunodeficiency virus (HIV) infection and a severe respiratory infection dies at the healthcare facility. Which of the following nursing procedures must the nurse perform for postmortem care of the client's body?
   a. Put on a pair of gloves before handling the client's body.
   b. Avoid changing the position of the client's body.
   c. Dispose of all the cards and flowers in the client's room.
   d. Close the client's mouth by placing a rolled towel under the chin.
2. A 95-year-old client diagnosed with intestinal carcinoma is admitted to a healthcare facility with respiratory complications. Which of the following nursing measures would the nurse perform when providing end-of-life care for the client?
   a. Encourage the client to frequently change positions.
   b. Apply a full code on the client's chart.
   c. Encourage the client to always lie on her back.
   d. Convince the client's family members to agree to organ donation.
3. A 55-year-old client was admitted to the healthcare center for cardiac bypass surgery. Before undergoing the surgery, the client had prepared an advance directive expressing his wish to donate his eyes in case of his death. The client died before the surgery. Which of the following should the nurse keep in mind when caring for the client's body?
   a. Harvest the eyes as soon as possible, based on the client's directive.
   b. Avoid placing heat or cold over the client's eyes.
   c. Avoid discussing the organ donation with the client's family members.
   d. Obtain legal permission from the client's next of kin.
4. A nurse is caring for an 80-year-old client who is in the stages of dying. The client asks the nurse, "Why is this happening to me?" Which of the following stages of dying is the client going through?
   a. Denial
   b. Anger
   c. Depression
   d. Detachment
5. An elderly client is admitted to the healthcare facility after a heart attack. The client tells the attending nurse that she wants to designate her eldest son to make the healthcare decisions if she becomes incompetent to do so. Which of the following advance directives is the client requesting?
   a. e-Health Key
   b. Advance living will
   c. Power of attorney
   d. Code blue

6. An 85-year-old client involved in a major motor vehicle accident is brought to the healthcare facility in a comatose state with severe blood loss and multiple injuries to his head. Brain death is diagnosed, and the client is being sustained on a ventilator. There is a disagreement among the family members of the client about the further course of action. Which of the following individuals or organizations must make the decisions in such a situation?
   a. Client's next of kin
   b. Attending nurse
   c. Ethics Committee
   d. Client himself

7. A nurse approaches the family of a 45-year-old male client after his death at the healthcare facility with the option of donating his kidneys to another client in the same facility. Which of the following must the nurse ensure during this procedure?
   a. Request the head nurse to assist the family in decision making.
   b. Talk to the client's relatives in private regarding the organ donation.
   c. Try to convince the family members to agree to the kidney donation.
   d. Place the client's body in an open casket until permission is obtained.

8. A 35-year-old client is rushed to the emergency unit of a healthcare facility after a motor vehicle accident. The client is not responding to sound and is lying still. Which of the following signs must the nurse use to confirm the brain death of the client?
   a. Lack of activity in the electroencephalogram
   b. Cessation of breathing
   c. Complete absence of pulse
   d. Complete unresponsiveness to stimulus

9. A 45-year-old client with human immunodeficiency virus (HIV) infection is admitted to the healthcare facility with severe respiratory infection. The client is in a semiconscious state, and her vital signs are gradually decreasing. Which of the following must the nurse do for the family members of the dying client?
   a. Restrict them from crying in front of the client.
   b. Tell them that the client is too weak to hear what they say.
   c. Explain to them the physical and emotional stages of dying.
   d. Restrict them from offering any fluids to the client.

10. A 45-year-old client who has liver carcinoma with extensive metastases to other parts of the body was admitted to a healthcare facility. The client was put on the ventilator. He was found to be unresponsive and was declared dead after examination. The client is survived by his wife. Which of the following decisions can the client's wife make? (Select all that apply.)
   a. Performance of an autopsy
   b. Donation of organs or tissues
   c. Details of the death certificate
   d. Choice of funeral home
   e. Switching off the ventilator

CHAPTER 60

# Review of Mathematics

## SECTION I: TESTING WHAT YOU KNOW

**Activity A** *Match the units of measurement in Column A with their systems of measurement in Column B.*

| Column A | Column B |
|---|---|
| ____ 1. Grain | a. Household system |
| ____ 2. Pint | b. Metric system |
| ____ 3. Microgram | c. Apothecary system |

**Activity B** *Match the terms related to mathematics in Column A with their descriptions in Column B.*

| Column A | Column B |
|---|---|
| ____ 1. Numerator | a. Refers to the number per hundred |
| ____ 2. Percentage | b. Refers to the total number of parts and is the bottom number in a fraction |
| ____ 3. Denominator | c. Refers to a part of the whole and is the top number in a fraction |
| ____ 4. Ratio | d. Refers to the relationship of one quantity to another |

**Activity C** *Mark each statement as either "T" (True) or "F" (False). Correct any false statements.*

1. T F The formula method is used to convert drug dosages from one system to another.
2. T F A trailing zero should not be used after a decimal point.
3. T F One thousand centimeters make one meter.
4. T F The safe administration of drugs is the vital responsibility of a pharmacist.
5. T F The United States monetary system is based on the metric system of measurement.

**Activity D** *Fill in the blanks.*

1. The denominator is always 100 when converting a percentage to a ____________.
2. A pill splitter can be used to divide tablets that are ____________.
3. The dilation of the cervix during childbirth is always measured in ____________.
4. The apothecary system of measurement is based on the average weight of one ____________ of wheat.
5. A milliliter is approximately equal to a cubic ____________.

**Activity E** ***A nurse can calculate the number of tablets to be administered using the ratio and proportion method when the prescribed dose of the tablet is different from the supplied dose. The steps for calculating the number of tablets to be administered are given below in random order. Write the correct sequence in the boxes provided.***

1. Set up a true proportion using a double colon.
2. Divide the product by the known extreme.
3. Convert the dosages into the same units of measurement.
4. Multiply the known means to get the product.

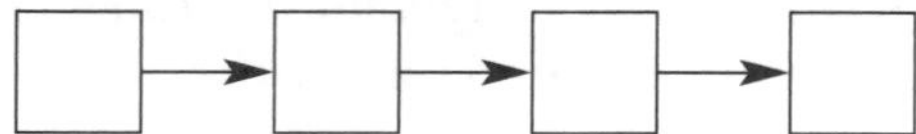

**Activity F** ***Briefly answer the following.***

1. Why is the metric system used exclusively in pharmacology?

   ______________________________

   ______________________________

2. Mention the three general rules applied in the ratio and proportion method.

   ______________________________

   ______________________________

3. What are significant figures?

   ______________________________

   ______________________________

4. How is a fraction converted to a percentage?

   ______________________________

   ______________________________

5. What is a fraction?

   ______________________________

   ______________________________

6. Which is the oldest system of measurement? What is it based on?

   ______________________________

   ______________________________

7. How is weight measured in pounds converted to kilograms?

   ______________________________

   ______________________________

## SECTION II: APPLYING WHAT YOU KNOW

**Activity G** ***Answer the following questions, which involve the nurse's role in drug dosage calculations.***

A nurse's role in safely dispensing and administering drug dosages involves accurate metric conversions. The nurse must be proficient in the use of the metric system to calculate drug dosages.

1. A client is to receive 1 L of dextrose in normal saline intravenously. The client is to be given 20% of this fluid in the first hour. How many milliliters should the nurse administer in the first hour?
   a. Name the method used by the nurse to calculate the dosage.
   b. List the steps involved in this calculation.
   c. Explain the steps involved in converting 20% into a fraction.
2. A client who is 158 cm tall weighs 76 kg on the scale in the healthcare facility. The client wants to know her height in feet and inches and her weight in pounds.
   a. Why are weights converted to pounds and ounces?
   b. List the steps involved in converting centimeters to feet and inches.
   c. List the steps involved in converting kilograms to pounds.
3. A primary healthcare provider prescribes 1¾ mg of Zithromax for a client with an upper respiratory tract infection. The medication is supplied as ½ mg scored tablets.
   a. How many tablets should the nurse give?
   b. How will the nurse divide the tablet?

## SECTION III: GETTING READY FOR NCLEX

**Activity H** *Answer the following questions.*

1. A client has been prescribed Lipitor 20 mg PO once daily. The medication is available as 10 mg/tablet. How many tablets should the nurse administer with each dose?
   a. ½ tablet
   b. 1 tablet
   c. 1½ tablets
   d. 2 tablets
2. What step should the nurse follow in converting larger units to smaller units in the metric system of measurement?
   a. Move the decimal point to the right
   b. Add a zero on the right-hand side
   c. Move the decimal point to the left
   d. Add a zero before the number
3. A nurse is calculating a drug dosage using the formula method. Which of the following criteria would the nurse use?
   a. The dosages should be in a different system and the same units of measurement.
   b. The dosages should be in the same system and the same units of measurement.
   c. The dosages should be in the same system and different units of measurement.
   d. The dosages should be in a different system and different units of measurement.
4. A nurse is calculating the number of tablets to be administered using the ratio and proportion method. How can the nurse avoid errors in dosage calculation?
   a. The nurse should know basic mathematical principles.
   b. The nurse should have an understanding of metric measurements.
   c. The nurse should be familiar with common units of measurement.
   d. All the calculations should be double-checked by another nurse.
5. A client is prescribed 0.25 g of Penicillin VK oral suspension three times a day for 10 days. The suspension is available as 125 mg/5 mL. How much medication will the nurse administer with each dose?
   a. 1 mL
   b. 5 mL
   c. 10 mL
   d. 15 mL
6. A client with pulmonary tuberculosis had a positive PPD test and a positive chest radiograph. Which unit of measurement should the nurse use to measure reactions to PPD tests?
   a. Milligrams
   b. Kilograms
   c. Millimeters
   d. Milliliters
7. A client is prescribed ¾ mg of Klonopin for anxiety and depression, and the medication is supplied as ½ mg tablets. How many tablets would the nurse give with each dose?
   a. 1¼ tablets
   b. 1½ tablets
   c. 1¾ tablets
   d. 2¼ tablets
8. What are the common Greek and Latin prefixes used by the nurse to describe various increments of metric units? (Select all that apply.)
   a. Milli
   b. Minim
   c. Deca
   d. Hecto
   e. Scruple
9. Given below are the nursing steps for multiplying fractions to calculate drug dosage, in random order. Arrange the steps in the correct order.
   a. Reduce the fraction to its lowest terms.
   b. Multiply the numerators.
   c. Write the given problem.
   d. Multiply the denominators.
10. Which of the following measurements will the nurse take in centimeters? (Select all that apply.)
    a. Skin ulcerations
    b. Oral fluid intake
    c. Surgical incisions
    d. Urinary output
    e. Height of newborns

CHAPTER 61

# Introduction to Pharmacology

## SECTION I: TESTING WHAT YOU KNOW

**Activity A** *Match the categories of medication names in Column A with their descriptions in Column B.*

**Column A**

____ 1. Chemical name

____ 2. Generic name

____ 3. Official name

____ 4. Trade name

**Column B**

a. Similar to the chemical name and assigned by the medication's first manufacturer

b. Copyrighted name assigned by the company manufacturing the medication and usually followed by the symbol®

c. Describes the medication's chemical composition

d. Name identified in the USP or NF or, in Canada, in Health Canada's publications

**Activity B** *Match the type of dose in Column A with its description in Column B.*

**Column A**

____ 1. Therapeutic dose

____ 2. Minimal dose

____ 3. Loading dose

____ 4. Maximal dose

____ 5. Toxic dose

____ 6. Lethal dose

**Column B**

a. Larger than the usual continuing dose; may be given as the first dose of a newly prescribed medication

b. Amount of medication that causes symptoms of poisoning or toxicity

c. Largest amount that can be given safely without causing an adverse reaction or toxic effect

d. Amount of medication required to obtain a desired effect in the majority of clients

e. Amount of medication that will cause death

f. Smallest amount of drug necessary to achieve a therapeutic effect

**Activity C** ***Mark each statement as either "T" (True) or "F" (False). Correct any false statements.***

1. T F A medication's form, properties, and desired effects determine its dosage and method of administration.
2. T F A client usually does not experience an adverse or allergic reaction on first exposure to a medication.
3. T F A medication that has an opposing effect, or acts against another medication, is called an agonist.
4. T F Semisolid medications used for systemic purposes are designed to melt at body temperature.
5. T F A suppository is stored at room temperature.

**Activity D** ***Fill in the blanks.***

1. A ___________ or drug is a medicinal agent that modifies body functions.
2. ___________ is the science that deals with the origin, nature, chemistry, effects, and uses of medications.
3. Liquid medications for topical use include instillations and ___________.
4. An oral ___________ is a medicated tablet that dissolves in the mouth.
5. When medications are absorbed via the oral mucosa or ___________ they bypass the gastrointestinal tract.

**Activity E** ***Consider the following figure.***

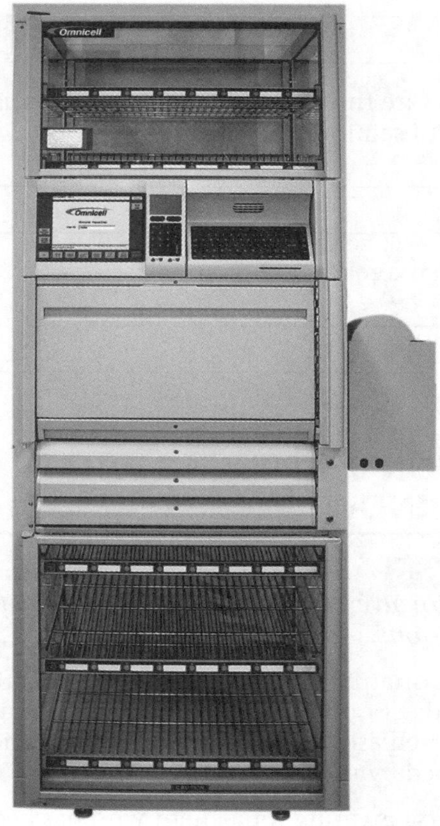


1. Identify the object in the figure.

_______________________________________

_______________________________________

2. What is it used for?

_______________________________________

_______________________________________

**Activity F** ***Briefly answer the following questions.***

1. What is the purpose of drug references?

_______________________________________

_______________________________________

2. List three drug references commonly used by nurses.

_______________________________________

_______________________________________

3. Which are the different routes of administration of a drug?

______________________________

______________________________

4. What are the different modes of administration of semisolid medications?

______________________________

______________________________

5. Who is a registered pharmacist?

______________________________

______________________________

## SECTION II: APPLYING WHAT YOU KNOW

**Activity G** ***Answer the following questions, which involve the nurse's role in administering medications.***

It is important for a nurse to have a general knowledge of pharmacology to be able to administer as well as teach clients about medications prescribed by the physician.

1. A nurse is caring for a client who has been prescribed a medication by the physician.
   a. What should the nurse know about the medication before administering it to the client?
   b. What details should the nurse know about the client before administering any medication to him?
2. A client admitted to the healthcare facility asks the nurse to administer the generic form of a medication prescribed for him.
   a. What are the client's rights related to administration of medication?
   b. What should the nurse do if the client refuses to take a medication?
3. A nurse is required to know all about the medications that are being administered to the client. What should the nurse do if in doubt regarding a medication?

## SECTION III: GETTING READY FOR NCLEX

**Activity H** ***Answer the following questions.***

1. A nurse has to administer diuretics to a client. Which of the following times of day is preferred for taking a diuretic?
   a. Before dinner
   b. Just before bedtime
   c. In the afternoon
   d. In the morning
2. A client has been prescribed a metered-dose inhaler. Which of the following is the advantage of using inhalers for administering medication to the client?
   a. The drug is absorbed into the body via the oral mucosa.
   b. It reduces systemic effects of the drug on the body.
   c. The drug is absorbed through the skin into the body.
   d. It dissolves instantly when placed on tongue.
3. A nurse who is administering a fat-soluble medication to a female client understands that women usually require smaller doses of this medication than men. Which of the following is the cause for this difference in medication dosage?
   a. Women have more body fluid.
   b. Women usually have less body fat.
   c. Women tend to be smaller in size.
   d. Women tend to absorb medication faster.
4. A nurse is assigned to administer medication to a client. Which of the following routes of administration takes the longest time to be effective?
   a. Sublingual medications
   b. Intramuscular injections
   c. Intravenous injections
   d. Rectally administered medications

5. A nurse is required to administer a controlled drug to a client. The nurse is expected to document the use of the drug. Which of the following is documented by the nurse on the form? (Select all that apply.)
   a. Time of administration
   b. Reason for administering dose
   c. Medication name and dose
   d. Physician's PIN number
   e. Signature of the licensed nurse

6. Which of the following actions can a nurse take with regard to a medication order for a client by the physician? (Select all that apply.)
   a. Make changes to the order.
   b. Consult a nursing supervisor.
   c. Question an order.
   d. Execute the order as given.
   e. Ignore the order if it is not legible.

7. A nurse working at a healthcare facility is required to understand a prescription thoroughly before carrying out the order. Which of the following is a valid prescription?
   a. A prescription that is 18 months old
   b. A prescription for a narcotic drug that is 1 year old
   c. A prescription that is written and signed by a physician
   d. A prescription that does not have a date on it

8. During discharge teaching, the nurse informs the client to avoid keeping the bottle containing medication near a window. Which of the following explanations should the nurse provide the client?
   a. Heat increases the speed of absorption.
   b. Exposure to light damages the medication.
   c. The medication may become too thick to drink.
   d. The medication may cause adverse side effects.

9. A client asks the nurse whether the medications that have been prescribed for him can be taken in a powdered form. Which of the following types of medications should the nurse tell the client that can be powdered and mixed with liquids or soft foods for oral administration?
   a. Enteric-coated tablets
   b. Orally disintegrating tablets
   c. Capsulated medication
   d. Immediate-release tablets

10. A nurse at the healthcare facility is in charge of the narcotic drugs cabinet. Which of the following should the nurse do when coming in for duty?
    a. Count the controlled drugs in the cabinet personally.
    b. Use a duplicate set of keys for the narcotics cabinet.
    c. Let the outgoing nurse count the number of remaining drugs.
    d. Record the narcotic drugs.

CHAPTER 62

# Classification of Medications

## SECTION I: TESTING WHAT YOU KNOW

**Activity A** *Match the class of drugs in Column A with its action in Column B.*

| Column A | Column B |
|---|---|
| ____ **1.** Ceruminolytics | **a.** Ophthalmic preparations used to dilate pupils |
| ____ **2.** Antiarrhythmics | **b.** Ophthalmic preparations used to constrict pupils |
| ____ **3.** Mydriatics | **c.** Medications used to loosen and remove impacted earwax |
| ____ **4.** Miotics | **d.** Medications that help to regulate heart rhythm |

**Activity B** *Match the drug in Column A with the class it belongs to in Column B.*

| Column A | Column B |
|---|---|
| ____ **1.** Digoxin | **a.** Narcotic analgesics |
| ____ **2.** Ibuprofen | **b.** Non-narcotic analgesics |
| ____ **3.** Morphine | **c.** Nonsteroidal anti-inflammatory drugs |
| ____ **4.** Aspirin | **d.** Cardiotonics |

**Activity C** *Mark each statement as either "T" (True) or "F" (False). Correct any false statements.*

**1.** T F Propranolol hydrochloride helps to reduce irritability of the myocardium and increases heart rate and the force of ventricular contraction.

**2.** T F Vasoconstrictors are used to control superficial hemorrhage.

**3.** T F Diuretics are medications that decrease the amount of urine excreted by the kidneys.

**4.** T F Diazoxide constricts the smooth muscles located in the arterial wall.

**5.** T F Epoetin alfa is a glycoprotein that stimulates red blood cell production.

**Activity D** *Fill in the blanks.*

**1.** The ____________ of tetracycline is influenced by the presence of aluminum in the stomach.

**2.** Tetracycline is a pregnancy category ____________ drug.

**3.** Antibiotics that retard the growth of bacteria are known as ____________ agents.

**4.** Aminoglycosides can damage the ____________ cranial nerve, leading to ototoxicity.

**5.** Analgesics are medications that relieve ____________.

**Activity E** ***The main action of digoxin is to strengthen the force of ventricular contractions and increase cardiac output. The increased cardiac output helps reduce the rate and workload of the heart to the desired level. The steps occurring during digoxin administration are given below in random order. Write the correct sequence in the boxes provided.***

1. The initial dose, called the digitalizing dose, is administered to reduce the heart rate to the desired rate of 60 to 80 beats per minute.
2. The apical pulse rate is counted for one full minute.
3. The client is placed on a maintenance dose, administered daily.
4. A stabilizing dose is administered to maintain the desired heart rate.

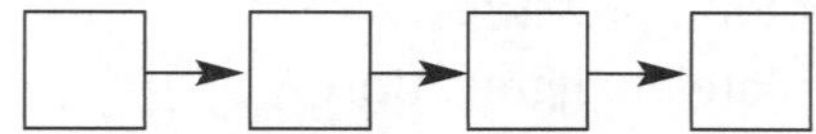

**Activity F** ***Briefly answer the following questions.***

1. What is the first sign of narcotic overdose?

______________________________

______________________________

2. What are nonsteroidal anti-inflammatory drugs? Give examples.

______________________________

______________________________

3. What are the side effects of barbiturates?

______________________________

______________________________

4. What is the action of a decongestant?

______________________________

______________________________

5. What are the toxic effects of aminoglycosides?

______________________________

______________________________

6. Briefly explain the causes of iron deficiency anemia.

______________________________

______________________________

## SECTION II: APPLYING WHAT YOU KNOW

**Activity G** ***Answer the following questions, which involve the nurse's role in administering medications.***

Administering the proper and scheduled dosages of drugs and observing the client for any adverse effects of the drugs are fundamental nursing responsibilities.

1. A nurse is required to administer tetracycline to a 40-year-old male client who is admitted to the healthcare facility with pneumonia and respiratory tract infection.
   a. What precautions should the nurse take to promote gastrointestinal absorption of tetracycline? Give reasons.
   b. What should the nurse instruct the client in regard to taking an antibiotic, such as tetracycline?
   c. What could be the possible side effects of tetracycline?
2. A client is prescribed sulfonamide for a urinary tract infection.
   a. What instructions should the nurse give the client?
   b. What could be the possible adverse effects of this drug?
3. A nurse is required to administer intravenous epinephrine to a client who has serious anaphylactic and hypersensitivity reactions.
   a. How should the nurse monitor a client who has been administered epinephrine?
   b. What are the effects of epinephrine when used parenterally?

## SECTION III: GETTING READY FOR NCLEX

**Activity H** *Answer the following questions.*

1. A nurse in the healthcare facility is caring for a client who has been administered warfarin to treat venous thrombosis. Which of the following side effects should the nurse monitor this client for?
   a. Potential for hemorrhage
   b. Dilated pupils
   c. Mental confusion
   d. Respiratory depression
2. A 60-year-old female client was prescribed methadone to relieve chronic pain of the knee joints. Which of the following vital signs should the nurse monitor in the client to prevent narcotic overdose?
   a. Respiration
   b. Blood pressure
   c. Heartbeat
   d. Pulse rate
3. Which of the following adverse effects should a nurse monitor for when administering albuterol to a client with asthma? (Select all that apply.)
   a. Palpitation
   b. Bradycardia
   c. Tremors
   d. Nervousness
   e. Urinary frequency
4. A 30-year-old client is prescribed a morphine-containing antitussive for a productive cough. Which of the following is an undesirable side effect of narcotic antitussives?
   a. Palpitation
   b. Habituation
   c. Tremors
   d. Hypotension
5. An 18-year-old female client with dysmenorrhea is prescribed ibuprofen. The client is on salicylate therapy for arthritis. The physician instructs her to stop taking the salicylate when on ibuprofen. What could be the reason for this?
   a. Salicylates may reduce absorption of ibuprofen.
   b. Salicylates may cause respiratory depression.
   c. Salicylates may reduce renal clearance of ibuprofen.
   d. Salicylates may cause drowsiness and sedation.
6. A 50-year-old client admitted with myocardial infraction has been prescribed a daily low dose of aspirin. How does aspirin help to reduce the incidence and severity of myocardial infraction?
   a. Reduces blood pressure
   b. Reduces platelet aggregation
   c. Constricts surface blood vessels
   d. Decreases cardiac output
7. A client who was admitted to the healthcare facility with morphine poisoning has a depressed respiratory rate. What action should be included in the emergency respiratory care measures?
   a. Reduce the dosage of morphine.
   b. Report this immediately to the physician.
   c. Document the respiration rate in client's chart.
   d. Initiate endotracheal intubation.
8. A pregnant client wants to know if she can take Migranal for her cluster headaches. Knowing that Migranal is a category X drug, the nurse informs the client that the drug should not be used during pregnancy, because it has demonstrated fetal risks. Which FDA pregnancy category suggests that no animal studies or adequate studies in humans have been done for the drug?
   a. Category A
   b. Category B
   c. Category C
   d. Category D

9. A 30-year-old female client is taking oral contraceptives with estrogen. Which of the following herbs may cause an adverse reaction if taken with hormonal contraceptives?
   a. Dandelion root
   b. Fenugreek
   c. Garlic
   d. Ginseng

10. A nurse is ordered to give grapefruit juice to a 50-year-old client. Grapefruit juice should not be combined with which of the following drugs? (Select all that apply.)
    a. Cortisol
    b. Warfarin
    c. Cyanocobalamin
    d. Erythromycin
    e. Folic acid

CHAPTER 63

# Administration of Non-Injectable Medications

## SECTION I: TESTING WHAT YOU KNOW

**Activity A** *Match the methods of medication administration in Column A with their descriptions in Column B.*

| Column A | Column B |
|---|---|
| ____ **1.** Topical method | **a.** Medication administration by way of the digestive tract |
| ____ **2.** Parenteral route | **b.** Placing the medication between the client's cheek and gum |
| ____ **3.** Enteral route | **c.** Administering medication into body parts by ways other than the digestive tract |
| ____ **4.** Buccal administration | **d.** Applying medications directly to the skin or mucous membranes |

**Activity B** *Mark each statement as either "T" (True) or "F" (False). Correct any false statements.*

**1.** T F The best way to identify the correct client for administration of medication is to ask the client his or her name.

**2.** T F Medications absorbed through the mucosa of the mouth are absorbed rapidly.

**3.** T F A medication's rate of absorption does not depend on its route of administration.

**4.** T F Discarding the first portion of ophthalmic ointment maintains the ointment's sterility.

**5.** T F Anaphylactic reactions are manifested by an increase in blood pressure.

**6.** T F All narcotics and other controlled substances are kept double-locked.

**Activity C** *Fill in the blanks.*

**1.** ____________ supply medications usually are those that can be sold over the counter.

**2.** A/An ____________ effect of medication is seen when the client's response is opposite to that which is desired.

**3.** Clients usually prefer ____________ administration, which is used most frequently.

4. A disadvantage of drugs administered orally is the ___________ absorption rate.
5. ___________ medications are placed on the tongue, where they are absorbed or dissolved.
6. An inhaler or nebulizer setup is used for ___________ clients only.

**Activity D** *Consider the following figure.*

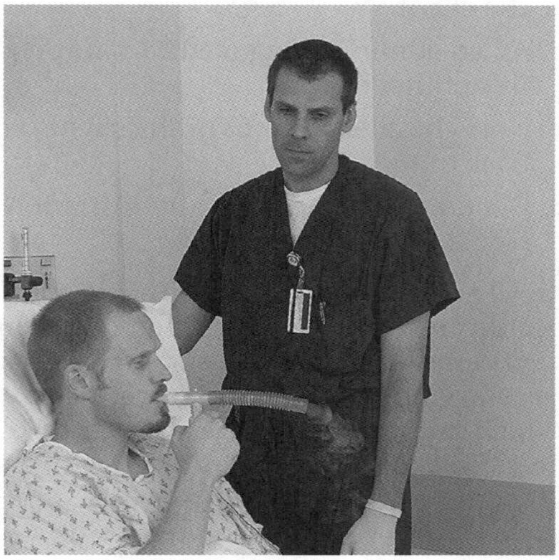

1. Identify the procedure shown in the figure.

___________________________________________

___________________________________________

2. State the basis for this procedure, and list some of the medications commonly administered by this procedure.

___________________________________________

___________________________________________

3. What important precautions should the nurse consider during this procedure?

___________________________________________

___________________________________________

**Activity E** ***The nurse needs to assist a client during the application of a nicotine patch to aid the client in smoking cessation. The steps followed during the application of a transdermal nicotine patch are given below in random order. Write the correct sequence in the boxes provided.***

1. Place the patch on a clean, dry, hairless area and press on all parts of the patch.
2. Take the patch from the package and remove the backing from the patch.
3. Wear gloves during the entire procedure, including the preparation of the patch.
4. Use a permanent marker to indicate the date and time the patch was applied.

☐ → ☐ → ☐ → ☐

**Activity F** ***Briefly answer the following questions.***

1. What are the advantages of storing medications in unit-dose systems?

___________________________________________

___________________________________________

2. What are self-administered medications? Give examples.

___________________________________________

___________________________________________

3. When are the three checks done to compare and confirm the medication's name and dosage with the client's medical administration record?

___________________________________________

___________________________________________

4. What are the common errors that occur during medication administration? How are they prevented?

___________________________________________

___________________________________________

5. What is meant by potentiation of drugs?

______________________________________

______________________________________

6. Describe the purpose of instilling eye drops and eye ointments.

______________________________________

______________________________________

## SECTION II: APPLYING WHAT YOU KNOW

**Activity G** ***Answer the following questions, which involve the nurse's role in safe medication administration.***

Administering medications is perhaps the single most important nursing function. Each nurse must be familiar with the recommended administration routes, dosages, desired actions, possible side effects, and nursing considerations for prescribed medications.

A 50-year-old client who underwent surgery for cervical spondylitis at a healthcare facility requests that the nurse provide the necessary medications that he must take after being discharged from the healthcare facility. On obtaining the prescribed medications, the client reports to the nurse that the shape of the medication provided by the nurse is different from the tablets that were given to him during his hospital stay.

1. What important teaching should the nurse provide the client before administering any medication?
2. What are the important assessments a nurse should make when a client asks for PRN medication?
3. How will the nurse reassure the client regarding the shape change of the medication?

## SECTION III: GETTING READY FOR NCLEX

**Activity H** ***Answer the following questions.***

1. A nurse is caring for a client admitted to the healthcare facility. Which of the following precautionary steps should the nurse follow when administering medications to the client?
   a. Leave the medication within the reach of the client.
   b. Avoid administering medications prepared by another nurse.
   c. Note the allergy status of the client on the back of the chart.
   d. Document medication administration before it is given.
2. An 11-year-old client is admitted to the healthcare facility with asthma. The client has been prescribed nasal spray, which has to be sprayed into each nostril twice daily. Which of the following measures should the nurse consider when administering the nasal spray to the client?
   a. Assist the client into a seated position with the head tilted back.
   b. Place the tip of the bottle as deep as possible inside the nares.
   c. Point the tip of the bottle away from the midline of the nose.
   d. Instruct the client to remain in the same position for 5 to 10 minutes.
3. A nurse is going to administer medications to a client. Which is a complete order for administration?
   a. Mr. Brown ibuprofen 400 mg 2100
   b. Mr. Brown aspirin 650 mg po 0900
   c. Mr. Brown acetaminophen 0900
   b. Mr. Brown multivitamin 2100
4. A nurse is administering a client's daily medications. When should the nurse document the medications?
   a. Before administering the medications
   b. Before or during the administering of each medication
   c. During or after administering the medications
   d. After administering the medications

**5.** A nurse receives an order to administer a rectal suppository to an adult client with active ulcerative proctitis. Which of the following steps should the nurse perform when administering a rectal suppository?

**a.** Assist the client into the Sims' position and cover the client.

**b.** Insert the suppository at least 2 inches into the anal canal.

**c.** Ask the client to maintain the Sims' position for 5 to 10 minutes.

**d.** Squeeze the suppository through the length of the foil.

**6.** A nurse is caring for a postoperative client who is anesthetized and intubated. The nurse is advised to administer medications to the client using a button-type gastrointestinal tube (G-tube). Which of the following measures should the nurse consider when caring for such clients?

**a.** Gently aspirate the G-tube for stomach contents.

**b.** Place the client in a high Fowler's position.

**c.** Flush the tube with water after giving all medications.

**d.** Keep the tube clamped for at least 10 minutes.

**7.** A 22-year-old client diagnosed with fungal infection of the skin has been prescribed ketoconazole. The nurse instructs the client to apply the medication topically. What should the nurse be aware of regarding topical medications?

**a.** Topical medications are absorbed into the general circulation.

**b.** Topical medications are transported throughout the entire body.

**c.** Topical applications reduce undesired systemic reactions.

**d.** Transdermal application is administered to achieve topical effects.

**8.** A nurse has been ordered to administer a medication STAT. Which of the following measures should the nurse employ in the proper time for administration of the medication?

**a.** Medication should be administered after breakfast

**b.** Medication should be given immediately

**c.** Medication should be given as needed

**d.** Medication should be given in the evening

**9.** A nurse is required to administer Ofloxacin solution to a 33-year-old client diagnosed with a middle ear infection. Given below in random order are the nursing steps for administering ear medications. Arrange the steps in the correct order.

**a.** Apply gentle pressure on the tragus.

**b.** Remove excess drainage with a dry wipe.

**c.** Make drops fall on the side of the canal.

**d.** Pull the ear lobe up, back, and outward.

**10.** An 8-year-old client diagnosed with attention deficit–hyperactivity disorder (ADHD) has been prescribed Ritalin by the healthcare provider. This is the client's first visit to the healthcare facility. What precautions should the nurse take before administering the medication? (Select all that apply.)

**a.** Determine the client's history of drug allergies.

**b.** Inquire about the client's history of allergic rhinitis.

**c.** Ask about the client's history of insect sting allergy.

**d.** Determine the client's allergies to tape and latex.

**e.** Inquire about the client's allergies to food products.

CHAPTER 64

# Administration of Injectable Medications

## SECTION I: TESTING WHAT YOU KNOW

**Activity A** *Match the injection preparation in Column A with their descriptions in Column B.*

**Column A**

____ 1. Ampule

____ 2. Vial

____ 3. Prefilled syringe

____ 4. Diluent

**Column B**

a. Provides a single medication dose prepared by a manufacturer or pharmacy

b. Some injectable medications are supplied as powders that must be reconstituted

c. Glass container equipped with a self sealing rubber stopper

d. Glass container that holds a premeasured, single medication dose

**Activity B** *Match the injection method in Column A with the process followed in Column B.*

**Column A**

____ 1. Subcutaneous injections

____ 2. Intradermal injections

____ 3. Intramuscular injections

____ 4. Intermittent infusions

**Column B**

a. Given using syringes with a needleless access tip/hub

b. Given using 1- or 2-mL syringes with ⅝- to 1-inch needles

c. Given using 2- to 3-mL syringes with 1- to 1½-inch needles

d. Given using 1-mL tuberculin syringes with needles of 25 to 26 gauge

**Activity C** *Mark each statement as either "T" (True) or "F" (False). Correct any false statements.*

1. T F Discard any unused portion of an ampule's contents, because no way exists to prevent contamination of an open ampule.

2. T F Parenteral administration of medications carries less risk than oral administration.

3. T F When choosing the correct type of needle for injection, only the length of the needle is important.

4. T F The nurse must be knowledgeable in drawing up and preparing medications for injection.

5. T F It is important to take precautions to prevent needle stick injuries.

6. T F It is important to seek assistance if there are any questions about IV administration.

**Activity D** *Fill in the blanks.*

1. Always dispose of all syringes and needles in the ____________ container provided.

2. ____________ injections typically are given using 1 mL tuberculin syringes.

3. The inner portion of the syringe that fits inside the barrel of the syringe is termed the ____________.

4. A ____________ is a glass container equipped with a self-sealing rubber stopper that contains a single premeasured or multidose medication.

5. Always ____________ injection sites for clients who receive injections on a regular basis.

6. When administering IM and subcutaneous injections insert and remove the needle ____________.

**Activity E** *Consider the following figures.*

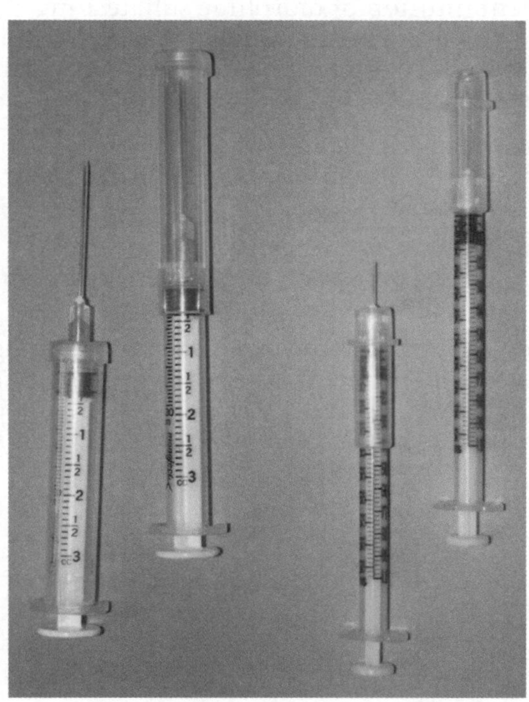

1. Identify the equipment in the figure.

______________________________________________

______________________________________________

2. State the purpose of this equipment.

______________________________________________

______________________________________________

3. What should the nurse with this equipment do when administering the medication?

______________________________________________

______________________________________________

4. Identify the figure.

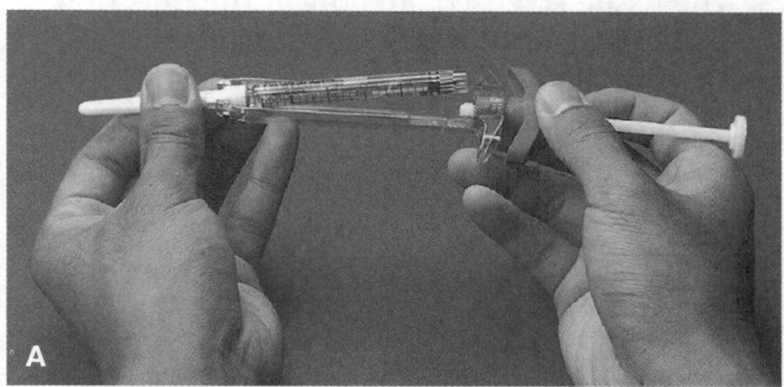

A

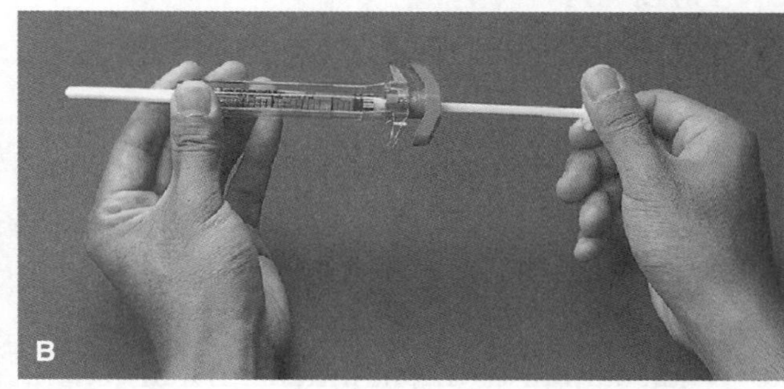

B

______________________________________________

______________________________________________

5. Explain the steps to set up the apparatus shown in the figure.

______________________________________________

______________________________________________

6. How is the correct quantity of medication obtained using this procedure?

______________________________________________

______________________________________________

**Activity F** *The nurse needs to administer an intramuscular injection using the Z track ("zig-zag" method. The steps followed during the Z track method are given below in random order. Write the correct sequence in the boxes provided.*

1. The tissues are slowly released while the needle is withdrawn. As each tissue plane slides by the other, the track is sealed.
2. The needle is inserted.
3. The tissue is tensed laterally at the injection site. This pulls the skin, subcutaneous tissue, and fat planes into a "Z" formation.

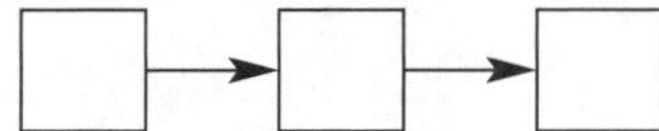

**Activity G** *Briefly answer the following questions.*

1. What are the most common signs of infiltration of an IV?

 ______________________________________

 ______________________________________

2. What are the common reasons that a medication may be administered by injection?

 ______________________________________

 ______________________________________

3. When administering an intradermal injection, why should the client not scratch or pinch the site?

 ______________________________________

 ______________________________________

4. There are a number of commonalities between the administration of subcutaneous and intramuscular injections. What are the major differences?

 ______________________________________

 ______________________________________

5. Name the commonly used intravenous (IV) solutions.

 ______________________________________

 ______________________________________

## SECTION II: APPLYING WHAT YOU KNOW

**Activity H** *Answer the following questions, which involve the nurse's role in safe medication administration.*

Administering medications is perhaps the single most important nursing function. Each nurse must be familiar with the recommended administration routes, dosages, desired actions, possible side effects, and nursing considerations for prescribed medications.

1. A nurse received a needle stick after the administration of an intramuscular injection into the ventrogluteal site of a client who is on MRSA precautions.
   a. To whom should the nurse immediately report the needle stick?
   b. Who is required to take blood tests? How often must the blood tests be obtained? Why?
2. A nurse is providing care for a 32-year-old client who recently underwent thoracotomy. The nurse is advised to provide an intermittent infusion of morphine sulfate 1 mg with 0.9% normal saline through an intravenous catheter for post-thoracotomy pain relief.
   a. What are the important nursing steps involved in administering an intermittent infusion?
   b. What measures should the nurse follow when caring for a client receiving intermittent infusion?
   c. What should the nurse document during the intermittent infusion of a medication?

## SECTION III: GETTING READY FOR NCLEX

**Activity I** *Answer the following questions.*

1. The primary care provider has ordered an influenza injection of 0.5 mL IM to be administered to a client. Which of the following size needle would the nurse select when preparing the injection for administration?
   a. 17 G
   b. 18 G
   c. 23 G
   d. 25 G

2. The nurse is getting ready to administer an intramuscular injection. The client tells the nurse that during a previous hospitalization the nurse hit the sciatic nerve during an intramuscular injection. Which of the following sites should the nurse avoid for this intramuscular injection?
   a. Dorsogluteal
   b. Ventrogluteal
   c. Deltoid
   d. Vastus lateralis

3. A severely anorectic client is prescribed treatment with intravenous hyperalimentation by an indwelling percutaneous intravenous central catheter (PICC). What special consideration should the nurse keep in mind during hyperalimentation using a PICC?
   a. The client can use the arm into which the PICC is inserted.
   b. PICC lines are generally flushed with normal saline.
   c. The PICC is inserted at the client's antecubital fossa.
   d. The PICC can remain in place for only about a week.

4. A client has been prescribed intramuscular injection of tetanus toxoid as a prophylactic measure after a minor traffic accident. At what angle should the nurse give an intramuscular injection?
   a. 45 degrees
   b. 60 degrees
   c. 75 degrees
   d. 90 degrees

5. The client has a primary IV infusion running at 150 mL/hour for severe dehydration following two days of continuous vomiting and diarrhea. Which of the following are signs of IV infiltration? (Select all that apply.)
   a. Swelling or puffiness
   b. Warmth
   c. Pain at the insertion site
   d. Feeling of sponginess in the area
   e. Leaking of fluid around the catheter

6. A nurse is monitoring an IV in a long term care setting which uses a microdrip IV set. The nurse needs to know the drops per milliliter of the intravenous set in order to properly monitor that the IV is running at the correct rate. Which of the following is the correct drops per milliliter for the microdrip intravenous set?
   a. 10
   b. 12
   c. 15
   d. 60

7. There is no infusion pump or controller available in the long-term care facility to administer IV fluid to the client. Which of the following factors would administer the IV fluid more rapidly? (Select all that apply.)
   a. Smaller, outer diameter bore catheter
   b. Lower the IV bag
   c. Place the IV bag up higher from the patient
   d. Larger, inner diameter bore catheter
   e. Position of the IV insertion site

8. A nurse has been ordered to discontinue the intravenous infusion of fluids to the client. Which of the following measures should the nurse employ on receiving an order to discontinue infusion? (Select all that apply.)
   a. Withdraw the catheter from the vein.
   b. Pinch the intravenous tubing.
   c. Apply pressure over the insertion site.
   d. Apply a bandage over the puncture site.
   e. Make sure that the catheter tip is intact.

**9.** A client has a PICC central line in place to administer large amounts of intravenous fluid and total parenteral nutrition. Which of the following accurately describes this type of central line?

**a.** Short (non-tunneled) triple lumen percutaneous central line catheter that is inserted into the subclavian vein and threaded up into the superior vena cava.

**b.** Inserted into the antecubital space and is long enough to be threaded up into the superior vena cava.

**c.** Implanted port allows for long term, intermittent access to the central vein, without the need for a catheter protruding from the skin.

**d.** Double lumen catheter with a Dacron cuff that helps hold it in place.

**10.** The nurse has to give an infant an intramuscular injection. Which of the following sites may be used in infants and children younger than three years of age?

**a.** Dorsogluteal

**b.** Ventrogluteal

**c.** Deltoid

**d.** Vastus lateralis

CHAPTER 65

# Normal Pregnancy

## SECTION I: TESTING WHAT YOU KNOW

**Activity A** *Match the terms related to pregnancy in Column A with their descriptions in Column B.*

**Column A**

____ 1. Gestation

____ 2. Fertilization

____ 3. Trimester

____ 4. Implantation

____ 5. Gravida

**Column B**

a. Total number of pregnancies a woman has had, including the present one if she is pregnant

b. Burrowing in and attachment of the blastocyst to the endometrium (or the decidua)

c. Union of two cells, the ovum and the sperm, which occurs in the outer third of the fallopian tube (oviduct)

d. Period of time from the moment the sperm fertilizes the ovum until the birth of the newborn

e. Distinct 3-month periods that pregnancy is divided into, during which fetal development takes place

**Activity B** *Match the signs in Column A with their descriptions in Column B.*

**Column A**

____ 1. Goodell's sign

____ 2. Chadwick's sign

____ 3. Hegar's sign

**Column B**

a. Softening of the lower uterine segment at about 6 weeks

b. Softening of the cervix during pregnancy

c. Blue or purple discoloration of the cervix, vulva, and vagina

**Activity C** *Mark each statement as either "T" (True) or "F" (False). Correct any false statements.*

1. T F The placenta produces human chorionic gonadotropin.
2. T F Fetal circulation differs from newborn and adult circulation.
3. T F The embryonic stage lasts until the 12th week after conception.
4. T F Pregnancy is considered an illness.
5. T F Pica is a normal craving for food items during pregnancy.

**Activity D** *Fill in the blanks.*

1. During pregnancy, women develop an inward curve of the lower back, known as ____________.
2. The zygote divides rapidly to form a ball of about 16 identical cells, which is called a/an ____________.

3. The fetus' chorionic villi eventually meet with an area of uterine tissue to form the ___________.

4. The ___________ is the inner membrane surrounding the fetus.

5. ___________ is the most common method used to evaluate fetal size.

**Activity E** *Consider the following figure.*

1. Label the diagram and list the order of circulation from mother to baby throughout the entire cycle.

_______________________________________________

_______________________________________________

2. Identify the features unique to fetal circulation in this figure.

_______________________________________________

_______________________________________________

3. What changes take place in the fetal circulation with the newborn's first few respirations?

_______________________________________________

_______________________________________________

4. How is fetal circulation different from adult circulation?

_______________________________________________

_______________________________________________

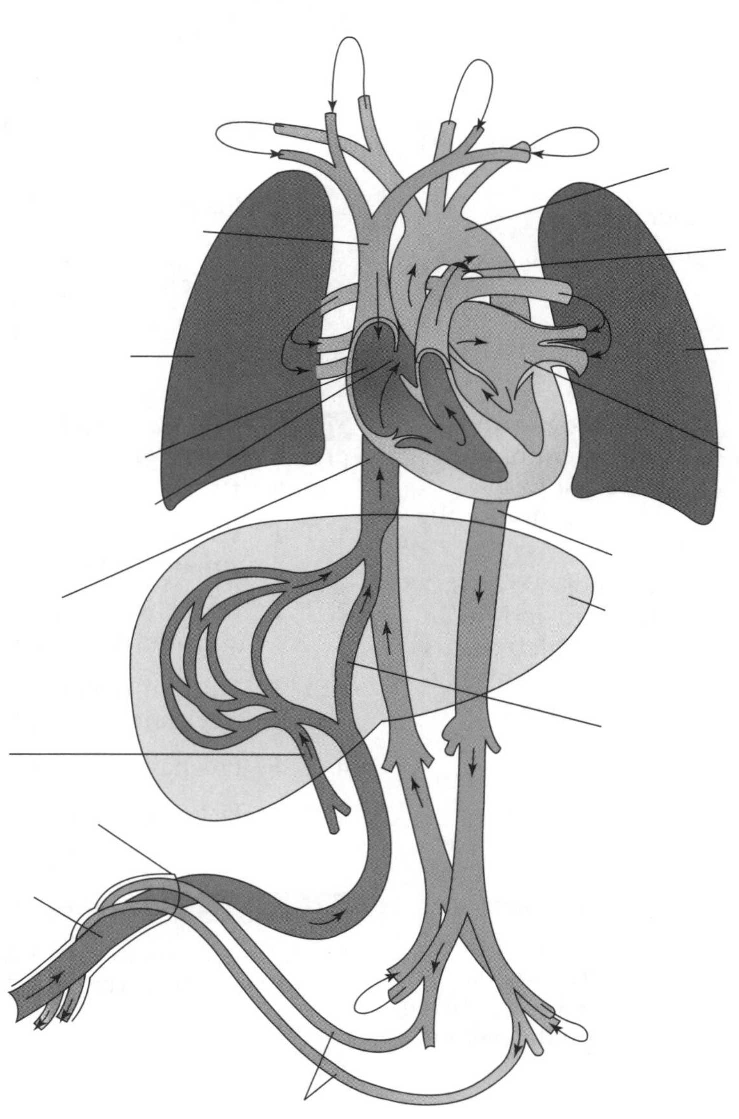

**Activity F** ***Pregnancy is dated from the first day of the woman's last normal menstrual period (LNMP). The steps for determining the estimated date of delivery by applying Nägele's rule are given below in random order. Write the correct sequence in the boxes provided.***

1. Determine the date of the first day of the last normal menstrual period.
2. The resulting date is the expected date of delivery.
3. Confirm that her last menstrual period was normal and on time.
4. Add 7 days and subtract 3 months from the date obtained.

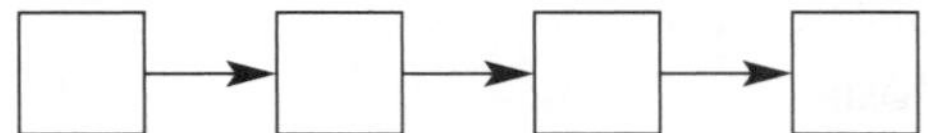

**Activity G** ***Briefly answer the following questions.***

1. What is hyperemesis gravidarum?

 ______________________________________

 ______________________________________

2. What is quickening, and when is it first experienced?

 ______________________________________

 ______________________________________

3. What pigment changes are seen during pregnancy?

 ______________________________________

 ______________________________________

4. Why does ballottement occur?

 ______________________________________

 ______________________________________

5. Why are beverages and foods that contain caffeine avoided during pregnancy?

 ______________________________________

 ______________________________________

## SECTION II: APPLYING WHAT YOU KNOW

**Activity H** ***Answer the following questions, which involve the nurse's role in managing pregnancy issues.***

A nurse's role in managing a pregnant client includes helping her adjust to her pregnancy, prepare for her baby, and maintain good health for herself and her child.

1. A woman in her eighth month of pregnancy is expecting her first child and is being prepared for childbirth.
   a. What is the goal of childbirth preparation?
   b. What are the common methods of childbirth preparation?
   c. What is the Lamaze method of childbirth preparation?
2. A primigravid client who plans to breastfeed is being educated about basics of infant care and preparations for infant feeding.
   a. What should the client education regarding general infant care include?
   b. What are the exceptions for breastfeeding?
   c. What topics regarding lactation should the nurse discuss with the client?

## SECTION III: GETTING READY FOR NCLEX

**Activity I** ***Answer the following questions.***

1. At a preconceptional visit a client whose husband's family has a history of a genetic defect says she is planning to have a baby. What should the nurse's response be?
   a. Reassure her that it is not a cause of concern.
   b. Refer the couple for genetic testing and counseling.
   c. Tell her that her husband's family history is unrelated to her pregnancy.
   d. Tell her that it is unadvisable to have a baby.

2. A primigravid client opts to formula-feed her infant after birth. What action should the nurse take?
   a. Educate her about formula preparation and storage.
   b. Tell her not to formula-feed her infant.
   c. Insist to her that only breastfeeding should be done.
   d. Tell her that it is a complicated decision and she should reconsider.

3. During her first trimester, a client experiences many physiologic changes. Which of the following changes should the nurse assure the client are normal for an 8-week pregnancy?
   a. Nausea and vomiting
   b. Dependent edema
   c. Colostrum production
   d. Visual changes

4. A pregnant client has had two previous pregnancies. She had a miscarriage at 6 weeks the first time. She also has a 4-year-old daughter, who was born at 40 weeks of gestation. Her pregnancy history could best be summarized as:
   a. G3, P0
   b. G2, P1
   c. G3, P1
   d. G3, P2

5. At what gestational age does the fetal stage begin?
   a. 2 weeks
   b. 5 weeks
   c. 7 weeks
   d. 9 weeks

6. A nurse is educating a 22-year-old primigravid client about the danger signs of pregnancy. Which of the following is a danger sign of pregnancy?
   a. Morning sickness
   b. Vaginal bleeding
   c. Shortness of breath
   d. Vaginal discharge

7. A nurse is auscultating a 22-week pregnant client with a fetoscope. Detection of the fetal heartbeat (fetal heart tones) by use of the fetoscope is a
   a. Possible sign of pregnancy
   b. Probable sign of pregnancy
   c. Presumptive sign of pregnancy
   d. Positive sign of pregnancy

8. A client in her 10th week of pregnancy with suspected pregnancy-induced hypertension has sudden development of edema. Which of the following symptoms may be signs of pregnancy-induced hypertension? (Select all that apply.)
   a. Visual changes
   b. Epigastric pain
   c. Lordosis
   d. Severe headache
   e. Breast enlargement

9. Many women do not keep an accurate record of their menstrual periods or may not have regular periods for many different reasons. In these cases, the estimated date of delivery is determined by
   a. Using the gestational wheel
   b. Applying Nägele's rule
   c. Estimating fetal age by ultrasound examination
   d. Adding 40 weeks to the date of detection

10. A nurse is auscultating for fetal heart tones in a client who is 20 weeks' pregnant. Given below are the steps for listening to fetal heart sounds using Doppler equipment, in random order. Arrange the steps in the correct order.
   a. Count the fetal heart tones for 15 seconds, and multiply by 4 to get the rate per minute.
   b. Exert a little pressure and place the instrument immediately above the pubic bone.
   c. Ask the woman to lie down on her back (supine position).
   d. Slowly rotate the Doppler instrument by 360 degrees until you hear the baby's heartbeat.

**11.** A client in her 19th week of gestation informs the nurse that she has been experiencing light, "fluttery" sensations which she refers to as fetal movements. The nurse knows that this sensation should be documented as which of the following? (Select all that apply.)

**a.** Feeling of life
**b.** Confirmed pregnancy
**c.** Quickening
**d.** Morning sickness
**e.** Presumptive sign of pregnancy

**12.** A 30-year old client has missed her menstrual period and is eager to know if she is pregnant. Which of the following signs ensures that the client is pregnant?

**a.** Positive home pregnancy test
**b.** Goodell's sign
**c.** Hearing a fetal heartbeat
**d.** Braxton Hicks contractions

**13.** A client in her first trimester visits the prenatal clinic. Which of the following should the nurse say is the pattern of future visits?

**a.** Once every week for the first 28 weeks
**b.** Once every 2 weeks for the first 28 weeks
**c.** Once every 3 weeks for the first 28 weeks
**d.** Once every 4 weeks for the first 28 weeks

CHAPTER 66

# Normal Labor, Delivery, and Postpartum Care

## SECTION I: TESTING WHAT YOU KNOW

**Activity A** *Match the different types of breech presentation in Column A with their descriptions in Column B.*

| Column A | Column B |
|---|---|
| ____ **1.** Complete | **a.** Either one or both legs are extended at both the hip and knee |
| ____ **2.** Frank | **b.** Either one or both legs are extended at the hip, flexed at the knee |
| ____ **3.** Kneeling | **c.** The fetus has the hips bent, but the knees are extended |
| ____ **4.** Footling | **d.** The fetus has both legs drawn up, bent at both the hip and the knee |

**Activity B** *Match the four main variables that affect labor in Column A with their descriptions in Column B.*

| Column A | Column B |
|---|---|
| ____ **1.** The passage | **a.** The contraction of the uterine muscles |
| ____ **2.** The passenger | **b.** The process of birthing, behavior of parents, and evaluation process of stages of labor |
| ____ **3.** The power | **c.** The diameter of the pelvis and its soft tissues |
| ____ **4.** The psyche | **d.** The fetus, umbilical cord, and placenta |

**Activity C** *Mark each statement as either "T" (True) or "F" (False). Correct any false statements.*

**1.** T F One of the most common methods of anesthesia used during labor and delivery is general anesthesia.

**2.** T F A birth plan is a written document in which the expecting mother expresses her desires about labor and birth.

**3.** T F Lochia rubra, which is yellow or white, starts on about day 10.

**4.** T F Complicated labor often occurs when body parts other than the fetal head present.

**5.** T F Postpartum is the time period during which labor and delivery take place.

**Activity D** ***Fill in the blanks.***

1. A/An ____________ is used to monitor the frequency of contractions.
2. After placental delivery, administration of a/an ____________ medication may be necessary to assist the uterus to contract and to minimize the risk of bleeding.
3. Brief increases in the fetal heart rate (FHR) of 15 beats per minute (BPM) or more are called ____________.
4. When the head of the fetus lies closest to the maternal pelvis, the presentation is said to be ____________.
5. If the uterine fundus is boggy, perform ____________ massage.

**Activity E** ***Consider the following figures.***

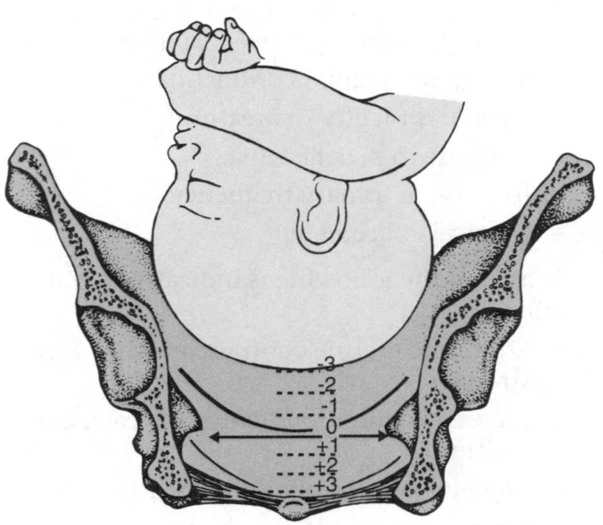


1. Identify what is shown in the figure.

_______________________________________

_______________________________________

2. What is station 0?

_______________________________________

_______________________________________

3. How is station measured?

_______________________________________

_______________________________________

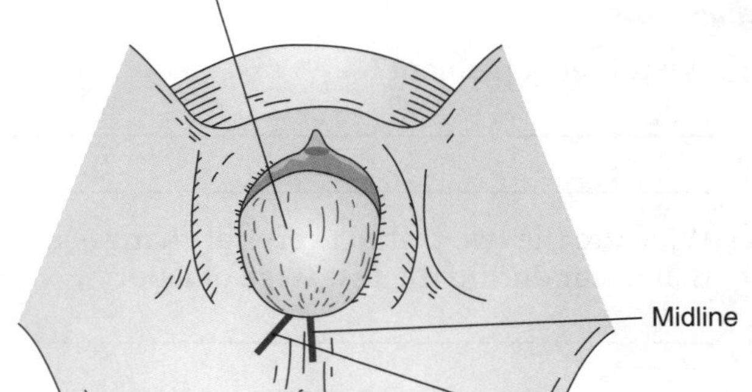


4. Identify the procedure shown in the figure.

_______________________________________

_______________________________________

5. What are its types?

_______________________________________

_______________________________________

6. What are the benefits?

_______________________________________

_______________________________________

**Activity F** ***The purpose of fundal massage is to encourage uterine muscle contraction and reduce blood loss. The steps occurring during fundal massage are given below in random order. Write the correct sequence in the boxes provided.***

1. Observe for passage of large clot; notify the healthcare practitioner if clots are numerous or frequent or if they indicate active hemorrhage.
2. Clean the female client's vulva and perineum. Apply a clean perineal pad.
3. Rotate the fundal hand gently and continue this massage until you feel that the uterus become a firm globe. Do not massage a contracted uterus.
4. Cup one hand around the uterine fundus. Place the other hand over the symphysis pubis to stabilize the uterus.

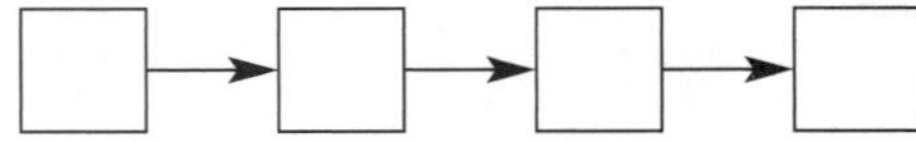

**Activity G** *Briefly answer the following questions.*

1. What is engorgement?

______________________________

______________________________

2. What are the two distinct cervical changes that occur during the first stage of labor?

______________________________

______________________________

3. What changes occur during crowning?

______________________________

______________________________

4. What are the disadvantages of delivery using epidural anesthesia?

______________________________

______________________________

5. What is colostrum?

______________________________

______________________________

## SECTION II: APPLYING WHAT YOU KNOW

**Activity H** *Answer the following questions, which involve the nurse's role in labor and delivery.*

A nurse's role in managing labor involves careful observations of the mother during delivery and of both mother and newborn after delivery. The nurse also functions as a teacher to provide knowledge that the family needs for maternal and newborn care.

1. A client is receiving epidural anesthesia during labor.
   a. What care should be exercised when administering epidural anesthesia during labor?
   b. What findings should the nurse report immediately when caring for a client receiving anesthesia during labor?
   c. Why is general anesthesia rarely used during labor?
2. A pregnant client has just experienced rupture of the membranes.
   a. What happens when the membranes break?
   b. Why should the nurse assess the baseline maternal temperature at the time the bag of waters ruptures?

## SECTION III: GETTING READY FOR NCLEX

**Activity I** *Answer the following questions.*

1. What nursing care should the nurse focus on during the first stage of labor?
   a. Assessment of client's vital signs
   b. Assessment of the placenta
   c. Administration of an oxytocic medication
   d. Assessment of the newborn
2. A pregnant client asks the nurse how she can identify whether she is in labor. Which of the following signs is most likely to indicate that labor is approaching? (Select all that apply.)
   a. Strong and regular contractions
   b. Greater difficulty in breathing
   c. Decrease in pedal edema
   d. Increase in urinary frequency
   e. Cervical effacement
3. Which of the following is indicative of false labor?
   a. Rhythmic uterine contractions that grow stronger
   b. Increase in duration (length) of each contraction
   c. Irregular pattern of uterine contractions
   d. Lower back pain that moves gradually around to the abdomen
4. A nurse is assessing a client in the postpartum period. Which of the following is normal in the postpartum period?
   a. Involution of the uterus
   b. Pain behind the knee on flexion of the feet
   c. Voiding of small amounts of urine
   d. Redness, pain, and swelling along a vein

**5.** A nurse is assessing a client to whom oxytocin is being given for labor augmentation. In which of the following situations should the nurse immediately report the observation of contractions?

**a.** If the contractions are rhythmic and becoming stronger

**b.** If the contractions come more often than every 2 minutes

**c.** If the uterine contractions are causing pain

**d.** If each contraction lasts less than 90 seconds

**6.** Which of the following characteristics of amniotic fluid is abnormal?

**a.** Clear and colorless

**b.** Slightly salty odor

**c.** Yellow, green, or cloudy

**d.** pH of 7.0 to 7.5

**7.** A client who is breastfeeding her baby complains of painful and swollen breasts. Which of the following measures help to relieve the nursing mother's breast engorgement?

**a.** Using medications (usually acetaminophen) as prescribed

**b.** Placing cold packs on her breasts three to four times a day

**c.** Avoiding manual expression or pumping of the breasts

**d.** Wearing a supportive bra and breastfeeding frequently

**8.** A nurse is assessing the progress of labor of a client. Which of the following stations indicates that the fetus is "floating"?

**a.** Station +5

**b.** Station 0

**c.** Station −5

**d.** Station −1

**9.** A nurse is assessing the lochia of a postpartum client. Which of the following are abnormal characteristics of lochia? (Select all that apply.)

**a.** Large clots are present in lochia.

**b.** Clear serous discharge occurs for the first 2 days.

**c.** Lochia does not change color and characteristics.

**d.** Lochia has a fleshy or metallic odor.

**e.** Lochia serosa has a slightly earthy odor.

**10.** Given below are the steps for application of an external monitor, in random order. Arrange the steps in the correct order.

**a.** Attach straps to the Doppler instrument and secure. Place tocodynamometer on the abdomen between umbilicus and top of fundus.

**b.** Review fetal heart rate and uterine assessment data with client and family. Use thorough descriptions of data.

**c.** Apply conductive jelly to Doppler instrument and place on client's abdomen until a strong fetal heart rate is heard and a consistent signal is obtained.

**d.** Elevate head of bed 15 to 30 degrees, or place the client in lateral position. Perform Leopold's maneuvers and place two straps under the client.

CHAPTER 67

# Care of the Normal Newborn

## SECTION I: TESTING WHAT YOU KNOW

**Activity A** ***Match the reflexes observed in newborns in Column A with their descriptions in Column B.***

| Column A | Column B |
|---|---|
| ____ **1.** Rooting reflex | **a.** Newborn's foot fans out when the foot is held and stroked up the lateral edge and across the ball of the foot |
| ____ **2.** Moro's reflex | **b.** Newborn turns head in the direction of the touch when lip or cheek is stroked |
| ____ **3.** Babinski's reflex | **c.** Newborn holds tightly onto an object that is placed in his or her hand |
| ____ **4.** Grasp reflex | **d.** Newborn throws out arms and draws up legs in response to sudden noise |

**Activity B** ***Match the conditions that may be seen in newborns in Column A with their descriptions in Column B.***

| Column A | Column B |
|---|---|
| 1. Cephalhematoma | **a.** Bluish discoloration of the arms and legs of the infant because of slowed peripheral circulation |
| 2. Hypospadias | **b.** Location of the urinary meatus on the underside of the penis |
| 3. Acrocyanosis | **c.** Accumulation of fluid within the newborn's scalp, making it puffy and edematous |
| 4. Caput succedaneum | **d.** Accumulation of blood between the bones of the skull and the periosteum in neonates |

**Activity C** ***Mark each statement as either "T" (True) or "F" (False). Correct any false statements.***

**1.** T F If the Apgar score is 4 to 6, the neonate does not need resuscitation.

**2.** T F Two identification bands are placed on the newborn—one around each wrist.

3. T F Normal hematocrit for the newborn is 45% to 60%.

4. T F The greenish-black, tarry first stool passed by the newborn is called vernix caseosa.

5. T F The newborn's sucking stimulates milk production.

**Activity D** *Fill in the blanks.*

1. The five criteria assessed by the Apgar score are Appearance, Pulse, Grimace, ____________ and Respiratory effort.
2. Vitamin K is administered to the neonate by the __________ route during the first hour after birth.
3. In many birth centers, a cap is placed on the newborn's head, because the infant loses a lot of ____________ from the head.
4. The ____________ are the "soft spots" in the newborn's skull, formed at the junction of the individual skull bones.
5. The fine, downy hair found on the face, shoulders, and back of a newborn is called ____________.

**Activity E** *Consider the following figure.*

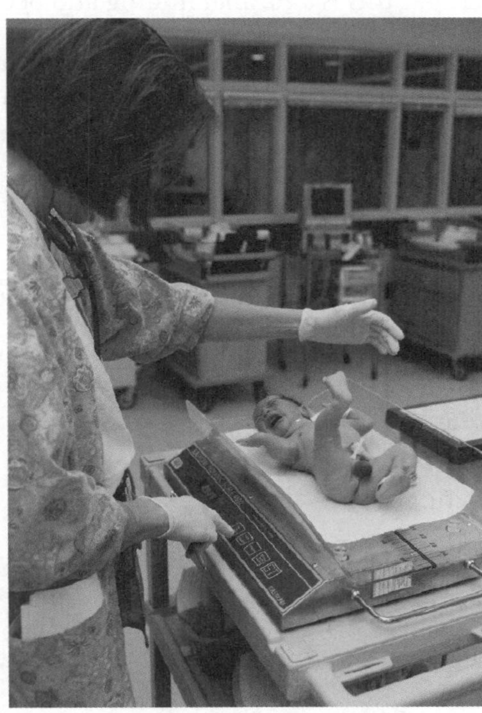

1. Identify the procedure shown in the figure.

____________________________________________

____________________________________________

2. How is the procedure conducted?

____________________________________________

____________________________________________

**Activity F** ***Steps that occur during and after the clamping and cutting of the umbilical cord are given below in random order. Write the correct sequence in the boxes provided.***

1. A plastic clamp is applied, and the Kelly clamp is removed.
2. The cord is cut between the two clamps.
3. The baby is dried and handed to the nurse or mother.
4. A cord blood sample is collected.

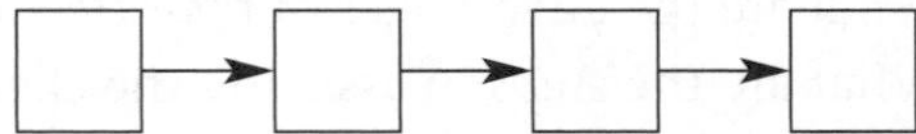

**Activity G** ***Briefly answer the following questions.***

1. What is an Apgar score? What does it indicate?

____________________________________________

____________________________________________

2. How is the newborn baby protected from developing eye infections after birth?

____________________________________________

____________________________________________

3. Why is vitamin K administered to most newborn infants?

____________________________________________

____________________________________________

4. What are the indications for bottle-feeding?

____________________________________________

____________________________________________

## SECTION II: APPLYING WHAT YOU KNOW

**Activity H** *Answer the following questions, which involve the nurse's role in newborn care.*

A nurse's role involves assisting the client with postdelivery care and caring for and managing the newborn.

1. A nurse assessing a newborn records an Apgar score of 5 and determines that the baby needs resuscitation.
   a. What is the importance of assessing the vital signs and physical condition of the newborn?
   b. What are the steps in performing neonatal resuscitation?
2. A nurse is required to guide and assist a client who has recently given birth in breastfeeding her baby.
   a. What are the advantages of breastfeeding?
   b. What are the steps in assisting the client to breastfeed her baby?
3. A nurse is required to instruct a client on how to give a tub bath to her newborn.
   a. What are the precautions to be taken?
   b. How is it performed?

## SECTION III: GETTING READY FOR NCLEX

**Activity I** *Answer the following questions.*

1. When inspecting a newborn, the nurse notices a flat, purple-red area with sharp borders on the infant's skin. Which of the following conditions does this indicate?
   a. Epstein's pearls
   b. Milia spots
   c. Stork bite
   d. Port-wine stain
2. A nurse is assigned to manage and care for a newborn immediately after delivery. Which of the following should be the immediate action of the nurse?
   a. Establish and maintain airway and respirations.
   b. Assist and guide the mother in nursing the baby.
   c. Give a warm water tub bath to the infant.
   d. Record the weight of the newborn infant.
3. A nurse is assessing a newborn baby. Which of the following characteristics indicate an abnormality in the newborn?
   a. Baby weighs 2,700 g.
   b. Baby's length is 50 cm.
   c. Head circumference is 35 cm.
   d. Chest circumference is 32 cm.
4. A client notices that her newborn has a slightly elongated skull. How should the nurse explain this to the client?
   a. Caput succedaneum
   b. Cephalhematoma
   c. Molding
   d. Ophthalmia neonatorum
5. A mother of a newborn baby notices that her baby appears cross-eyed. The nurse reassures her that this is a normal finding and occurs because the neonate's eyes are unable to focus. What other finding should the nurse reassure the client is normal in a newborn?
   a. Flattened ears
   b. Protruding chin
   c. Pointed nose
   d. Flat abdomen
6. When inspecting a newborn, a nurse notices that the child's urinary meatus is on the underside of the penis (near the scrotum). Which of the following conditions does this indicate?
   a. Prepuce
   b. Phimosis
   c. Epispadias
   d. Hypospadias

**7.** A mother has just finished bottle-feeding her otherwise healthy baby. The baby is still crying and is believed to have swallowed air from the bottle. What step should the nurse instruct the mother to take?

**a.** Give gentle but firm pressure on the abdomen.

**b.** Hold the baby, rock, and pat lightly on the back.

**c.** Give a little water so that the air settles down.

**d.** Eliminate milk from the diet for 2 weeks.

**8.** When inspecting the skin of a 2-day-old newborn, the nurse notices a white, thick, cheesy material in the hair and skin folds. Which of the following should the nurse consider this to be?

**a.** Erythema toxicum

**b.** Lanugo

**c.** Vernix caseosa

**d.** Acrocyanosis

**9.** Which of the following routes is contraindicated for recording body temperature in the newborn?

**a.** Rectal route

**b.** Axillary route

**c.** Oral route

**d.** Tympanic route

**10.** A nurse is informing a new mother about the various types of immunizations that the baby may need. Which of the following forms a part of the recommended regimen for vaccination against hepatitis B?

**a.** First dose within 24 hours after birth

**b.** Second dose at 3 months

**c.** Third dose at 6 months

**d.** Fourth dose at 1 year

CHAPTER 68

# High-Risk Pregnancy and Childbirth

## SECTION I: TESTING WHAT YOU KNOW

**Activity A** ***Match the health conditions in Column A with their descriptions in Column B.***

**Column A**

____ **1.** Mastitis

____ **2.** Cystitis

____ **3.** Puerperal infection

____ **4.** Thrombophlebitis

**Column B**

**a.** An infection in any part of the reproductive tract occurring after childbirth

**b.** A clot in a blood vessel, with resultant inflammation

**c.** A breast infection most commonly caused by *Staphylococcus aureus*

**d.** An inflammation of the bladder caused by a microorganism

**Activity B** ***Match the fetal assessment tests in Column A with their descriptions in Column B.***

**Column A**

____ **1.** Oxytocin challenge test

____ **2.** Nonstress test

____ **3.** Amniocentesis

____ **4.** Chorionic villus sampling

**Column B**

**a.** Invasive test that is performed if a client is considering abortion because of a serious genetic defect

**b.** Test that detects fetal abnormalities and establishes fetal lung maturity

**c.** Test that provides information on the fetal heart rate in response to fetal activity

**d.** Test done to evaluate the response of the fetal heart to uterine contractions

**Activity C** ***Mark each statement as either "T" (True) or "F" (False). Correct any false statements.***

**1.** T F In a pregnant client with a cardiac disorder, cesarean delivery is safer than vaginal delivery.

**2.** T F ABO incompatibility is not detectable before birth.

3. T F Placenta previa is a condition in which the placenta tears abruptly and prematurely from the uterus.

4. T F Precipitate labor most often occurs in induced labor or in primipara.

5. T F Dystocia is prolonged, painful labor that does not result in effective cervical dilation or effacement.

**Activity D** ***Fill in the blanks.***

1. A/an ___________ abortion occurs when the fetus has died but remains in the uterus.
2. If the pregnant client contracts rubella early in pregnancy, fetal ___________ or abnormality is a strong possibility.
3. Phototherapy is often useful in treating neonatal ___________.
4. Labor that occurs before the end of the 37th week of gestation is called ___________.
5. ___________ agents may be given to stop the contractions.

**Activity E** ***Consider the following figures.***

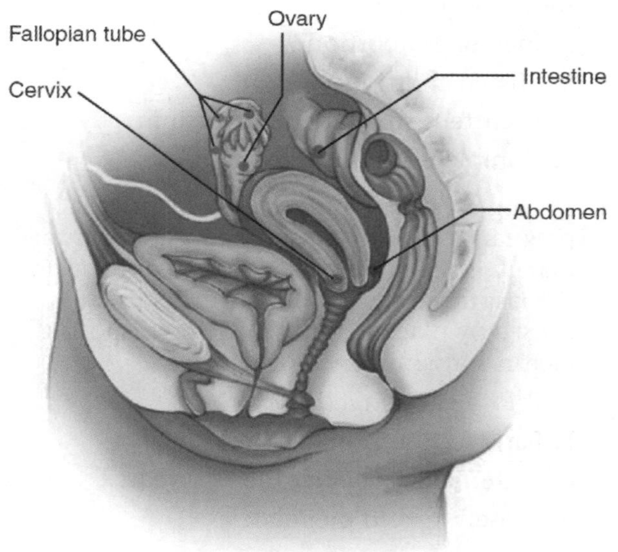


1. Identify the figure.

___________________________________________

___________________________________________

2. What is the most common type?

___________________________________________

___________________________________________

3. What are the predisposing factors?

___________________________________________

___________________________________________

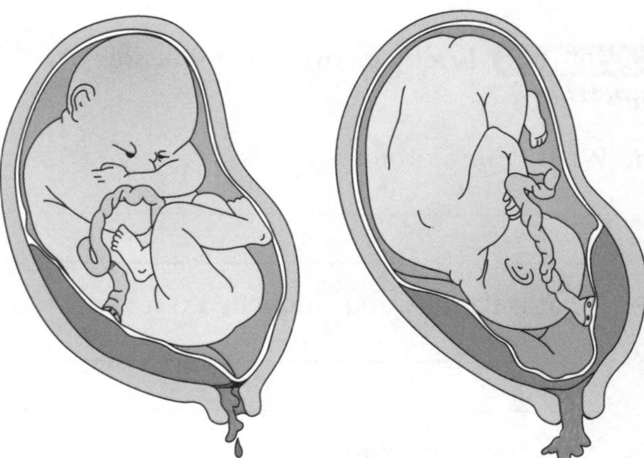

4. Identify the figure.

___________________________________________

___________________________________________

5. What are the predisposing factors?

___________________________________________

___________________________________________

6. What is the primary symptom?

___________________________________________

___________________________________________

**Activity F** ***Sometimes not enough time is available for a woman to get to the healthcare facility for delivery. In this case, police officers, rescue personnel, or nurses may be asked to assist with emergency childbirth. Steps for assisting in an emergency delivery are given below in random order. Write the correct sequence in the boxes provided.***

1. Keep the newborn warm. Tie off the umbilical cord in two places, but do not cut the umbilical cord.
2. Have the mother hold the newborn and initiate breast feeding. Get medical assistance as soon as possible.
3. Follow aseptic technique as closely as possible, and make sure the membranes have ruptured.

4. Make sure the newborn's airway is clear before the first breath. Initiate respiration in the newborn.

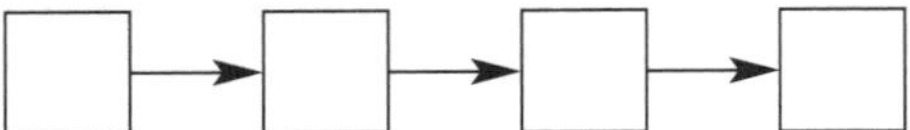

**Activity G** *Briefly answer the following questions.*

1. What is amniotomy?

______________________________

______________________________

2. What is Bandl's ring, and when is it seen?

______________________________

______________________________

3. What is nuchal cord?

______________________________

______________________________

4. How is vacuum extraction done?

______________________________

______________________________

5. What is done in internal version?

______________________________

______________________________

## SECTION II: APPLYING WHAT YOU KNOW

**Activity H** *Answer the following questions, which involve the nurse's role in management of high-risk pregnancy.*

A nurse's role in managing high-risk pregnancy and childbirth involves careful observations of the mother and fetus during pregnancy and of both mother and newborn during and after delivery. The nurse also functions as a teacher to provide knowledge and the necessary precautions that the family needs for maternal and newborn care.

1. A nurse is caring for a pregnant client with diabetes.
   a. What client and family teachings should a nurse provide for this client?
   b. Why is it important to take special care of pregnant women with diabetes?
2. An adolescent client is in labor in the 36th week of gestation.
   a. Define preterm labor.
   b. How should preterm labor be managed?
   c. Why should the nurse assess for signs and symptoms of labor frequently in adolescent clients who are pregnant?

## SECTION III: GETTING READY FOR NCLEX

**Activity I** *Answer the following questions.*

1. During an emergency delivery, a client had a laceration that involved the anal sphincter. What degree of laceration should the nurse document it as?
   a. First degree
   b. Second degree
   c. Third degree
   d. Fourth degree
2. A pregnant client has spontaneously lost three successive pregnancies previously. Which of the following terms best describes these abortions?
   a. Inevitable abortion
   b. Missed abortion
   c. Recurrent spontaneous abortion
   d. Complete abortion
3. During an assessment, a nurse instructs a pregnant client to consult a physician immediately if she has any vaginal bleeding during the last trimester. Such bleeding is usually caused by placenta previa, the predisposing factors for which include
   a. Previous vaginal delivery
   b. Early fertilization of the ovum
   c. Maternal age greater than 40 years
   d. Closely spaced pregnancies
4. After delivery, a client's placenta has failed to separate. What is the most appropriate action in this condition?
   a. Ultrasound examination
   b. Manual removal of the placenta
   c. Postpartum uterine D&C
   d. Support and monitoring of vital signs

5. A client has premature rupture of membranes. Interventions for this condition are listed below in random order. Arrange the interventions according to priority.
   a. Induction of labor
   b. Admission of the client
   c. Ultrasound examination
   d. Amniocentesis

6. Which of the following complications is more likely in an adolescent pregnancy?
   a. Placenta previa
   b. Hydramnios
   c. Preterm labor
   d. Hypotonic dystocia

7. A client who is breastfeeding her baby complains of painful and swollen breasts and is febrile. Which of the following should the nurse ask the client to do in order to prevent mastitis complications?
   a. Nurse the baby on the unaffected breast only.
   b. Place cold packs on the breasts.
   c. Follow the antibiotic therapy regimen strictly.
   d. Move around as much as possible.

8. A client is diagnosed with pregnancy-induced hypertension. Which of the following precautions should the nurse tell the client and her family to take?
   a. Keep the client's room well lit.
   b. Avoid sedating the client.
   c. Ask the client to ambulate.
   d. Decrease external stimuli and stress.

9. A client in labor is admitted to a healthcare facility with a prolapsed cord. What actions should the nurse take? (Select all that apply.)
   a. Notify the physician at once and prepare for resuscitation.
   b. Place the woman in the left lateral position.
   c. Perform a sterile vaginal examination immediately.
   d. Cover cord with moistened sterile towels.
   e. Hold the presenting part away from the cord.

10. A client is being given preoperative care for cesarean delivery. What is the nurse's role in preoperative care?
    a. Assess for symptoms of fetal distress.
    b. Administer general anesthesia to the client.
    c. Administer perineal care and oxytocic drugs.
    d. Perform external version to turn the fetus.

CHAPTER 69

# The High-Risk Newborn

## SECTION I: TESTING WHAT YOU KNOW

**Activity A** *Match the health conditions in Column A with their descriptions in Column B.*

**Column A**

____ 1. Erythroblastosis fetalis

____ 2. Pyloric stenosis

____ 3. Spina bifida

____ 4. Choanal atresia

**Column B**

a. Obstruction/closure of the nostrils at the entrance to the throat

b. Neural tube defect in which the vertebral spaces fail to close

c. Increase in size of the musculature at the junction of the stomach and small intestine

d. Hemolytic disease of the newborn caused by Rh sensitization

**Activity B** *Match the infections in Column A with their complications in newborns in Column B.*

**Column A**

____ 1. Gonorrhea

____ 2. Syphilis

____ 3. Cytomegalovirus

____ 4. Rubella

**Column B**

a. Cataracts, deafness, congenital heart defects, cardiac disease, and mental retardation

b. Bilateral conjunctivitis and blindness (ophthalmia neonatorum)

c. Premature labor and delivery, congenital disorders, and stillbirth

d. Small for gestational age, microcephaly, hydrocephaly, and mental retardation

**Activity C** *Mark each statement as either "T" (True) or "F" (False). Correct any false statements.*

1. T F An asymptomatic pregnant woman can transmit cytomegalovirus to her fetus through the placenta or through contact during delivery.

2. T F Marijuana, if used during pregnancy, may cause shortened gestation or precipitate labor of fewer than 3 hours.

3. T F Thrush is a bacterial infection in which milk-like spots form in the newborn's mouth.
4. T F Postterm newborns are those born after the completion of the 41st week of gestation.
5. T F The "H" in TORCH stands for hepatitis.

**Activity D** ***Fill in the blanks.***

1. The virus that causes German measles is called ___________.
2. ___________ is a catarrhal discharge from the nasal mucous membrane of newborn infants with syphilis.
3. The "C" in TORCH stands for ___________.
4. When the urethra opens on the bottom side of the penis, the condition is called ___________.
5. ___________ is a genetic disorder in which the newborn is incapable of metabolizing galactose.

**Activity E** ***Consider the following figures.***

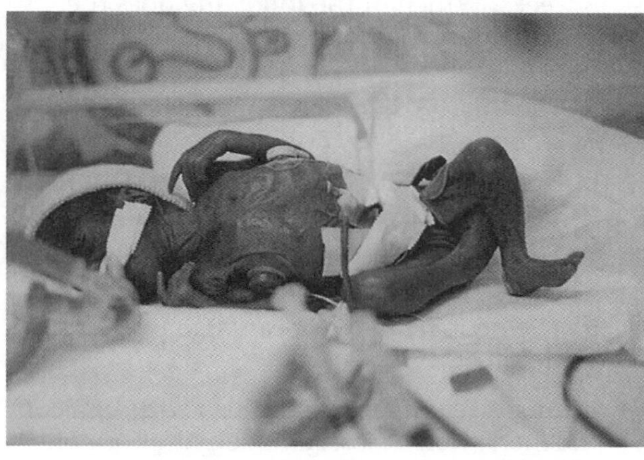

1. Identify the procedure in the figure.

___________________________________________

___________________________________________

2. Explain the need for the cap.

___________________________________________

___________________________________________

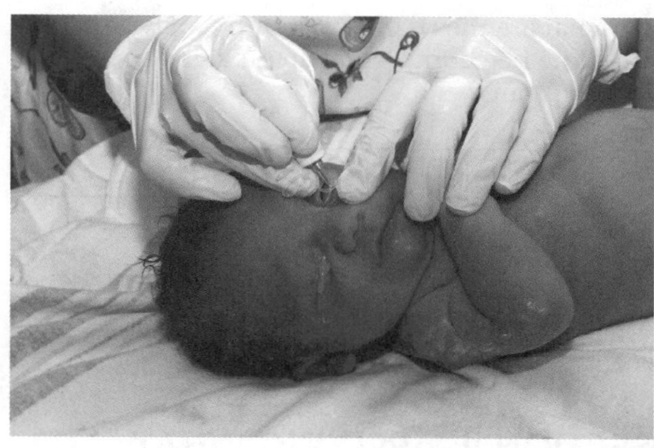

3. Identify the procedure shown in the figure.

___________________________________________

___________________________________________

4. Why is this procedure done?

___________________________________________

___________________________________________

**Activity F** ***Steps that occur during the treatment for dehydration in a newborn with diarrhea are given below in random order. Write the correct sequence in the boxes provided.***

1. Obtain stool cultures.
2. Give intravenous fluids.
3. Replace lost electrolytes.
4. Administer antibiotics (if necessary).

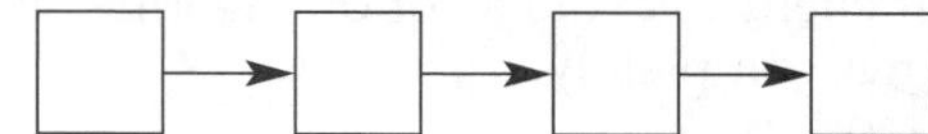

**Activity G** ***Briefly answer the following questions.***

1. What is respiratory distress syndrome?

___________________________________________

___________________________________________

2. How is physiologic jaundice caused in infants?

___________________________________________

___________________________________________

3. What is phototherapy? Explain the procedure.

___________________________________________

___________________________________________

4. What are the risk factors for hypoglycemia in the newborn? What are its signs and symptoms?

_______________________________________________

_______________________________________________

5. What is Down syndrome?

_______________________________________________

_______________________________________________

## SECTION II: APPLYING WHAT YOU KNOW

**Activity H** ***Answer the following questions, which involve the nurse's role in management of high-risk newborns.***

A nurse's role in managing high-risk newborns involves assisting clients in the care and management of preterm infants with developmental and congenital disorders.

1. An 18-year old client has just delivered a preterm baby. When assessing the condition of the baby, the nurse notices that the neonate is gradually losing body temperature.
   a. What interventions should the nurse take to ensure that the body temperature returns to normal? Explain with rationales.
   b. How is the return of body temperature in newborns evaluated?
2. As a part of client teaching, a nurse instructs a pregnant client to avoid alcohol, nicotine, and other drugs completely.
   a. Why should a pregnant client avoid these substances?
   b. What suggestions should a nurse provide for handling an addicted newborn?

## SECTION III: GETTING READY FOR NCLEX

**Activity I** ***Answer the following questions.***

1. A 19-year-old client gave birth to a postterm newborn at the healthcare facility. The baby's weight is below the 10th percentile for gestational age. How should this newborn be classified?
   a. Very low birth weight infant
   b. Small-for-gestational-age infant
   c. Normal birth weight infant
   d. Large-for-gestational-age infant
2. A client who recently gave birth to a low birth weight newborn rushes her child to the healthcare facility with frequent vomiting and diarrhea. Which of the following should the nurse monitor in such a case?
   a. Dehydration
   b. Jaundice
   c. Necrotizing enterocolitis
   d. Hypoglycemia
3. A 35-year-old client is overdue for delivery by 3 weeks. Which of the following does the nurse expect to find in the postterm newborn?
   a. The infant's skin may appear wet and smooth.
   b. Excess vernix caseosa may be seen on the skin.
   c. The infant may have aspirated meconium into the lungs.
   d. The neonate may appear large for gestational age.
4. A nurse is caring for a newborn with signs of fussiness, weight loss, and dehydration. The infant first vomited a milky substance after an initial feed, and then the vomiting was projectile. Which of the following conditions do these symptoms indicate?
   a. Pyloric stenosis
   b. Tracheoesophageal fistula
   c. Imperforate anus
   d. Cleft palate

5. When caring for a preterm newborn, the nurse notices milk-like spots or monilial infection in the newborn's mouth. Which of the following nursing considerations should the nurse employ when caring for the newborn?
   a. Use an antibiotic solution to swab the affected area.
   b. Administer humidified oxygen to the newborn.
   c. Maintain the newborn on parenteral nutrition.
   d. Isolate the newborn and treat with nystatin.
6. A client with a previous history of syphilis infection recently gave birth. The newborn has acquired syphilis infection and has rose spots, blebs (blisters) on the soles and palms, and catarrhal discharge from the nasal mucous membrane. Which of the following interventions should the nurse implement when caring for the newborn?
   a. Isolate the newborn and begin treatment with antibiotics as ordered.
   b. Treat the newborn with 1% to 2% aqueous solution of gentian violet.
   c. Wipe the newborn's mouth with a sterile gauze sponge after each feeding.
   d. Administer oxygen, vitamin K, anticonvulsive medications, and sedatives as required.
7. A nurse is assessing a 26-year-old pregnant client with a history of marijuana and alcohol abuse. Which of the following complications of such abuse should the nurse warn the client about?
   a. Postterm birth
   b. Hypoglycemia
   c. Low birth weight
   d. Prolonged labor
8. When assessing the condition of a preterm baby, the nurse notices a deep crease that runs horizontally across the infant's hands. The baby has slanted eyes and a large protruding tongue. Which of the following conditions should the nurse suspect in such a child?
   a. Anencephaly
   b. Down syndrome
   c. Spina bifida
   d. Hydrocephalus
9. A nurse is caring for a 2-day-old infant with signs of seizures, respiratory distress, cyanosis, a shrill cry, and muscle weakness. The child is diagnosed with intracranial hemorrhage. Which of the following procedures must the nurse employ when caring for the child?
   a. Position the head of the bed slightly lowered.
   b. Administer vitamin K immediately.
   c. Subject the newborn to phototherapy.
   d. Avoid using a gavage tube for feeding.
10. A nurse caring for a newborn notices an abnormal breathing pattern. The newborn shows signs of dyspnea and cyanosis along with tachycardia and an expiratory grunt. Which of the following does the nurse suspect in the newborn?
    a. Fetal alcohol syndrome
    b. Respiratory distress syndrome
    c. Down syndrome
    d. Congenital rubella syndrome

CHAPTER 70

# Sexuality, Fertility, and Sexually Transmitted Infections

## SECTION I: TESTING WHAT YOU KNOW

**Activity A** *Match the type of sexual orientation in Column A with its description in Column B.*

**Column A**

____ 1. Heterosexuals

____ 2. Homosexuals

____ 3. Bisexuals

____ 4. Asexuals

**Column B**

a. Individuals who are attracted to both sexes

b. Individuals who are attracted to the opposite sex

c. Individuals who are not particularly attracted to either sex

d. Individuals who are attracted to persons of the same sex

**Activity B** *Match the sexually transmitted infection in Column A with its causative agent in Column B.*

**Column A**

____ 1. Condylomata acuminata

____ 2. Moniliasis

____ 3. Chancroid

____ 4. Pediculosis pubis

**Column B**

a. *Candida albicans*

b. Pubic lice

c. Human papillomavirus

d. *Haemophilus ducreyi*

**Activity C** *Mark each statement as either "T" (True) or "F" (False). Correct any false statements.*

1. T F The only 100% effective method of birth control and protection against sexually transmitted infections is continual abstinence.

2. T F Artificial insemination can be used if the man's sperm count is low.

3. T F Syphilis is caused by a virus.

4. T F The most common sexual dysfunction in males is impotence.

5. T F Hormonal methods of contraception interfere with conception by physically preventing sperm from fertilizing ova.

**Activity D** *Fill in the blanks.*

1. Involuntary contraction of the vaginal outlet muscles, preventing penile penetration, is called ___________.
2. ___________ contraception is sometimes inaccurately referred to as the "morning-after pill."
3. Gonorrhea is caused by invasion of the bacteria ___________ *gonorrhoeae.*
4. A radiographic study called a ___________ looks for problems within the fallopian tubes and uterus.
5. ___________ contraceptives are also called birth control pills.

**Activity E** *Consider the following figure.*

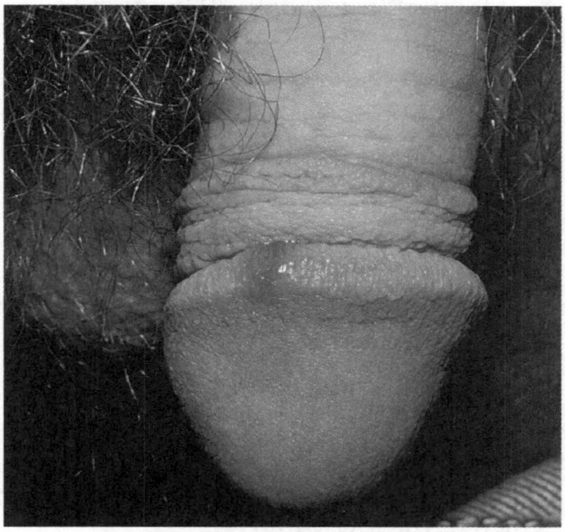

1. Identify the figure.

___________________________________

___________________________________

2. How does this condition spread?

___________________________________

___________________________________

3. What are the blood tests for this condition?

___________________________________

___________________________________

**Activity F** ***Methods of birth control are effective only if the individuals who use them do so correctly. Steps that occur when a nurse is instructing a client who has requested information about birth control are given below in random order. Write the correct sequence in the boxes provided.***

1. Teach the couple about the method selected, including any specific instructions.
2. Encourage participation of both client and husband. Determine the couple's knowledge level.
3. Review various methods of contraception that are available. Allow the couple to ask questions.
4. Provide information using different forms, including diagrams, charts, and pictures.

☐ → ☐ → ☐ → ☐

**Activity G** ***Briefly answer the following questions.***

1. What are the types of assisted reproductive technology?

___________________________________

___________________________________

2. What is the rhythm method?

___________________________________

___________________________________

3. What is Lunelle?

___________________________________

___________________________________

4. Why is tubal ligation referred to as the "Band-Aid tubal"?

___________________________________

___________________________________

5. What is emergency contraception?

___________________________________

___________________________________

## SECTION II: APPLYING WHAT YOU KNOW

**Activity H** *Answer the following questions, which involve the nurse's role in sexual healthcare.*

A nurse's role is to provide the client with pertinent information related to sexual concerns and birth control. The nurse should provide effective and accurate communication to make clients feel comfortable discussing personal issues and to ensure that they have correct knowledge.

1. A female client has come in for insertion of an intrauterine device (IUD).
   a. What is an IUD?
   b. What instructions should the nurse give the client?
   c. What are the three brands of IUDs that are available in the United States?
2. A female client who is infertile has come to the fertility clinic for an artificial insemination.
   a. What is infertility?
   b. How will the nurse determine whether the client is ovulating?
   c. What is artificial insemination?

## SECTION III: GETTING READY FOR NCLEX

**Activity I** *Answer the following questions.*

1. A 24-year-old client approaches a nurse for information on the use of oral contraceptives. Which of the following health problems can occur from the use of oral contraceptives?
   a. Increased rate of pelvic inflammatory disease
   b. Increased rate of cancers of the endometrium
   c. Increased rate of recurrent ovarian cysts
   d. Increased rate of cerebrovascular accidents
2. A 40-year-old client is planning to undergo a vasectomy. What is the information that the nurse should impart to the client?
   a. The procedure is relatively easy and has few complications.
   b. The client need not use any birth control measures after vasectomy.
   c. The client may lose his sexual potency or drive.
   d. The client should get a sperm count again after 1 year.
3. A client who delivered a baby 2 weeks ago asks the nurse about the use of the Today Sponge. During client education, the nurse should tell the client which of the following?
   a. Its effectiveness is higher in women who have had children.
   b. It is effective for up to 30 hours after insertion.
   c. It protects against sexually transmitted infections.
   d. It is kept in place for at least 6 hours.
4. Which of the following is a symptom of chlamydial infection in the male client?
   a. Chancre on the penis
   b. Yellowish-white discharge from the penis
   c. Pain and swelling in the testicles
   d. Numerous warts in the genital area
5. A nurse is informing a pregnant client about the contraceptives she can use in the postpartum period. Benefits of Depo-Provera include which of the following?
   a. It provides protection against sexually transmitted diseases.
   b. It ensures fewer chances of having an ectopic pregnancy.
   c. It can be used in clients with cardiac disorders.
   d. It is 99% effective in preventing pregnancy.
6. An 18-year-old male client is diagnosed with genital herpes. What client teaching should the nurse give the client?
   a. Keep the area moist to promote healing.
   b. Do not share food or engage in kissing.
   c. Wear synthetic underwear.
   d. Use a condom to prevent spread of the disease.

**7.** A 17-year-old female client has been admitted to the healthcare facility after a sexual assault. Which of the following nursing interventions are involved in caring for this client?

**a.** Instruct the client to take a shower first.

**b.** Instruct the client to douche before examination.

**c.** Provide emotional support.

**d.** Perform a pelvic examination immediately.

**8.** A 22-year-old female client who has had unprotected sex is apprehensive and wants to know more about emergency contraception. What instructions would the nurse give her about emergency contraception?

**a.** It does not offer protection against sexually transmitted diseases.

**b.** It must be taken 72 hours after unprotected sex.

**c.** It must be taken in two doses, 24 hours apart.

**d.** It offers 100% protection against pregnancy.

**9.** A 34-year-old male client who has a history of hypertension is being evaluated at the fertility clinic. Which of the following are likely to reduce his fertility? (Select all that apply.)

**a.** The client smokes marijuana regularly.

**b.** The client consumes alcohol daily.

**c.** The client has hypertension.

**d.** The client works as a clerk.

**e.** The client had an attack of mumps 5 years ago.

**10.** A nurse is assessing a female client diagnosed with gonorrhea. Which of the following is a symptom of gonorrhea? (Select all that apply.)

**a.** Yellow-green vaginal discharge

**b.** Purulent anal discharge

**c.** Cervical tenderness

**d.** Intense vulval itching

**e.** Multiple vulval warts

CHAPTER 71

# Fundamentals of Pediatric Nursing

## SECTION I: TESTING WHAT YOU KNOW

**Activity A** *Match the method of oxygen administration in Column A with its nursing consideration in Column B.*

**Column A**

____ 1. Isolette

____ 2. Hood

____ 3. Nasal cannula

____ 4. Tent

**Column B**

a. Monitor placement so that gas does not blow directly onto the baby's face.

b. Change linen and clothing frequently.

c. Observe child for dryness, because the oxygen is not humidified.

d. Make sure nares are clear of mucus.

**Activity B** *Match the restraints in Column A with their purpose in Column B.*

**Column A**

____ 1. Mummy restraint

____ 2. Papoose board

____ 3. Mitt

____ 4. Sleeve restraint

**Column B**

a. Used to keep the child from bending the arm, pulling on tubes or other devices, or disrupting a facial suture line

b. Used to restrain the entire body with a small blanket, exposing only the head

c. Commonly used for circumcising infants

d. Prevents the child from scratching or pulling on tubes

**Activity C** *Mark each statement as either "T" (True) or "F" (False). Correct any false statements.*

1. T F The nurse should use an infant seat for a child in respiratory distress.

2. T F A rubber-tipped bulb syringe may be used to administer an enema to an infant.

3. T F Oral hygiene for an infant involves wiping the baby's gums with a damp washcloth or gauze pad.

4. T F Twelve-year-olds who do not have a reliable history of chickenpox need not be immunized.

5. T F The occipital-frontal circumference (OFC) reflects intracranial volume pressure.

**Activity D** *Fill in the blanks.*

1. ___________ is a scaly scalp condition in infants that is also known as cradle cap.
2. The preferred site for venipuncture in infants is the femoral or ___________ area.
3. Catheterization can introduce ___________ into the bladder, causing urinary tract infections.
4. Pediatrics requires knowledge of developmental ___________ to help determine developmental delays in children.

**Activity E** *Consider the following figure.*

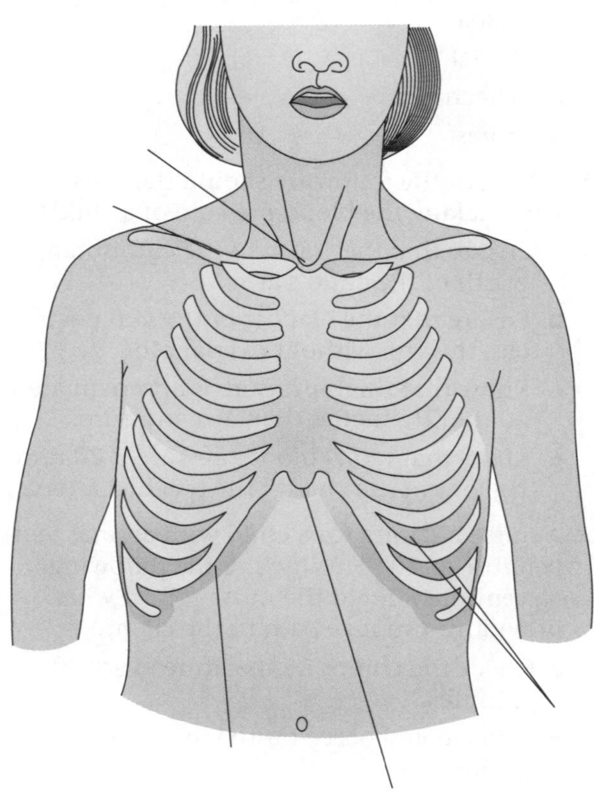

1. Label the sites of respiratory retraction.

______________________________________

______________________________________

2. What are the signs of pediatric respiratory distress?

______________________________________

______________________________________

**Activity F** *Steps that occur when a blood sample is to be taken from the jugular vein of a very young child are given below in random order. Write the correct sequence in the boxes provided.*

1. Restrain the child with the head extended over the table's edge.
2. Note any signs of swelling or bleeding.
3. Assist the physician by holding the child.
4. Pad the table edge and hold the child perfectly still.

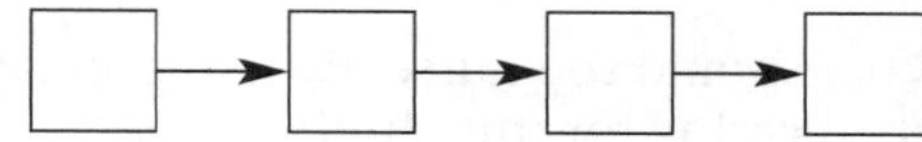

**Activity G** *Briefly answer the following questions.*

1. What is the goal of pediatric nursing?

______________________________________

______________________________________

2. Why is immunization needed?

______________________________________

______________________________________

3. What cross-cultural considerations should the nurse keep in mind when communicating with children at the healthcare facility?

______________________________________

______________________________________

4. What is gavage feeding?

______________________________________

______________________________________

## SECTION II: APPLYING WHAT YOU KNOW

**Activity H** *Answer the following questions, which involve the nurse's role in pediatric healthcare.*

The nurse understands that pediatric healthcare involves health maintenance and promotion as well as disease prevention. A nurse will encounter children of all ages in various health conditions at various healthcare settings.

1. A mother arrives at the healthcare facility with her 1-month-old infant for a checkup.
   a. What should the nurse observe generally when caring for this child?
   b. What specific observations should the nurse make?
2. A nurse is required to care for a 3-year-old child who is admitted to the healthcare facility.
   a. How can the nurse help the family and the child during their hospital experience?
   b. What factors affect the reactions of family caregivers?
3. A nurse is caring for a toddler at the healthcare clinic during one of his well-child visits.
   a. What should the nurse document during the well-child checkup?
   b. What teaching should the nurse provide the family caregivers?
   c. What observations should the nurse make during the visit?

## SECTION III: GETTING READY FOR NCLEX

**Activity I** *Answer the following questions.*

1. Which of the following should the nurse do when applying the clove hitch restraint to a child?
   a. Apply the restraint directly to the arm.
   b. Check the extremity every 2 hours.
   c. Take off the restraint every 4 hours.
   d. Tie a knot when applying the device.
2. A nurse is caring for an 8-year-old child with diarrhea. Which of the following interventions should the nurse perform when caring for the child?
   a. Observe the feet for signs of edema.
   b. Observe the child for skin excoriation.
   c. Take a rectal temperature for accuracy.
   d. Provide plenty of solids to prevent dehydration.
3. A child has been admitted to the healthcare facility for surgery. The nurse observes that the child is inactive, miserable, and clutching her blanket. The nurse understands that the child is in which of the following stages of anxiety?
   a. Despair
   b. Denial
   c. Detachment
   d. Protest
4. Which of the following should the nurse do when taking the blood pressure of a child?
   a. Ensure that the width of the cuff is half the width of the child's arm.
   b. Ensure that the bladder of the cuff encircles the arm without overlapping.
   c. Know that thigh pressure is approximately 10 mm Hg higher than arm pressure.
   d. Know that radial blood pressure is 20 mm Hg lower than that of the brachial artery.
5. A nurse is caring for a child with an oral temperature of 103°F. Which of the following interventions should the nurse follow when providing a sponge bath to the client?
   a. Check the child's temperature every 30 minutes.
   b. Add alcohol or ice for the tepid sponge bath.
   c. Maintain the water temperature at 70° to 85°F.
   d. Stop the sponge bath if the child shows signs of chilling.
6. Which of the following interventions should the nurse perform with regard to an infant's bath?
   a. Provide a tub bath every day.
   b. Wash the eyes after washing the face.
   c. Provide daily shampoo to prevent cradle cap.
   d. Probe the outer ear canals of the infant.

7. A 10-year-old child has just been brought to the nursing unit after abdominal surgery. Which of the following nursing interventions must the nurse perform for the child? (Select all that apply.)
   a. Assist the child to a side position.
   b. Check for return of peristalsis.
   c. Evaluate pain and discomfort.
   d. Ask the child not to move from bed.
   e. Prevent the child from deep breathing.
8. Which of the following interventions should the nurse consider when administering medications to a child? (Select all that apply.)
   a. Tell the child that she has been "good."
   b. Reassure the child that an injection will not hurt.
   c. Reassure the child that crying is okay.
   d. Keep the time of administration to a minimum.
   e. Ensure accuracy in medication administration.
9. A nurse in the pediatric unit of the healthcare facility may be required to assist in resuscitating a child. Which of the following should the nurse know if required to assist in the procedure?
   a. Emergency drugs are calculated according to a child's age.
   b. Drugs are administered based on the circumference of the child's head.
   c. A Broselow tape is used to measure the circumference of the child's chest.
   d. The Broselow system of length may be substituted for weight.
10. A nurse is evaluating the respiratory status of a child. Which of the following symptoms may indicate pediatric respiratory distress? (Select all that apply.)
   a. Head bobbing
   b. Fever
   c. Nasal flaring
   d. Wheezing
   e. Running nose

CHAPTER 72

# Care of the Infant, Toddler, or Preschooler

## SECTION I: TESTING WHAT YOU KNOW

**Activity A** ***Match the inflammatory diseases in Column A with their symptoms in Column B.***

| Column A | Column B |
|---|---|
| ____ 1. Glomerulonephritis | a. Nuchal rigidity |
| ____ 2. Meningitis | b. Lower back ache |
| ____ 3. Pyelonephritis | c. Hematuria |
| ____ 4. Epiglottitis | d. Drooling of saliva |

**Activity B** ***Match the neurologic disorders in Column A with their descriptions in Column B.***

| Column A | Column B |
|---|---|
| ____ 1. Meningocele | a. Congenitally small brain size with intellectual impairment |
| ____ 2. Hydrocephalus | b. Malformation in which one layer of the meninges protrudes through an opening in the vertebral column |
| ____ 3. Microcephaly | c. Collection of spinal fluid that causes head swelling and brain damage |

**Activity C** ***Mark each statement as either "T" (True) or "F" (False). Correct any false statements.***

1. T F Rickets is a disease caused by vitamin C deficiency.
2. T F Celiac disease occurs due to intolerance to the protein collagen.
3. T F In paralytic strabismus, the muscles of one eye are underactive.
4. T F Passive smoke inhalation is a primary cause of otitis media.
5. T F In megacolon disorder, the child's colon lacks a sympathetic nerve supply.
6. T F Ventricular septal defect is the most frequent congenital anomaly of the circulatory system.

**Activity D** ***Fill in the blanks.***

1. Reconstruction of the eardrum, usually with a graft of temporalis fascia, is known as ____________.
2. Phenylketonuria (PKU) is caused by the absence of the enzyme phenylalanine ____________.
3. Surgical repair of the cleft lip is called ____________.
4. Acute ____________ of the meninges of the brain is known as meningitis.

5. Narrowing of the right ventricular outflow tract of the heart, including the valve, is known as ____________ stenosis.
6. Tricuspid atresia is an ____________ of an opening between the right atrium and the right ventricle allowing no blood to flow from the right atrium to the right ventricle greatly decreasing pulmonary blood flow.

**Activity E** ***Consider the following figures.***

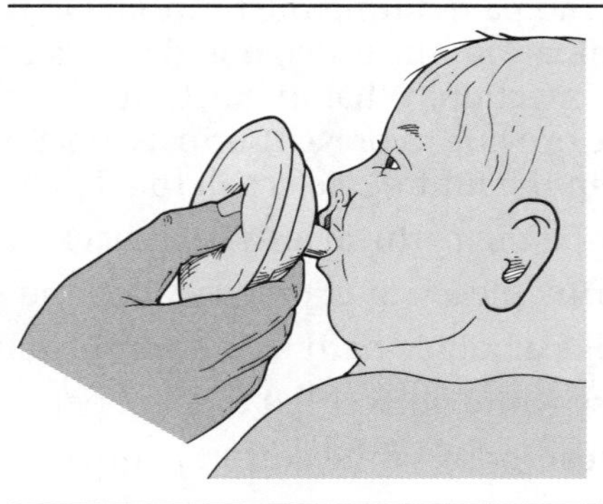

1. Identify the equipment in the figure.

______________________________

______________________________

2. Explain the use of this equipment.

______________________________

______________________________

3. Identify the equipment shown in the figure in the next column.

______________________________

______________________________

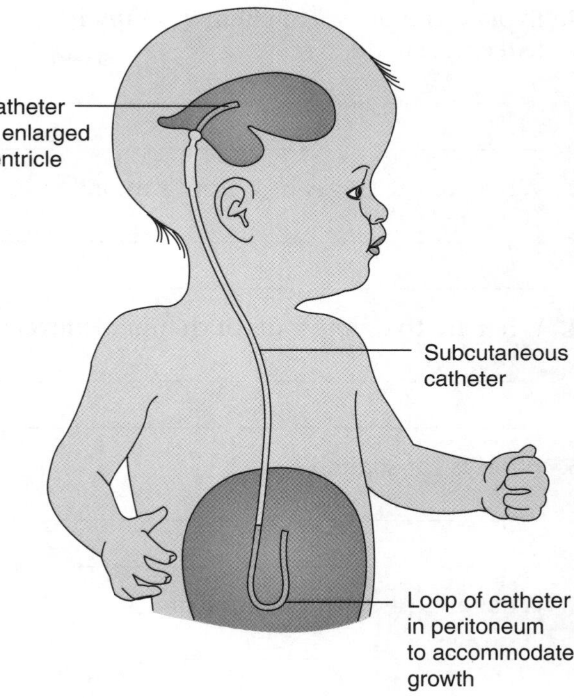


4. Explain the use of the equipment.

______________________________

______________________________

**Activity F** ***Ribavirin is the medication used for the treatment of bronchiolitis. Some of the steps that occur during the administration of ribavirin are given below in random order. Write the correct sequence in the boxes provided.***

1. Set up the equipment and medication.
2. Administer ribavirin using the hood.
3. Auscultate the lung fields thoroughly.
4. Disinfect the hands thoroughly.

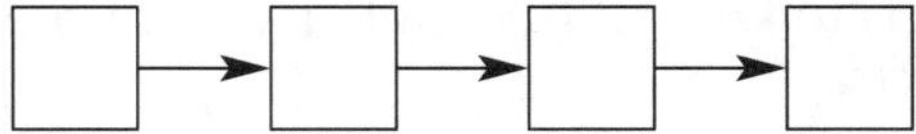

**Activity G** ***Briefly answer the following questions.***

1. How does leukemia affect children?

______________________________

______________________________

2. Explain the phases of chemotherapy for leukemic clients.

_______________

_______________

3. What are the stages of Wilms' tumor?

_______________

_______________

4. What are the symptoms of rheumatic fever?

_______________

_______________

5. What is cat-scratch fever?

_______________

_______________

6. What are the signs of sexual abuse?

_______________

_______________

## SECTION II: APPLYING WHAT YOU KNOW

**Activity H** ***Answer the following questions, which involve the nurse's role in infant, toddler, and preschooler healthcare.***

A nurse's role in caring for an infant, toddler, or preschooler involves monitoring signs and symptoms of any diseased condition, preventing diseases, and providing proper nourishment for the child.

1. During a routine visit to the healthcare clinic, a mother tells the nurse that her 2-year-old child is still in the habit of bottle feeding. She wants to know if this could have any adverse effects.
   a. What could be the possible adverse effects of baby-bottle syndrome?
   b. What instructions should the nurse give the parents to prevent this condition?
2. An 8-year-old child is brought to the primary healthcare facility with symptoms of easy bruising and frequent nosebleeds. The healthcare provider diagnoses the condition as idiopathic thrombocytopenic purpura.
   a. What symptoms should the nurse monitor for in such a case?
   b. What are the nursing considerations to be employed when caring for the client?

## SECTION III: GETTING READY FOR NCLEX

**Activity I** ***Answer the following questions.***

1. A 10-year-old girl complains of frequent urination and pain during micturition. On further examination, she is diagnosed with a urinary tract infection. What instruction should the nurse provide to prevent urinary tract infection in the future? (Select all that apply.)
   a. Wipe the perineal area from back to front.
   b. Drink plenty of cranberry juice and water.
   c. Take a bubble bath to prevent irritation.
   d. Use white, unscented toilet paper.
   e. Wear loose, white cotton panties.
2. A 7-year-old child was admitted to the healthcare facility because of frequent passage of loose and watery stools. The healthcare provider diagnoses it as a case of diarrhea. Which of the following should be included in the nursing care plan for the child?
   a. Encourage the late reintroduction of regular nutrients.
   b. Provide only clear fluids and juices to the child.
   c. Observe the child for any signs of dehydration.
   d. Cover the child's buttocks to prevent contact with air.
3. A 5-year-old child is diagnosed with iron deficiency anemia. The physician has prescribed administration of iron-containing preparations. Which of the following should be taken into consideration when administering iron-containing preparations to the client?
   a. Administer the preparation along with food to enhance absorption.
   b. Dilute the liquid iron preparation with water before administration.
   c. Avoid rinsing of the mouth after ingestion of the preparation.
   d. Avoid giving orange juice along with the medicine.

**4.** A nurse is required to care for a 4-year-old child who has sickle cell anemia. Which of the following should the nurse include in the parent teaching?

**a.** Avoid cold environments and high altitudes.

**b.** Practice handwashing to prevent disease transmission.

**c.** Give oral rehydration supplements to prevent dehydration.

**d.** Avoid gluten-containing food supplements.

**5.** A nurse is required to care for a 9-year-old child who has a Wilms' tumor. Which of the following nursing care measures should be employed when caring for the child?

**a.** Take tympanic temperatures to reduce hemorrhage.

**b.** Gently touch or move the child to prevent injury.

**c.** Avoid palpating the abdomen preoperatively.

**d.** Give gavage feedings or parenteral nutrition.

**6.** A 2-year-old child with a distended abdomen and absence of stool is diagnosed with cystic fibrosis. The client is prescribed a pancreatic enzyme preparation and some fat-soluble vitamin supplements. Which of the following nursing care measures should be followed when caring for the child? (Select all that apply.)

**a.** Administer water-soluble forms of fat-soluble vitamins.

**b.** Restrict salt in client's diet plan.

**c.** Monitor the weight of the client frequently.

**d.** Provide a low-calorie, low-protein, moderate-fat diet.

**e.** Give a pancreatic enzyme preparation along with cold milk.

**7.** A 7-year-old boy is brought to the healthcare facility with complaints of painful enlargement of the scrotum. Which of the following terms should be used to describe this condition?

**a.** Encephalocele

**b.** Meningocele

**c.** Hydrocele

**d.** Meningomyelocele

**8.** A 10-month-old baby who had a facial deformity has undergone cheiloplasty. Which of the following should be included in the postoperative care plan? (Select all that apply.)

**a.** Apply a tongue-blade arm restraint.

**b.** Use a straw to feed the baby.

**c.** Give the child water after the formula feed.

**d.** Cleanse the suture line after each feeding.

**e.** Position the child on the abdomen.

**9.** A nurse is required to care for a 5-year-old child who is in a cast with traction after a fracture of the right femur. Which of the following should the nurse monitor to check the blood circulation toward the injured area?

**a.** Heartbeat

**b.** Urine color

**c.** Skin color

**d.** Blood pressure

**10.** A nurse is required to care for a 10-month-old baby who has undergone palatoplasty for repair of a cleft palate. Which of the following nursing care measures should be employed when caring for the child?

**a.** Avoid positioning the child on the abdomen or the side.

**b.** Discourage the child from sucking and blowing.

**c.** Avoid feeding the child using a spoon.

**d.** Always use a nipple or straw to feed the child.

CHAPTER 73

# Care of the School-Age Child or Adolescent

## SECTION I: TESTING WHAT YOU KNOW

**Activity A** *Match the childhood disorders in Column A with their symptoms in Column B.*

| Column A | Column B |
|---|---|
| ____ 1. Lyme disease | a. Honey-colored crust |
| ____ 2. Impetigo contagiosa | b. Flu-like symptoms |
| ____ 3. Scoliosis | c. Ring-shaped rash |
| ____ 4. Mononucleosis | d. S-shaped spine |

**Activity B** *Match the diseases seen in school-age children or adolescents in Column A with their causes in Column B.*

| Column A | Column B |
|---|---|
| ____ 1. Acne vulgaris | a. Epstein-Barr virus |
| ____ 2. Mononucleosis | b. Hormonal changes |
| ____ 3. Encephalitis | c. Tick-borne bacteria |
| ____ 4. Lyme disease | d. Mosquito-borne pathogens |

**Activity C** *Mark each statement as either "T" (True) or "F" (False). Correct any false statements.*

1. T F Lordosis is an abnormal curvature of the thoracic spine that results in a "hunchback" appearance.
2. T F Structural scoliosis is a lateral curvature of the spine caused by poor posture.
3. T F The goal of treatment for Legg-Calve-Perthes disease is to maintain the head of the femur in the acetabulum.
4. T F Chronic ulcerative colitis can also lead to delay in the appearance of secondary sexual characteristics, if the disease occurs before puberty.
5. T F Somnambulism is more common in girls than in boys and is more common when children are excited or anxious.

**Activity D** *Fill in the blanks.*

1. Bone ____________ is the characteristic dark retinal pigmentation seen in people with retinitis pigmentosa.
2. ____________ is the term used to describe an attack of muscular weakness and lack of muscle tone.
3. The correction of tooth positioning and jaw deformities is known as ____________.
4. ____________ is the term used to describe involuntary bowel movements in school-age children.
5. The feeling of abnormal thirst is known as ____________.

**Activity E** *Consider the following figures.*

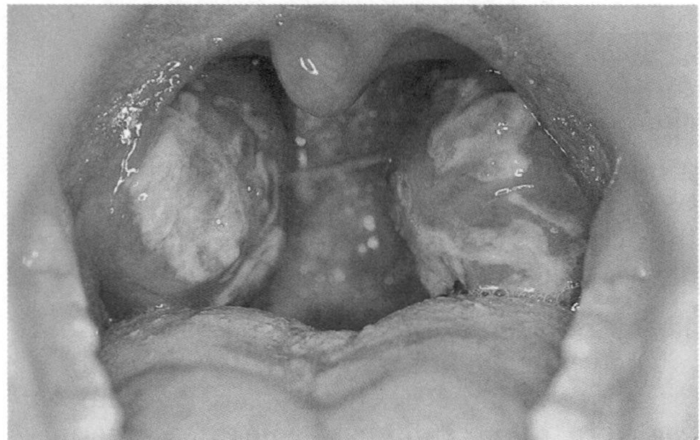

1. Identify what is shown in the figure.

______________________________

______________________________

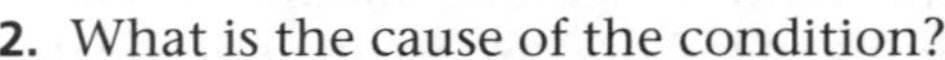

2. What is the cause of the condition?

______________________________

______________________________

3. Mention the various other signs and symptoms of this condition.

______________________________

______________________________

4. How is a client with this condition cared for?

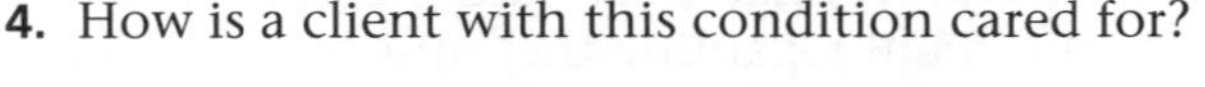

______________________________

______________________________

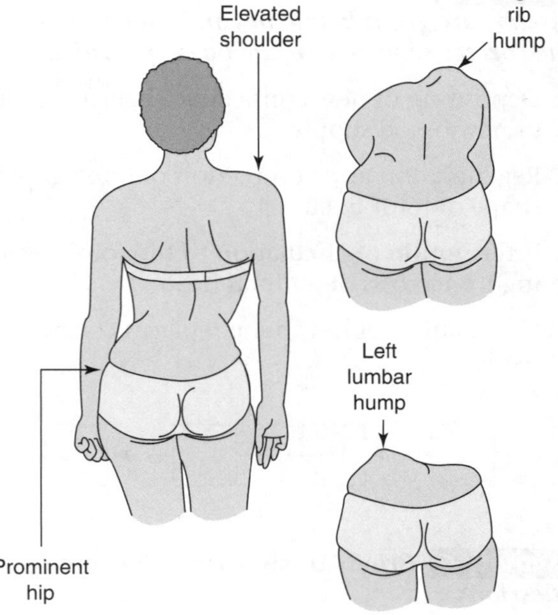


5. Identify what is shown in the figure.

______________________________

______________________________

6. Mention its various types.

______________________________

______________________________

7. What device is used to treat postural defects in clients with this condition?

______________________________

______________________________

8. What nursing diagnoses may be seen on the nursing care plan?

______________________________

______________________________

**Activity F** *The stages of Legg-Calve-Perthes disease are given below in random order. Write the correct sequence in the boxes provided.*

1. Depositing of new connective tissue because of new blood supply
2. Regeneration and completion of bone growth; shape of joint fixed
3. Interruption of circulation to hip joint, resulting in necrosis of femoral head
4. Granulation of new bone replaces connective tissue

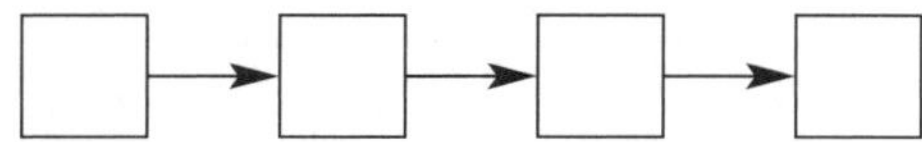

**Activity G** *Briefly answer the following questions.*

1. What is juvenile glaucoma?

___

___

2. What are the common elimination disorders of childhood?

___

___

3. What is gorge-purge syndrome?

___

___

4. What is hypersomnia?

___

___

5. What is dental malocclusion?

___

___

## SECTION II: APPLYING WHAT YOU KNOW

**Activity H** *Answer the following questions, which involve the nurse's role in school-age child or adolescent healthcare.*

A nurse's role in managing the care of the school-age child or adolescent involves assisting the clients in prevention and symptomatic care of various childhood diseases.

1. During a routine examination of a 7-year-old client, the parents of the client are concerned about a rash on the client's face. They are worried that their child has Lyme disease, because his elder brother had developed this condition a few years earlier.
   a. What explanation would the nurse provide the client's parents about the symptoms of Lyme disease?
   b. What preventive measures should the client and family members take to prevent the development of Lyme disease?
   c. What should the family members do when faced with a tick bite?
2. A 15-year-old male client is apprehensive about the development of acne on his face for the past few days. He wants to know why these eruptions are occurring on his face.
   a. What information should the nurse provide the client regarding the cause and development of acne?
   b. What instructions should the nurse give the client regarding acne care?

## SECTION III: GETTING READY FOR NCLEX

**Activity I** *Answer the following questions.*

1. Which of the following statements are true about children with school phobia?
   a. This condition is more common in boys than in girls.
   b. These children are usually very good students.
   c. This condition usually occurs before summer vacations.
   d. These children do not get physically ill in reality.

**2.** A 15-year-old client is brought to the healthcare facility with complaints of loss of control during overeating, followed by purging. Which of the following signs and symptoms must the nurse expect to find in the client during routine examination and care?

- **a.** Feelings of guilt and depression are rare.
- **b.** The client is usually underweight due to excessive vomiting.
- **c.** The client has a higher incidence of dental caries.
- **d.** Severe electrolyte imbalance is rarely seen.

**3.** An 11-year-old client with somniloquism is referred to the healthcare facility by the family physician. Which of the following symptoms would the nurse expect to find in the client during initial examination and case history recording?

- **a.** Cessation of breathing for short durations during sleep.
- **b.** Logical conversation or talking while sleeping.
- **c.** Difficulty in falling asleep due to an emotional problem.
- **d.** Walking, usually during the later stages of non-REM sleep.

**4.** Which of the following statements about narcolepsy is true?

- **a.** It is associated with seizures and convulsions.
- **b.** Girls are affected more often than boys.
- **c.** It is not associated with hallucinations.
- **d.** It may be precipitated by an emotional disturbance.

**5.** A 9-year-old client with chronic ulcerative colitis is being cared for at the healthcare facility. Which of the following would the nurse expect to find in such a client? (Select all that apply.)

- **a.** Weight loss
- **b.** Growth delays
- **c.** Constipation
- **d.** Anorexia
- **e.** Precocious puberty

**6.** Which of the following symptoms are seen in clients with diabetes mellitus type 1?

- **a.** Increased thirst
- **b.** Decreased urine output
- **c.** Increased weight gain
- **d.** Decreased hunger

**7.** A client diagnosed with Ewing's sarcoma is admitted to the healthcare facility with excruciating pain in his left leg. Which of the following facts should the nurse provide to the client's family members?

- **a.** The growth of tumors is often slow in children.
- **b.** Cancer cells rarely spread to the lungs in children.
- **c.** This cancer can also involve flat bones in the body.
- **d.** This cancer is more often seen in children younger than 6 years of age.

**8.** A 5-year-old client is brought to the healthcare facility with symptoms of intermittent limp on the left side and hip pain or soreness and stiffness. After further examinations, the client is diagnosed with Legg-Calvé-Perthes disease. Which of the following teachings must the nurse provide for the client's family members?

- **a.** The client should be on bed rest for an extended period.
- **b.** The disorder is self-limited and often resolves spontaneously.
- **c.** The client needs to move his leg frequently during bed rest.
- **d.** Application of heat in the form of whirlpool treatment is helpful.

9. A 14-year-old client is admitted to the health-care facility with complaints of headaches, low-grade fever, anorexia, and cervical lymphadenopathy. On further evaluation, the client is diagnosed with acute infectious mononucleosis. Which of the following facts about mononucleosis must the nurse keep in mind when caring for the client?
   a. Mononucleosis is caused by a bacterial infection.
   b. Upper airway obstruction can occur in clients with mononucleosis.
   c. Systemic steroids are always avoided in clients with mononucleosis.
   d. Mononucleosis often spreads though food and water.

10. Which of the following symptoms would the nurse expect to find in the client with Lyme disease? (Select all that apply.)
    a. Intellectual impairment
    b. Watery blisters that burn and itch
    c. Arthritis resembling rheumatoid arthritis
    d. Honey-colored crust over the face and hands
    e. Psychiatric disturbances

CHAPTER 74

# The Child or Adolescent with Special Needs

## SECTION I: TESTING WHAT YOU KNOW

**Activity A** *Match the syndromes in Column A with their characteristic features in Column B.*

| Column A | Column B |
|---|---|
| ____ **1.** Down syndrome | **a.** Large, protruding ears |
| ____ **2.** Fetal alcohol syndrome | **b.** Involuntary movements |
| ____ **3.** Fragile X syndrome | **c.** Tetralogy of Fallot |
| ____ **4.** Tourette syndrome | **d.** Small, low-set ears |

**Activity B** *Match the major classifications of cerebral palsy in Column A with their characteristic features in Column B.*

| Column A | Column B |
|---|---|
| ____ **1.** Spastic cerebral palsy | **a.** Spasticity and athetoid movements |
| ____ **2.** Dyskinetic cerebral palsy | **b.** Increased muscle tone or spasticity |
| ____ **3.** Ataxic cerebral palsy | **c.** Muscle weakness and lack of coordination |
| ____ **4.** Mixed cerebral palsy | **d.** Slow, writhing involuntary movements |

**Activity C** *Mark each statement as either "T" (True) or "F" (False). Correct any false statements.*

**1.** T F Macrocephaly is a distinguishing characteristic feature in children with fetal alcohol syndrome.

**2.** T F A child with Duchenne muscular dystrophy exhibits a waddling gait.

**3.** T F Dysarthria is difficulty with reading, spelling, or writing words.

**4.** T F The process of inhaling chemicals that produces a feeling of delirium or a "high" is known as huffing.

**5.** T F Breastfeeding is contraindicated in HIV-positive mothers.

**Activity D** *Fill in the blanks.*

**1.** ____________ is characterized by "cafe-au-lait" spots.

**2.** The nucleus of every human cell contains 23 pairs of ____________.

**3.** The type of spastic cerebral palsy that involves only one side of the body is termed spastic ____________.

**4.** A/An ____________ line is an abnormal crease running straight across the palms of children with Down syndrome.

**5.** Obsessive–____________ disorder is an anxiety disorder characterized by an intense need to repeat actions.

**Activity E** *Consider the following figures.*

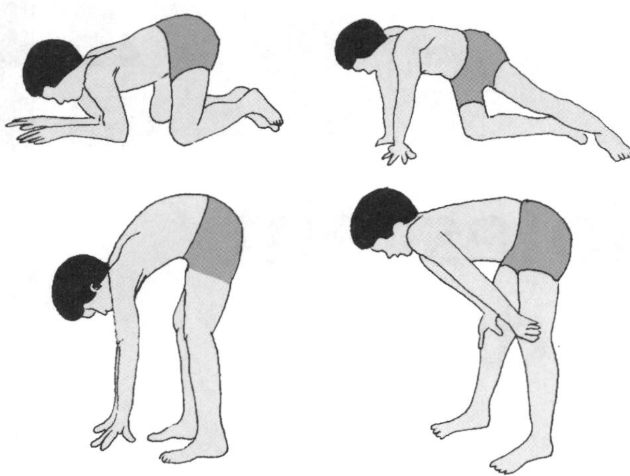

1. Identify the figure.

2. In which condition is this commonly seen?

3. What are the common clinical features of this condition?

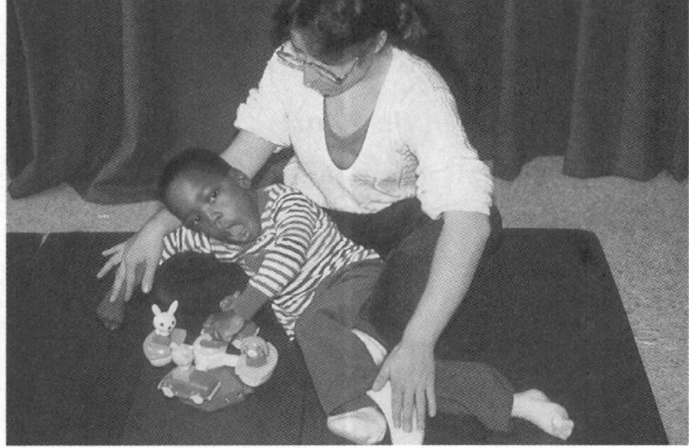

4. Identify the procedure shown in the figure.

5. What is the purpose of this procedure?

6. What devices can be used to aid ambulation in a child with cerebral palsy?

**Activity F** ***The nurse needs to assist a mentally disabled child with feeding because he or she may have difficulty sucking. The steps for feeding a mentally disabled child are given below in random order. Write the correct sequence in the boxes provided.***

1. Teach the child to suck by massaging the cheeks or using a special nipple.
2. Encourage the child to use the lips to remove food from the spoon.
3. Place food in the side of the mouth, not in the center, to prevent choking.
4. Ensure correct positioning to close the larynx, preferably in a sitting position.

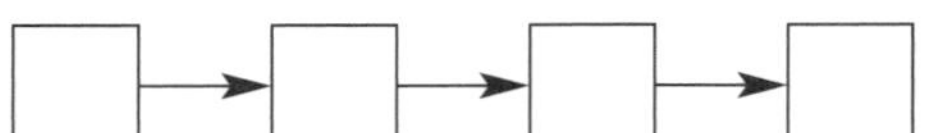

**Activity G** *Briefly answer the following questions.*

1. What are congenital disorders? Give four examples of congenital disorders.

2. What are developmental disabilities?

3. What is the importance of the alpha-fetoprotein test?

4. Name at least three maternal infections that result in long-term consequences in fetuses.

5. What is a suicide gesture?

______________________________________

______________________________________

6. Describe the features of children with a profound level of mental impairment.

______________________________________

______________________________________

## SECTION II: APPLYING WHAT YOU KNOW

**Activity H** ***Answer the following questions, which involve the nurse's role in the management of such situations.***

Children with special needs, such as those with physical or emotional disorders, have additional challenges. Family caregivers of such children also go through a grieving process. The nurse's role includes providing support and education to the client as well as the family.

1. A 10-year-old boy with Down syndrome is prescribed an adenoidectomy. This is the client's first hospitalization.
   a. What are the various observations and data collections a nurse should make in this client?
   b. What are the nursing actions required to help the client develop trust in the nurse?
   c. How will the nurse assist the client in making his needs known to the nurse?
2. A 12-year-old girl is brought to the psychiatric healthcare facility by her grandfather. It is reported that the girl's parents died in a recent motor vehicle accident. The grandfather reports depression and a marked change in the behavior of the child. The provider instructs the nurse to keep the child under observation.
   a. What are the common risk factors the nurse should be aware of while caring for this client?
   b. What behavioral changes should the nurse monitor for in the client, which could indicate a need for intervention?
   c. What measures must the nurse take to promote self-esteem in suicidal clients?

## SECTION III: GETTING READY FOR NCLEX

**Activity I** ***Answer the following questions.***

1. A neonate born to a client who used narcotic analgesics during the last trimester of her pregnancy is diagnosed with neonatal abstinence syndrome. Which of the following features would the nurse observe in the baby?
   a. Blue-black line on the gums
   b. Hyperactive Moro reflex
   c. Positive Gowers' sign
   d. White spots on the iris
2. An 11-year-old child with Down syndrome is hospitalized to undergo minor dental surgery. Which of the following nursing measures should the nurse perform when caring for the client?
   a. Assist with all activities of daily life.
   b. Avoid using the child's personal items.
   c. Note any verbal or nonverbal expressions.
   d. Give a detailed explanation of the surgery.
3. A nurse is caring for children with specific disabilities in a pediatric rehabilitation center. What special consideration should the nurse keep in mind when helping in behavior modification of these children?
   a. Teach feeding skills in a group.
   b. Use baby talk with those who have speech impairments.
   c. Praise them for all work that is done well.
   d. Do not allow family members to interfere.
4. A newborn infant is diagnosed with Down syndrome. Where would the nurse find Brushfield's spots in the infant?
   a. Irises
   b. Hands
   c. Tongue
   d. Cheeks
5. A nurse is caring for a 9-year-old boy diagnosed with attention deficit–hyperactivity disorder (ADHD). Which of the following features will the nurse notice in this client?
   a. Takes good care of belongings
   b. Continuously clears his throat
   c. Has a poor attention span
   d. Has difficulty talking

6. A 12-year-old client with degenerative disorder of the basal ganglia and cerebellum is admitted to the hospital for special nursing care and attention. The client is instructed to stay in the hospital for an extended period. Which of the following is most important during the long-term care of such clients?
   a. Allow two to three nurses to assist in caring for the client.
   b. Allow the client to learn self-care gradually.
   c. Explain treatments just before they are done.
   d. Keep the client away from social contacts.
7. A 2-year-old child with significant behavioral changes, lack of response to verbal stimuli, and a dislike of being touched or cuddled is diagnosed as autistic. Which of the following are features of autism spectrum disorder (ASD)?
   a. It is not actually a disease but a syndrome of specific behaviors.
   b. Autism spectrum disorder usually has a well-identified cause.
   c. Compared to boys, more girls are affected with autism.
   d. Autistic children typically demonstrate a profound loss of hearing.
8. Which of the following distinctive physical features should the nurse associate with fragile X syndrome in a client? (Select all that apply.)
   a. Long face
   b. Small head
   c. Large ears
   d. Broad nose
   e. Low palate
9. An 18-year-old client is admitted to the rehabilitation center for polysubstance abuse. The client was addicted to smoking marijuana and tobacco and was regularly consuming alcohol. What damage could marijuana abuse cause to the client's central nervous system? (Select all that apply.)
   a. Disturbed equilibrium
   b. Tactile hallucinations
   c. Myocardial infarction
   d. Perceptual difficulties
   e. Personality changes
10. An 8-year-old client has been diagnosed with attention deficit–hyperactivity disorder (ADHD) by the healthcare provider. The client lives with her grandparents, who are very old and have a low family income. What special nursing considerations should be kept in mind when providing care for such clients? (Select all that apply.)
   a. Be aware of the client's economic condition.
   b. Encourage homebound education.
   c. Encourage participation in age-appropriate activities.
   d. Emphasize the importance of regular follow-up care.
   e. Observe and document functional level of the child.

CHAPTER 75

# Skin Disorders

## SECTION I: TESTING WHAT YOU KNOW

**Activity A** ***Match the dermatologic condition in Column A with its description in Column B.***

**Column A**

____ 1. Vitiligo

____ 2. Angioma

____ 3. Furuncle

____ 4. Psoriasis

**Column B**

a. A chronic, noncontagious, proliferative skin disorder characterized by red papules covered with silvery, yellow-white scales

b. A condition characterized by depigmented areas of the skin

c. Vascular skin tumor that involves the underlying tissues and blood vessels

d. A firm, red, tender nodule also called a boil

**Activity B** ***Match the type of graft in Column A with its description in Column B.***

**Column A**

____ 1. Autograft

____ 2. Homograft

____ 3. Xenograft

**Column B**

a. Graft in which cadaver skin or skin from another person is used

b. Graft using another animal's skin/hide

c. Graft using the client's own skin

**Activity C** ***Mark each statement as either "T" (True) or "F" (False). Correct any false statements.***

1. T F Special precautions should be taken if there are boils on the face, because the skin area drains directly into the cranial venous sinuses.

2. T F Clear indications of smoke inhalation are singed nasal hairs, facial burns, and soot-stained sputum.

3. T F Bedbug bites appear as groups of eight to nine nodules.

4. T F Inadequate moisture in the skin contributes to folliculitis, a staphylococcal infection of the hair follicle.

5. T F Skin and eyes are commonly affected by chemical burns.

**Activity D** ***Fill in the blanks.***

1. Urticaria is characterized by the sudden appearance of edematous, raised pink areas, called ____________, that itch and burn.

2. Nail loosening at the beginning of the fingertips is called ____________.

3. ____________ are small, brown papules caused by the human papillomavirus (HPV).

4. In ____________ dermatitis, there is scaling, primarily of the scalp and often associated with itching.

5. Mafenide acetate is associated with burning after application and also with development of metabolic ____________.

**Activity E** *Consider the following figure.*

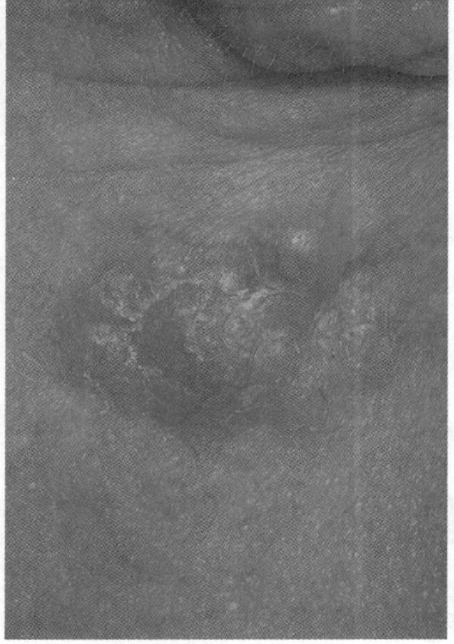

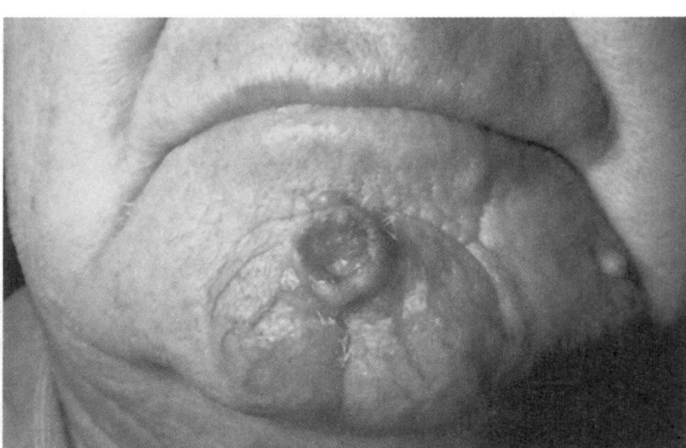

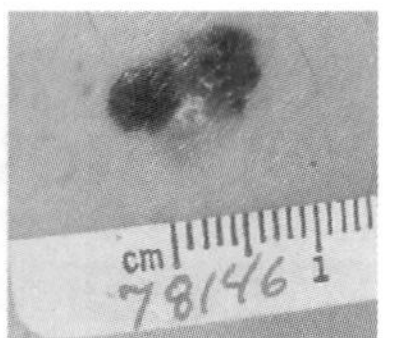


1. Identify the figure and list the individuals who are at risk of developing this condition.

 ______________________________

 ______________________________

2. What changes in a mole or wart warrants notification of a healthcare provider?

 ______________________________

 ______________________________

**Activity F** ***The steps that are undertaken during management of a burn injury are given below in random order. Write the correct sequence in the boxes provided.***

1. Wound dressing
2. Physical therapy
3. Vital signs assessment
4. Pain management

☐ → ☐ → ☐ → ☐

**Activity G** ***Briefly answer the following questions.***

1. What is the purpose of Tzanck's smear? How is it performed?

 ______________________________

 ______________________________

2. List some of the systemic disorders that cause pruritus.

 ______________________________

 ______________________________

3. What precautions need to be undertaken when caring for clients with skin problems?

 ______________________________

 ______________________________

4. What is the purpose of applying moist packs?

 ______________________________

 ______________________________

## SECTION II: APPLYING WHAT YOU KNOW

**Activity H** ***Answer the following questions, which involve the nurse's role in the management of burn injuries.***

A nurse's role in the management of a burn injury during the resuscitative phase involves monitoring vital signs and noting any changes, monitoring the client's respiratory status, and measuring pulse oximetry, blood gases, and pH frequently. The nurse also assesses for infection and helps in pain management.

1. A client has been brought to the emergency department with third-degree burns after an accidental oil spillage.
   - **a.** What are the three phases of burn injury management?
   - **b.** What are the standard precautionary measures taken when caring for a client with burns?
   - **c.** What precautionary measures should a nurse take when caring for a client with extensive burns?
2. A nurse, when assessing a client with burns, notices singed nasal hairs and soot-stained sputum.
   - **a.** What do singed nasal hairs and soot-stained sputum indicate?
   - **b.** What assessments should a nurse perform in this case?

## SECTION III: GETTING READY FOR NCLEX

**Activity I** ***Answer the following questions.***

1. A client with complaints of itching is prescribed diphenhydramine HCl (Benadryl) by the healthcare provider. What client teaching should the nurse provide with regard to the use of antihistamines?
   - **a.** Limit intake of fluids.
   - **b.** Avoid taking with milk.
   - **c.** Avoid use of sunscreen.
   - **d.** Avoid intake of alcohol.
2. A client has been admitted to a healthcare facility with extensive burns. Which of the following should the nurse perform soon after admission?
   - **a.** Assessment of vital signs
   - **b.** Application of synthetic dressing
   - **c.** Preparation for wound debridement
   - **d.** Preparation for whirlpool treatment
3. A 5-year-old client is brought to a healthcare facility with complaints of head lice infestation. Which of the following characteristics of lice infestation should the nurse monitor this client for?
   - **a.** Row of blackish dots with tiny vesicles
   - **b.** Groups of eight to nine nodules
   - **c.** Presence of nits inhabiting the hair
   - **d.** Presence of red macular lesions
4. Which of the following methods is used for the removal of filiform warts?
   - **a.** Debridement
   - **b.** Electrodessication
   - **c.** Escharotomy
   - **d.** Photochemotherapy
5. What teaching should the nurse impart to clients with eczema?
   - **a.** Use soaps that are more alkaline.
   - **b.** Use lotions containing lanolin.
   - **c.** Use a lotion containing menthol.
   - **d.** Take starch baths daily.
6. A client with psoriasis is prescribed a topical application of Dovonex (calcipotriene). Which of the following is achieved through the use of Dovonex?
   - **a.** It slows the development of skin cells.
   - **b.** It softens the scales.
   - **c.** It reduces the skin edema.
   - **d.** It retards skin inflammation.
7. A client admitted to a healthcare facility with urticaria has developed angioedema. Which of the following findings should the nurse notify the healthcare provider of? (Select all that apply.)
   - **a.** Small pruritic vesicles
   - **b.** Respiratory distress
   - **c.** Scaly patches on the skin
   - **d.** Swelling around the eyes
   - **e.** Extreme swelling of the lips

**8.** A nurse is caring for a client with severe burns who has developed skin ulcers. Which of the following are other complications associated with burn injury? (Select all that apply.)

**a.** Hypostatic pneumonia

**b.** Kidney failure

**c.** Asthma

**d.** Curling's ulcers

**e.** Angioma

**9.** Which of the following are precautionary measures to be followed to prevent an accident when handling electric equipment?

**a.** Always use multiple outlet plugs.

**b.** Tape the frayed cord of equipment before use.

**c.** Ensure cords are concealed under a rug.

**d.** Keep water heater's thermostat set lower than 120°F.

**10.** A client with second-degree burns has been prescribed moist dressing applications. Given below, in random order, are the steps undertaken during the application of moist dressings for a client with burn injury. Write the correct sequence.

**a.** Apply dressing according to specific protocol.

**b.** Premedicate with analgesics and anxiolytics.

**c.** Document the observations made during the procedure.

**d.** Premoisten existing dressings with normal saline.

CHAPTER 76

# Disorders in Fluid and Electrolyte Balance

## SECTION I: TESTING WHAT YOU KNOW

**Activity A** *Match the type of edema in Column A with its description in Column B.*

| Column A | Column B |
|---|---|
| ____ **1.** Pulmonary edema | **a.** Observable edema that dents under slight finger pressure |
| ____ **2.** Pitting edema | **b.** Edema that occurs in an area that hangs down |
| ____ **3.** Dependent edema | **c.** Edema of the sacral area in the bedridden client |
| ____ **4.** Sacral edema | **d.** Accumulation of interstitial fluid in the lungs |

**Activity B** *Match the acid–base balance disturbance in Column A with its possible cause in Column B.*

| Column A | Column B |
|---|---|
| ____ **1.** Metabolic acidosis | **a.** Kyphoscoliosis |
| ____ **2.** Respiratory acidosis | **b.** Mechanical ventilation |
| ____ **3.** Metabolic alkalosis | **c.** Alcoholic ketoacidosis |
| ____ **4.** Respiratory alkalosis | **d.** Diuretic therapy |

**Activity C** *Mark each statement as either "T" (True) or "F" (False). Correct any false statements.*

**1.** T F High protein levels cause fluid retention and edema.

**2.** T F Decreased sodium levels cause water to be drawn out of the circulation and into the tissues.

**3.** T F Excessive administration of sodium bicarbonate causes respiratory alkalosis.

**4.** T F Prolonged fever can cause fluid volume deficit leading to dehydration.

**5.** T F Hypernatremia occurs in diabetes insipidus.

**Activity D** *Fill in the blanks.*

**1.** Excess production of antidiuretic hormone results in ____________ retention.

**2.** Potassium is primarily excreted by the ____________.

**3.** ____________ is the term used for tingling in the fingers and toes.

**4.** Excess calcium excretion in urine is called ____________.

**5.** Fasting and starvation result in ____________ acidosis.

**Activity E** *Consider the following figures.*

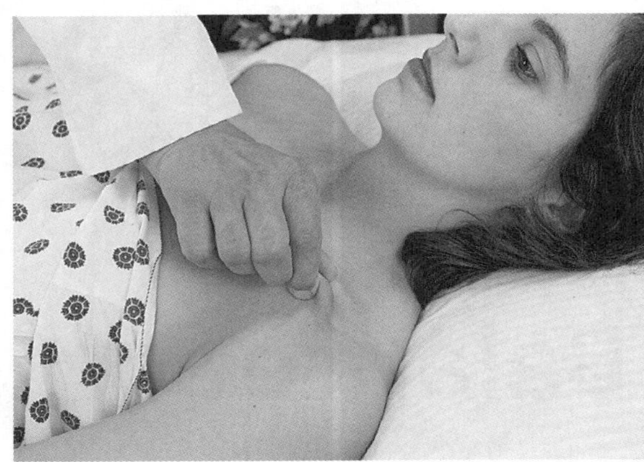

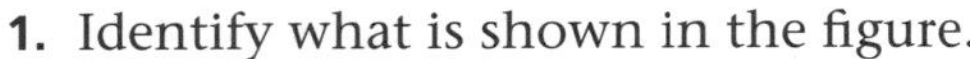

1. Identify what is shown in the figure.

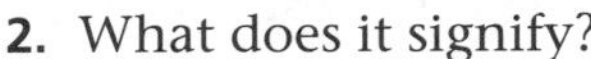

2. What does it signify?

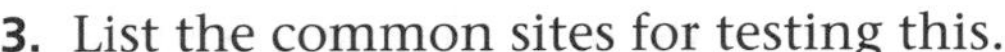

3. List the common sites for testing this.

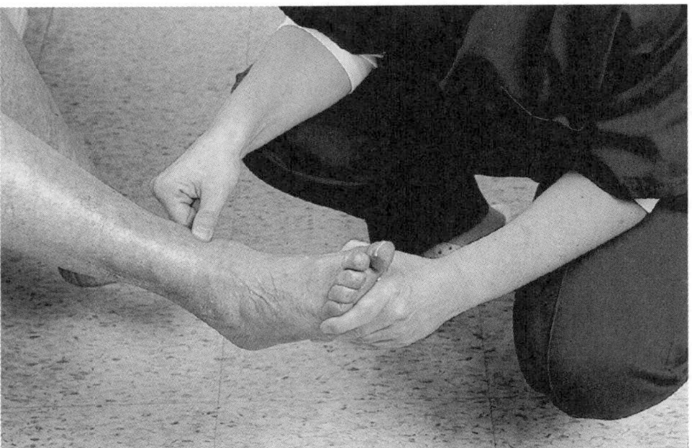

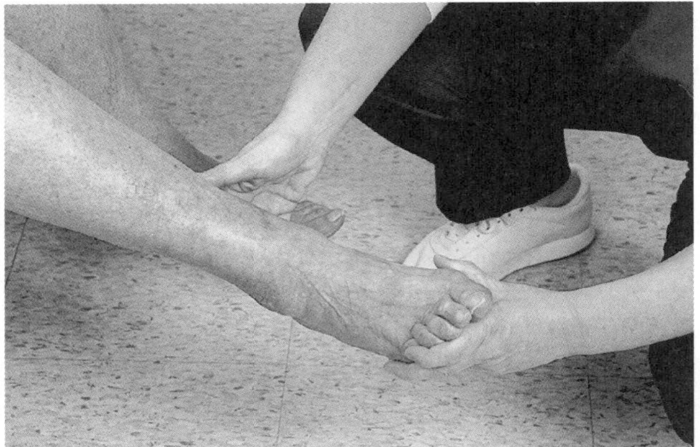

4. Identify what is shown in the figure.

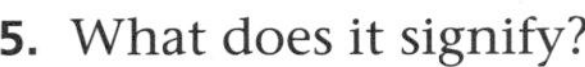

5. What does it signify?

**Activity F** ***A condition called respiratory acidosis may occur with administration of large doses of certain drugs, such as barbiturates and narcotic analgesics, that cause hypoventilation. Steps that occur during the nursing management of a client with a narcotic overdose are given below in random order. Write the correct sequence in the boxes provided.***

1. Administer oxygen to the client as ordered.
2. Notify the healthcare provider of respiratory changes.
3. Give stimulants or narcotic antagonists as ordered.
4. Elevate the head end of the bed as ordered.

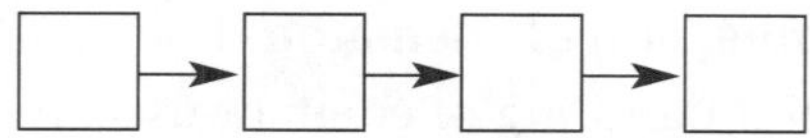

**Activity G** ***Briefly answer the following questions.***

1. What is meant by the term "homeostasis"?
2. When are electrolytes administered intravenously?
3. What is the unit of measure for electrolytes?
4. What are the functions of sodium in the body?
5. What are the causes of hypophosphatemia?

## SECTION II: APPLYING WHAT YOU KNOW

**Activity H** ***Answer the following questions, which involve the nurse's role in maintaining fluid–electrolyte balance.***

A nurse's role in managing fluid–electrolyte balance disturbances involves collecting and documenting data about a client's fluid and electrolyte balance. The nurse also assists clients with mouth and skin care.

1. A nurse is providing assistance with mouth and skin care in a 25-year-old client who is admitted to a healthcare facility with complaints of persistent watery diarrhea for the past 5 days.
   a. What should the nurse observe for when collecting and documenting data about the fluid and electrolyte balances of the client?
   b. What is the most likely nursing diagnosis?
   c. Why should the nurse provide assistance with mouth and skin care in this client?
2. A nurse is caring for a 35-year-old client who was admitted to a healthcare facility with complaints of decreased urination for the past month. The client has hypotension, has been losing weight rapidly over the past month, and has dry skin.
   a. What is the most likely nursing diagnosis?
   b. What are the requirements of a client with fluid or electrolyte imbalance?
   c. How is fluid balance assessed?

## SECTION III: GETTING READY FOR NCLEX

**Activity I** ***Answer the following questions.***

1. Which of the following hormones is known to control the level of potassium in the body?
   a. Aldosterone
   b. Calcitonin
   c. Parathormone
   d. Antidiuretic hormone
2. A nurse is assessing a client with a chronic liver disorder. The client has hypertension, ascites, and extremity edema on examination. Which of the following is the most probable nursing diagnosis?
   a. Excess fluid volume
   b. Impaired urinary elimination
   c. Deficient fluid volume
   d. Impaired tissue integrity
3. A nurse is assessing a client who has developed a pathologic fracture of the right tibia due to primary hypoparathyroidism. Which of the following electrolyte disturbances should the nurse monitor for?
   a. Hypokalemia
   b. Hypocalcemia
   c. Hypochloremia
   d. Hyponatremia

4. A nurse is giving dietary recommendations to a client who is diagnosed with vitamin D deficiency and complains of tingling in the fingers and toes and muscle twitching. Which of the following should be increased in the diet?
   a. Chloride
   b. Sodium
   c. Magnesium
   d. Calcium

5. A client admitted to a healthcare facility for salicylate overdosage has deep respirations with rapid breathing, lightheadedness, dizziness, and paresthesia. On examination, Chvostek's and Trousseau's signs are positive. The client's pH is increased and $PCO_2$ is decreased on arterial blood gas evaluation. Which of the following acid–base imbalances should the nurse document for this client?
   a. Respiratory alkalosis
   b. Respiratory acidosis
   c. Metabolic acidosis
   d. Metabolic alkalosis

6. A client who self-medicated for constipation presents to a healthcare facility with complaints of weakness and has diminished deep-tendon reflexes and hypotension on examination. The laboratory results reveal a serum magnesium level of 3 mEq/L. What immediate action should the nurse take?
   a. Decrease magnesium intake
   b. Connect to cardiac monitor
   c. Give calcium gluconate
   d. Increase oral fluids

7. A client diagnosed with left-sided heart failure develops rapid, shallow respirations, shortness of breath, and cough. What immediate action should the nurse take?
   a. Give the client a cough expectorant.
   b. Ask the client to breathe into a paper bag.
   c. Auscultate chest and report to physician.
   d. Start intravenous fluids and monitor.

8. A client is receiving long-term thiazide diuretic therapy for hypertension. What should the nurse monitor for in this client? (Select all that apply.)
   a. Signs of potassium deficit
   b. Signs of fluid volume excess
   c. Signs of acid–base imbalance
   d. Signs of dehydration
   e. Signs of hypernatremia

9. A nurse is teaching a client with chronic renal failure who is being cared for at home and the client's family about how to handle edematous areas. Which of the following should be included in the client and family teaching? (Select all that apply.)
   a. Compression of edematous body part
   b. Careful handling of edematous skin
   c. Frequent position changing
   d. Monitoring for tenting of skin
   e. Elevation of edematous body part

10. Which of the following clinical features should a nurse look for in a client with metabolic alkalosis? (Select all that apply.)
   a. Hyperreflexia
   b. Rapid breathing
   c. Convulsions
   d. Tetany
   e. Hypertension

CHAPTER 77

# Musculoskeletal Disorders

## SECTION I: TESTING WHAT YOU KNOW

**Activity A** *Match the diagnostic procedure in Column A with its definition in Column B.*

**Column A**

____ 1. Arthrogram

____ 2. Myelogram

____ 3. Arthrocentesis

____ 4. Arthroscopy

**Column B**

a. X-ray exam of spinal cord after injection of a contrast medium or air

b. Aspiration of synovial fluid, blood, or pus from a joint cavity

c. An invasive procedure using a special endoscope to view joints

d. X-ray study of a joint after injection of a contrast medium or air

**Activity B** *Match the musculoskeletal disorder in Column A with its definition in Column B.*

**Column A**

____ 1. Gout

____ 2. SLE

____ 3. Scleroderma

____ 4. Rickets

**Column B**

a. Autoimmune skin disorder leading to the formation of immune-complex and tissue damage

b. Accumulation of uric acid crystals in the joints

c. Disease that results from a deficiency of vitamin D during childhood

d. Collagen disorder that involves chronic hardening and shrinking of connective tissues

**Activity C** *Mark each statement as either "T" (True) or "F" (False). Correct any false statements.*

1. T F A wrist fracture in an elderly client caused by the act of getting up out of a chair is called a pathologic fracture.

2. T F Women are more prone to fractures than men until the age of 45 years.

3. T F Osteogenic sarcoma, chondrosarcoma, and multiple myeloma are examples of primary benign bone tumors.

4. T F Compartment syndrome results from inadequate or obstructed blood flow to muscles, nerves, and tissues.

5. T F Pulmonary embolism is the most common embolism associated with fractures.

**Activity D** *Fill in the blanks.*

1. ____________ of the spine is known as Pott's disease.
2. The process of loosening of fragments of dead bone is called ____________.
3. Repair or replacement of a joint is called ____________.
4. The halo device is a form of ____________ fixation device.
5. The procedure of covering the rough edges of a cast with tape is called ____________.

**Activity E** *Consider the following figures.*



1. Identify the condition shown in the figure.

______________________________________________

______________________________________________

2. What are the other complications of this condition?

______________________________________________

______________________________________________

3. How is the condition caused?

______________________________________________

______________________________________________

4. Identify the type of traction and splint in the figure.

______________________________________________

______________________________________________

5. What is the purpose of the trapeze?

______________________________________________

______________________________________________

**Activity F** ***Steps that occur during open reduction and internal fixation are given below in random order. Write the correct sequence in the boxes provided.***

1. Reduction of the fracture ends.
2. Insertion of a pin, wire, or screw into the bone.
3. Debridement of the dead and damaged tissue.
4. Splinting of the fractured area.

☐ → ☐ → ☐ → ☐

**Activity G** ***Briefly answer the following questions.***

1. What are hip fractures, and what are their common complications in the elderly?

______________________________________________

______________________________________________

2. What are the advantages of a synthetic cast?

______________________________________________

______________________________________________

3. What are strains, and how are they treated?

______________________________________________

______________________________________________

4. What is the difference between rickets and osteomalacia?

_______________________________________________

_______________________________________________

5. What are the signs and symptoms of gout?

_______________________________________________

_______________________________________________

## SECTION II: APPLYING WHAT YOU KNOW

**Activity H** *Answer the following questions, which involve the nurse's role in the management of musculoskeletal disorders.*

A nurse's role in managing musculoskeletal disorders involves assisting clients in the symptomatic care of the condition.

1. A 56-year-old client is diagnosed with arthritis. The client and family are apprehensive about the condition and want to know how they can assist in reducing the pain. They would also like to know how to exercise with arthritis.
   a. What are the clinical features of arthritis?
   b. What explanation should the nurse give regarding management of pain in a client with arthritis?
   c. What information should the nurse provide this client with regard to exercising?
2. A 25-year-old client involved in an accident is diagnosed with a simple fracture in the tibia of the left leg. A plaster cast is applied to the client's left leg. The client is apprehensive about the cast being applied and complains of discomfort.
   a. What information should the nurse provide regarding the advantages of applying a cast to a fractured limb?
   b. What instructions should the nurse provide to the client about care of the cast?
   c. What instructions should the nurse provide to the client before removal of the cast?

## SECTION III: GETTING READY FOR NCLEX

**Activity I** *Answer the following questions.*

1. A client is diagnosed with an oblique fracture to the ulna. A cast is applied to the client's arm to immobilize the fractured area. What assessment would indicate complications of pressure due to immobilization?
   a. Warmer temperature in the fingers of the affected hand
   b. Rapid return of color when the nail bed is compressed
   c. Lack of distal pulsation in the affected arm
   d. Elevated temperature and hypotension
2. A nurse is caring for an elderly client who has undergone hip replacement surgery. What measures must the nurse employ when caring for the client? (Select all that apply.)
   a. Turn the client every 1 to 2 hours from the unaffected side to the back.
   b. Support the client with pillows or sandbags and trochanter rolls.
   c. Avoid elevating the head of the bed when the client is on her back.
   d. Place a trapeze on the overhead frame over the client's bed.
   e. Discourage early mobility in the client after the surgery.
3. A young client is diagnosed with a dislocation of the hip joint after a motorcycle accident. The dislocated segment is repositioned and stabilized with traction. What measures must the nurse employ when caring for a client with traction?
   a. Ensure that the weights on the traction rest on the floor.
   b. Ensure that the footpiece is touching the pulleys at the bottom of the bed.
   c. Place a pillow under the extremity in traction.
   d. Encourage the client to frequently position the ankles in a neutral position.

4. An adult client who has undergone spinal fusion surgery is put in a body cast. The client complains of frequent abdominal pains and a bloated feeling. What considerations must the nurse employ when caring for a client in a body cast?
   a. Avoid frequent turning of the client lying in bed.
   b. Report the symptoms to the healthcare provider.
   c. Stabilize the client's cast by placing a plastic wedge inside it.
   d. Discourage the client from performing isometric exercises.
5. What type of traction would be used for a 2-year-old client with a fracture of the femur?
   a. Bryant's traction
   b. Pelvic traction
   c. Dunlop's traction
   d. Balanced traction
6. Which of the following statements is true about a client with malignant bone tumor?
   a. Malignant tumors spread slowly and rarely involve the lungs.
   b. Sarcomas tend to metastasize to bone more commonly than do carcinomas.
   c. Malignant bone tumors can lead to pathologic fractures.
   d. Primary bone tumors travel to the bone from some other part of the body.
7. A young client with a cast on his fractured arm visits the healthcare facility with complaints of pain that is unrelieved by medications and aggravated by passive stretching of the arm. The client also exhibits signs and symptoms of swelling, tightness, and paresthesia of the affected extremity. What do these symptoms indicate?
   a. Compartment syndrome
   b. Hemorrhage
   c. Deep vein thrombosis
   d. Atelectasis
8. An adult female client diagnosed with scleroderma comes to a healthcare facility with complaints of joint pains. What considerations must the nurse employ when caring for a client with scleroderma?
   a. Teach the client isometric exercises for the quadriceps.
   b. Evaluate the client's neurologic function at frequent intervals.
   c. Instruct the client to avoid smoking and exposure to cold.
   d. Teach the client never to reach or stretch for items.
9. What considerations must the nurse employ when caring for a client with ankylosing spondylitis?
   a. Instruct the client not to bend more than 90 degrees.
   b. Assist the client in the turning procedures.
   c. Apply antiembolism stockings and pneumatic compression devices.
   d. Teach the client to refrain from lying on her side.
10. A 45-year-old client diagnosed with sciatica undergoes lumbar decompression surgery to relieve the pressure over the nerve. A thoracic-lumbar-sacral orthosis brace is applied to the client to support his back. What considerations must the nurse employ when caring for the client?
   a. Avoid covering the client's skin before applying the brace.
   b. Smooth all wrinkles over the skin before applying the brace.
   c. Lift the client gently when placing a fracture bedpan.
   d. Encourage client to perform reach or stretch exercises.

CHAPTER 78

# Nervous System Disorders

## SECTION I: TESTING WHAT YOU KNOW

**Activity A** *Match the medication in Column A with the nursing considerations employed during its administration in Column B.*

| Column A | Column B |
|---|---|
| ____ **1.** Medicines for migraine headache | **a.** Avoid high-protein foods and foods high in vitamin $B_6$ |
| ____ **2.** Medicines for status epilepticus | **b.** Administer at the first sign to be most effective |
| ____ **3.** Medicines for Parkinson's disease | **c.** Observe for CNS signs and monitor kidney function |

**Activity B** *Match the disorder in Column A with its signs and symptoms in Column B.*

| Column A | Column B |
|---|---|
| ____ **1.** Bell's palsy | **a.** Impaired bowel and bladder function and loss of sensation |
| ____ **2.** Autonomic dysreflexia | **b.** Temporary one-sided facial paralysis and weakness |
| ____ **3.** Huntington's disease | **c.** Abnormal involuntary movements called chorea |
| ____ **4.** Acute transverse myelitis | **d.** Sudden and dangerous elevation of blood pressure |

**Activity C** *Mark each statement as either "T" (True) or "F" (False). Correct any false statements.*

**1.** T F After positron emission tomography, the client is made to lie flat in bed for 15 to 20 minutes.

**2.** T F When moving a client from the bed to the neuro chair, the bed and chair should be placed in a flat position, and both should be raised to a high setting.

**3.** T F Individuals with amyotrophic lateral sclerosis (ALS) have impaired intellectual and sensory function throughout the course of the disease.

**4.** T F The Glasgow coma scale (GCS) is most commonly employed as a broad indicator of the severity of brain injury.

**5.** T F Routine immunization with the Hib vaccine in schoolchildren has prevented the most common cause of meningitis.

**Activity D** *Fill in the blanks.*

**1.** ____________ epilepsy is a form of focal seizure in which rhythmic jerking movements start in one muscle group and spread to another.

**2.** A ____________ hematoma is caused by the accumulation of blood on the brain's surface as the result of a torn vein.

**3.** ____________ is a sensation of rotation of self or one's surroundings without true dizziness.

4. An acute spasm in which the body is bowed forward with the head and heels bent backward, seen in meningitis, is known as ____________.

5. Difficulty in maintaining balance and coordination, seen commonly in individuals with Parkinson's disease, is referred to as ____________.

**Activity E** *Consider the following figure.*

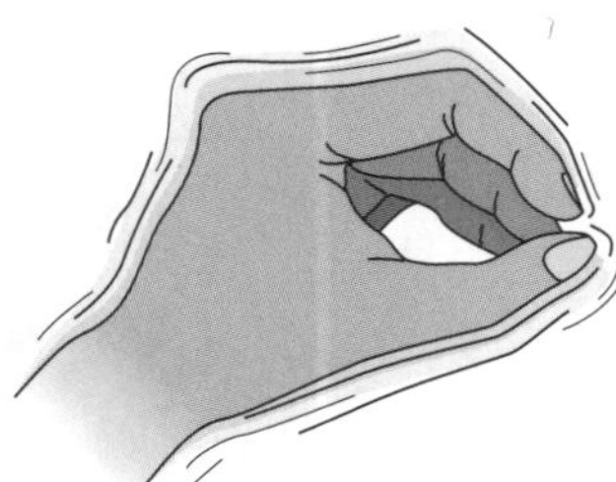

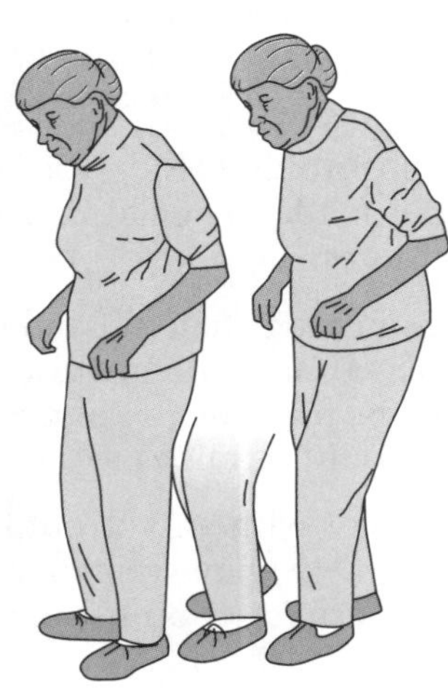

1. Identify the disorder shown in the figure.

______________________________________

______________________________________

2. Describe the type of tremors seen in this disease.

______________________________________

______________________________________

3. Describe the type of posture and gait in this disease condition.

______________________________________

______________________________________

**Activity F** ***Steps that are followed when assisting the physician to obtain a sample of cerebrospinal fluid (CSF) using the lumbar puncture procedure are given below in random order. Write the correct sequence of steps in the boxes provided.***

1. Note the beginning CSF pressure, color, and clarity, as measured by the physician.
2. Position the client on the side with the lower part of the back at the edge of the bed.
3. Place equipment within the physician's reach, and provide extra lighting as necessary.
4. Keep the client's head flat (supine) for at least 6 hours or as otherwise ordered.

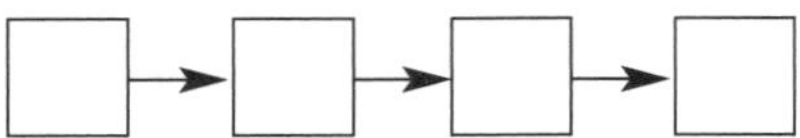

**Activity G** ***Briefly answer the following questions.***

1. What are the common signs and symptoms of a brain tumor?

______________________________________

______________________________________

2. Describe the characteristic features of a depressed skull fracture.

______________________________________

______________________________________

3. Name the vaccines available to prevent poliomyelitis.

______________________________________

______________________________________

4. Discuss the important nursing considerations involved in the treatment of encephalitis.

______________________________________

______________________________________

5. What is meant by myasthenic crisis?

______________________________________

______________________________________

## SECTION II: APPLYING WHAT YOU KNOW

**Activity H** ***Answer the following questions, which involve the nurse's role in the management of nervous system disorders.***

The medical specialty dealing with the nervous system is referred to as neurology. Neuroscience nurses are registered nurses who specialize in the care of people with nervous system disorders.

1. A client is brought into the emergency department with a head injury after a motor vehicle accident. The client is conscious and well oriented to place and time at the time of admission. The neurosurgeon admits the client to the intensive care unit to monitor his ICP.
   a. What ICP value should be considered an increased ICP?
   b. What signs of increased ICP should the nurse look for in the client?
   c. What should the nurse consider during ICP monitoring?
2. A 32-year-old female client with paralysis from the neck down is admitted to the neurology department of the healthcare facility. A nurse is advised to provide care and monitor this client.
   a. What measures should the nurse employ when caring for a client with paralysis?
   b. What client teaching should the nurse provide for female clients with paralysis?
   c. What special skin care should the nurse provide the client?

## SECTION III: GETTING READY FOR NCLEX

**Activity I** ***Answer the following questions.***

1. A nurse is caring for a 55-year-old client with a left-sided cerebrovascular accident. Which of the following measures should the nurse use to prevent footdrop in this client?
   a. Trapeze bar
   b. Splints
   c. Sandbags
   d. Tilt table
2. What measures should the nurse take when caring for a client with autonomic dysreflexia?
   a. Be vigilant in monitoring the client for possible triggers.
   b. Discourage active exercises, to prevent fatigue and exertion.
   c. Assist the client with all activities of daily living.
   d. Keep an oral suction machine at the client's bedside.
3. A general neurologic examination of a client with complaints of fever, chills, neck stiffness, and irritability confirms meningitis. Which of the following measures should the nurse employ when caring for this client?
   a. Elevate the head of the bed to at least 60 degrees.
   b. Encourage the client to flex his neck often.
   c. Monitor the client's respiratory status.
   d. Observe for signs of urinary retention.
4. A 50-year-old client was admitted to a healthcare facility after a traffic accident. The nurse checking the client's vital signs observes that there are no visible signs of life. Respiration has ceased, and there is no heartbeat. Which of the following tests should the nurse expect the physician to order to confirm brain death in this client?
   a. Positron emission tomography (PET)
   b. Radioisotope brain scan
   c. Cerebral angiography
   d. Electroencephalography (EEG)
5. A nurse is assisting a neurosurgeon in performing positron emission tomography. What should the nurse observe for in the client during the procedure?
   a. Signs of anaphylaxis
   b. Signs of ptosis
   c. Respiratory distress
   d. Goose bumps on skin

6. A rehabilitation nurse is caring for an elderly client with a neurologic disorder. The nurse is assisting the client in using the Clinitron special bed. What is this special bed mostly used for?
   a. To help change the client's position frequently
   b. To prevent skin breakdown and alleviate pain
   c. To help maintain proper body alignment
   d. To assist in easy transfer in and out of the bed
7. A nurse is caring for a client with Guillain-Barré syndrome. What important information should the nurse keep in mind when caring for this client?
   a. Total or near-total recovery is not possible.
   b. Asymmetrical pain and weakness is often evident.
   c. Muscle function should be maintained to prevent atrophy.
   d. Bacterial infection typically precedes the syndrome.
8. A nurse is providing care for a client who recently underwent craniotomy for surgical resection of a brain tumor. Which of the following measures should the nurse employ when providing postoperative care for this client? (Select all that apply.)
   a. Elevate the head of the bed.
   b. Place the client in a supine position.
   c. Check the client's hands for ability to grasp.
   d. Perform nasogastric suction.
   e. Warn the client about headache.
9. A nurse is required to document the neurologic assessment of a client with recent head trauma. Which of the following should the nurse document as a part of a neurologic nursing assessment? (Select all that apply.)
   a. Protective reflexes
   b. Muscle strength
   c. General appearance
   d. Vital signs
   e. Speech patterns
10. An 11-year-old client is admitted to the healthcare facility with loss of sensation, generalized weakness of the extremities, and impaired bowel and bladder function. The physician confirms the diagnosis of acute transverse myelitis. What should a nurse be alert for when caring for such a client? (Select all that apply.)
    a. Urinary retention
    b. Severe diarrhea
    c. Vertigo and dizziness
    d. Thrombus formation
    e. Skin breakdown

CHAPTER 79

# Endocrine Disorders

## SECTION I: TESTING WHAT YOU KNOW

**Activity A** *Match the disorder in Column A with the related hormone in Column B.*

| Column A | Column B |
|---|---|
| ____ 1. Cushing's syndrome | a. Insulin |
| ____ 2. Graves' disease | b. Antidiuretic hormone |
| ____ 3. Diabetes insipidus | c. Thyroxine |
| ____ 4. Diabetes mellitus | d. Cortisol |

**Activity B** *Match the disease in Column A with its characteristic feature in Column B.*

| Column A | Column B |
|---|---|
| ____ 1. Hirsutism | a. Benign tumor that originates in the adrenal medulla |
| ____ 2. Pheochromo cytoma | b. Appearance of facial hair in women |
| ____ 3. Colloid goiter | c. Autoimmune condition in which the body builds up antibodies against thyroid tissue |
| ____ 4. Hashimoto's thyroiditis | d. Enlargement of thyroid gland and filling of the distended spaces with a gelatinous material |

**Activity C** *Mark each statement as either "T" (True) or "F" (False). Correct any false statements.*

1. T F The radioactive iodine uptake (RAIU) test helps to evaluate parathyroid gland activity.
2. T F The Somogyi phenomenon occurs when hyperglycemia is followed by a compensatory period of rebound hypoglycemia.
3. T F Humulin-L is an example of intermediate-acting insulin.
4. T F Increased basal hepatic glucose production is one of the major mechanisms that cause blood glucose level elevation in clients with type 2 diabetes.
5. T F Hypothyroidism is caused by an increase in the metabolic process due to increased thyroxine production.

**Activity D** *Fill in the blanks.*

1. The condition of breaking down of fat tissue with scarring and malabsorption is called ____________.
2. Diabetes that develops spontaneously or without an identifiable cause is called ____________ diabetes.
3. The condition of excessive hunger is called ____________.
4. Hypoglycemia is caused by an excess of ____________ hormone.
5. Surgical removal of the pituitary gland is called ____________.

**Activity E** *Consider the following figures.*

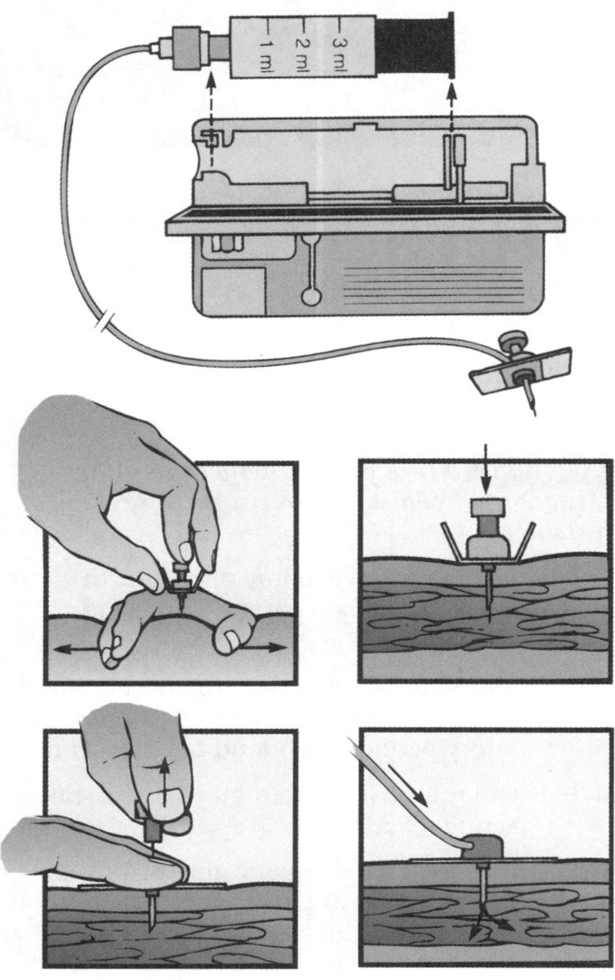


1. Identify the equipment shown in the figure.

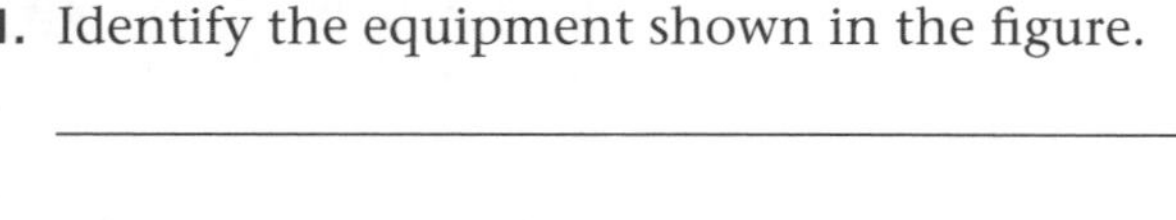

2. Explain the working of this equipment.

3. Name the health condition in which this equipment is used.

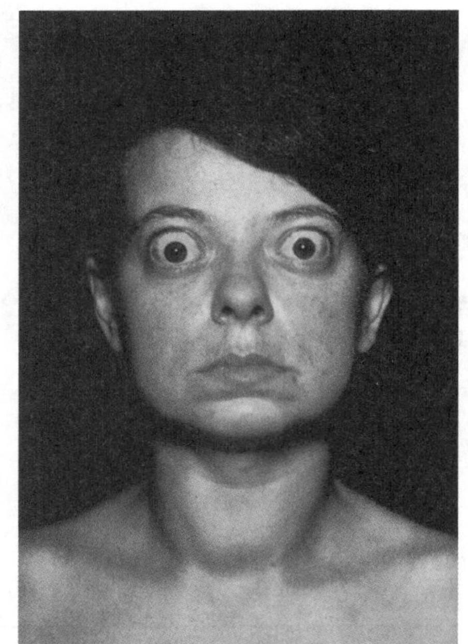

4. Identify the disorder shown in the figure.

5. Describe the symptoms of this disorder.

6. Explain the nursing considerations followed when caring for a client with this disorder.

**Activity F** ***A glucose testing meter is an instrument used for testing blood glucose levels in diabetic clients. A few of the steps involved in testing blood glucose levels with a glucose testing meter are given below in random order. Write the correct sequence in the boxes provided.***

1. Put on sterile disposable gloves.
2. Gently massage and keep finger in dependent position.
3. Clean the puncture site with alcohol.
4. Prepare the lancet by twisting off the cap.

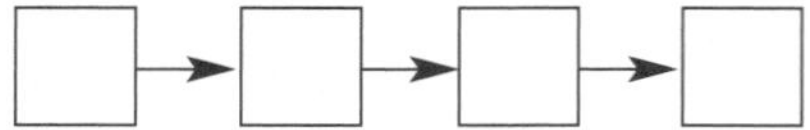

**Activity G** ***Briefly answer the following questions.***

1. What are the signs and symptoms of diabetes mellitus?

______________________________________

______________________________________

2. What are the signs and symptoms of hypoparathyroidism?

______________________________________

______________________________________

3. Name the laboratory tests that are conducted to evaluate the function of the parathyroid gland.

______________________________________

______________________________________

4. Explain the complications associated with angiogram or venogram tests used to evaluate adrenal function.

______________________________________

______________________________________

5. Name the classes of diabetes mellitus.

______________________________________

______________________________________

## SECTION II: APPLYING WHAT YOU KNOW

**Activity H** ***Answer the following questions, which involve the nurse's role in the management of endocrine disorders.***

A nurse's role in managing endocrine disorders involves monitoring the symptoms of the disorder and providing proper nursing care. The nurse also helps clients with activities of daily living (ADL).

1. A 30-year-old client with hypothyroidism is admitted to the healthcare facility.
   a. What data should the nurse collect from clients with endocrine disorders?
   b. What are the nursing considerations employed when caring for a client with hypothyroidism?
2. A 55-year-old male client with diabetes was brought to a healthcare facility with complaints of weakness and sudden exhaustion. He experienced dizziness, confusion, and excessive sweating. He was diagnosed as having a hypoglycemic attack.
   a. What information should the nurse provide to the client to help him control his hypoglycemic condition?
   b. What are the foot care measures that should be employed when caring for a diabetic client?

## SECTION III: GETTING READY FOR NCLEX

**Activity I** ***Answer the following questions.***

1. A nurse is caring for a client in the late stage of ketoacidosis. The nurse notices that the client's breath has a characteristic fruity odor. Which of the following substances is responsible for the fruity smell in the breath?
   a. Iodine
   b. Acetone
   c. Alcohol
   d. Glucose
2. A nurse is caring for a client with Addison's disease. Which of the following nursing considerations should be employed when caring for this client?
   a. Avoid sodium in the client's diet.
   b. Monitor and protect skin integrity.
   c. Document the specific gravity of urine.
   d. Monitor increases in blood pressure.
3. A nurse is assigned to care for and monitor any complications in a 40-year-old client with chronic diabetes. Which of the following is a macrovascular complication of diabetes?
   a. Neuropathy
   b. Retinopathy
   c. Nephropathy
   d. Arteriosclerosis

4. A nurse is instructing a 50-year-old diabetic client about the steps to be followed for self-administration of insulin. Which of the following instructions should be included in the client teaching?
   a. Instruct the client to avoid taking injections in the abdomen.
   b. Encourage client to always inject insulin in the same site.
   c. Inform the client about the type of syringe to use.
   d. Encourage the client to do active exercise after injection.
5. A nurse is preparing a diet plan for a 50-year-old client with a simple goiter. Which of the following should be included in the client's diet to decrease the enlargement of the thyroid gland?
   a. Iodine
   b. Sodium
   c. Potassium
   d. Calcium
6. A nurse is caring for a 60-year-old client affected with hypoparathyroidism. When checking the laboratory report, the nurse finds that the client's calcium level was very low. Which of the following vitamins regulates the calcium level in the body?
   a. Vitamin A
   b. Vitamin D
   c. Vitamin E
   d. Vitamin K
7. A nurse is asked to check the blood glucose level of a diabetic client using a Glucometer. Which of the following guidelines should be followed for blood glucose monitoring? (Select all that apply.)
   a. Use the lateral aspect of the fingertip for testing.
   b. Avoid the use of alcohol to disinfect the fingertips.
   c. Check the calibration number on the strip bottle with the meter.
   d. Expose the strips to 40°C before use.
   e. Rotate the site of lancing for each test.
8. A 30-year-old client is diagnosed with syndrome of inappropriate antidiuretic hormone (SIADH). Which of the following statements is true regarding SIADH? (Select all that apply.)
   a. The disorder is caused by a deficiency of ADH hormone.
   b. Clients with SIADH usually have concentrated urine.
   c. Sodium levels in the client's body are higher than normal.
   d. Chemotherapy may be a possible cause of this disease.
   e. Weight gain may occur due to fluid retention.
9. A nurse is administering a Lantus insulin injection to a 50-year-old diabetic client. Which of the following precautions should the nurse keep in mind when administering the insulin injection? (Select all that apply.)
   a. Avoid mixing Lantus with other types of insulin.
   b. Store the medicine at −4°C in the freezer.
   c. Roll the syringe before administration of the medicine.
   d. Shake the vial before taking the medicine into the syringe.
   e. Check the color of the vial or prefilled syringes before using them.
10. A diabetic client is admitted to the healthcare facility in a stage of insulin shock. Which of the following can lead to insulin shock?
   a. Decreasing the insulin below the optimum level
   b. Mixing of different types of insulin injections
   c. Consuming alcohol along with insulin injections
   d. Lowering of the blood glucose level to 80 mg/dL

CHAPTER 80

# Sensory System Disorders

## SECTION I: TESTING WHAT YOU KNOW

**Activity A** *Match the sensory system disorder in Column A with the corresponding description in Column B.*

| Column A | Column B |
|---|---|
| ____ 1. Hordeolum | a. Abnormal curvature of the cornea or the lens |
| ____ 2. Hyphema | b. Hearing loss due to advancing age |
| ____ 3. Astigmatism | c. Hemorrhage into the anterior chamber of the eye |
| ____ 4. Presbycusis | d. Acute inflammation of the sweat gland of the eyelid |

**Activity B** *Match the surgical procedure in Column A with its description in Column B.*

| Column A | Column B |
|---|---|
| ____ 1. Keratoplasty | a. Partial-thickness incisions made in the cornea to correct the refractive error |
| ____ 2. Tympanoplasty | b. Replacement of damaged corneal tissue to restore vision |
| ____ 3. Enucleation | c. Removal of the eyeball when disease or injury has destroyed the eye |
| ____ 4. Radial keratotomy | d. Plastic reconstruction of the tiny ossicles of the middle ear |

**Activity C** *Mark each statement as either "T" (True) or "F" (False). Correct any false statements.*

1. T F Most electroretinogram recording is performed in a bright, well-lit room.
2. T F Ear irrigation is done only on a physician's order.
3. T F Pure-tone audiometry tests sensorineural hearing deficits only.
4. T F Contact lenses may provide better vision than eyeglasses by abolishing minification or magnification of objects.
5. T F Ectropion is the condition of inward turning of the eyelid margin common in older individuals.

**Activity D** *Fill in the blanks.*

1. A ___________ is an instrument that simulates various corrective lenses.
2. ___________ is defined as an uncontrolled, rapid, rhythmic movement of the eyes.
3. A/An ___________ is responsible for grinding lenses and fitting spectacles as specified by the ophthalmologist.
4. A ___________ is an accumulation of fatty material from a chronically obstructed meibomian gland present on the eyelid.
5. ___________ is the surgical removal of a portion of the iris to allow uninhibited flow of aqueous humor from the posterior chamber of the eye to the anterior chamber.

**Activity E** *Consider the following figures.*

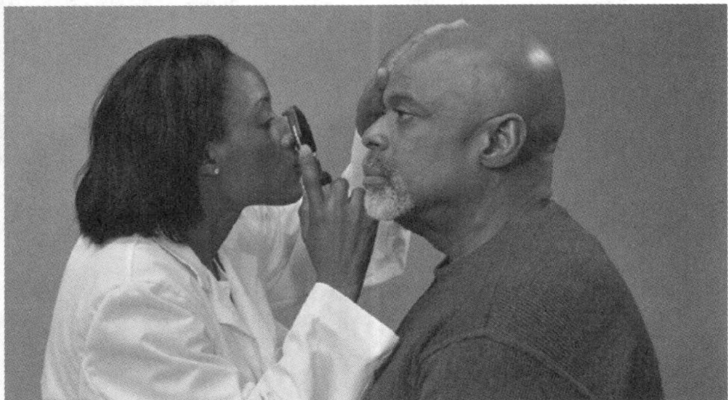

1. Identify the procedure in the figure.

2. What is the purpose of this procedure?

3. How is this procedure performed?

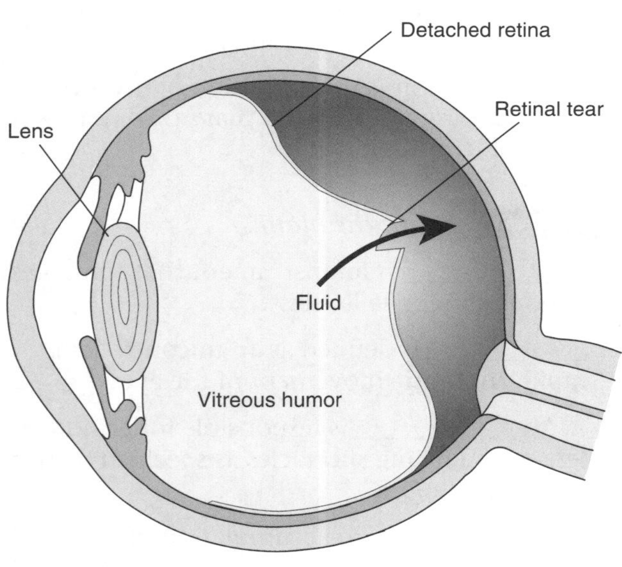


4. Identify the figure.

5. Explain the disease process involved.

6. What are the signs and symptoms of this condition?

**Activity F** ***Nursing steps that are followed during irrigation of the external auditory canal are given below in random order. Write the correct sequence in the boxes provided.***

1. Allow the client to lie on the affected side.
2. Have the client hold a large emesis basin under the ear to be irrigated.
3. Warm the solution to body temperature.
4. Dry the canal and ear.
5. Expel air from the sterile syringe, and draw up the irrigating solution.
6. Straighten the ear canal.
7. Irrigate gently with the prescribed solution.

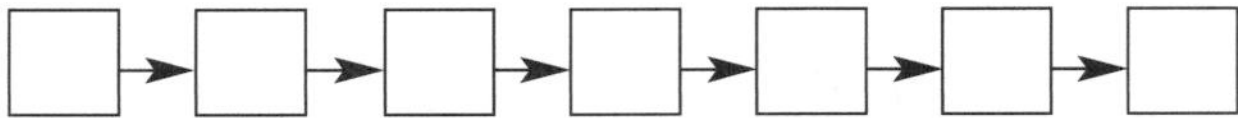

**Activity G** ***Briefly answer the following questions.***

1. What are furuncles?

2. What is labyrinthitis?

3. List the types of otitis media.

4. How are corneal abrasions diagnosed?

5. What is phacoemulsification?

## SECTION II: APPLYING WHAT YOU KNOW

**Activity H** *Answer the following questions, which involve the nurse's role in the management of sensory deficits.*

Nursing considerations for clients with sensory deficits include approaches to effective care for both the client and the family caregivers. The primary role of a nurse in the treatment of sensory deficits is to create short-term and long-term goals and to help clients to understand more about the disorder, its prognosis, and its treatment.

1. A client with profound deafness in his left ear underwent ear surgery. The client was prescribed hearing aids after the surgery.
   a. What nursing considerations should the nurse undertake when caring for a client with hearing impairment?
   b. What information should the nurse provide the client regarding the use of hearing aids?
   c. What goals should the nurse include in the plan of care to encourage the client to use the hearing aid?
2. A 60-year-old client with a history of cataracts is admitted to a healthcare facility to undergo extracapsular cataract extraction. A nurse is required to prepare the client for the surgery. The client is anxious about the surgery.
   a. What measures should the nurse employ to gain the client's cooperation?
   b. What preoperative care should the nurse provide in such a case?
   c. What instructions should the nurse provide the client to prevent disruption of the suture line?

## SECTION III: GETTING READY FOR NCLEX

**Activity I** *Answer the following questions.*

1. A nurse is required to prepare a client for eye surgery. Which of the following measures should the nurse take when clipping the eyelashes?
   a. Apply sticky strips of tape over the lashes.
   b. Use blunt scissors coated with petrolatum.
   c. Apply a soft, padded metal clip over the lashes.
   d. Use a padded plastic clip coated with boric acid.
2. Which of the following activities should the nurse help a client who has a hearing impairment with? (Select all that apply.)
   a. Communication
   b. Preparation of meals
   c. Maintenance of balance
   d. Recreational needs
   e. Rehabilitation care
3. A nurse is caring for a client with conjunctivitis. Which of the following measures should the nurse employ to help remove discharge from the client's eye?
   a. Apply cold soaks over the eye.
   b. Apply a simple single patch.
   c. Use boric acid irrigations.
   d. Ask the client to blink frequently.
4. A nurse is caring for a client with blepharitis. Which of the following should the nurse expect to find in the client?
   a. Drooping of the eyelid
   b. Spasms of the eyelid
   c. Cloudiness of the lens
   d. Redness of lid margins
5. A nurse is required to irrigate a client's ear for cerumen removal. To what temperature should the nurse heat the irrigating solution?
   a. 95.6°F
   b. 98.6°F
   c. 101.6°F
   d. 103.6°F
6. A nurse is caring for a client with inner ear disorder. Which of the following is true for this client?
   a. He has had long-term medication with streptomycin.
   b. He has been involved in activities such as swimming.
   c. He has previously undergone surgery of the ear.
   d. He has been experiencing crackling sensations and fullness in the ear.

7. A nurse is caring for a client with glaucoma. What information should the nurse provide this client?
   a. Encourage increased fluid intake.
   b. Give hourly antibiotic drops.
   c. Encourage annual eye examination.
   d. Caution against atropine medications.

8. A nurse is caring for a visually impaired client who is receiving eye medications. For which of the following side effects should the nurse observe the client? (Select all that apply.)
   a. Nausea
   b. Bradycardia
   c. Dizziness
   d. Hearing loss
   e. Syncope

9. A nurse is caring for a client with a hearing aid. What information should the nurse provide this client? (Select all that apply.)
   a. Tell the client to wear the hearing aid occasionally.
   b. Inform the client that adjusting to the hearing aid takes time and patience.
   c. Caution the client against washing the ear pieces.
   d. The client may use a pipe cleaner to clean and dry the cannula.
   e. Ask the client to check the batteries in the hearing aid regularly.

10. A nurse is caring for a postoperative client who underwent an extracapsular cataract extraction. What instructions should the nurse provide the client to prevent disruption of the suture line?
    a. Avoid sudden movements.
    b. Press on the operated eye gently.
    c. Do not bend over with the head below the waist for 24 hours after surgery.
    d. Avoid lifting 10 to 20 pounds for 2 weeks after surgery.

CHAPTER 81

# Cardiovascular Disorders

## SECTION I: TESTING WHAT YOU KNOW

**Activity A** *Match the type of peripheral vascular disorder in Column A with its appropriate description in Column B.*

**Column A**

____ **1.** Raynaud's phenomenon

____ **2.** Telangiectasia

____ **3.** Buerger's disease

____ **4.** Varicose veins

**Column B**

**a.** First sign is cramps in the calf muscles, brought on by exercise, which disappear with rest.

**b.** Dark, tortuous, superficial veins that become more prominent when the person stands and appear as dark protrusions

**c.** Extremities are blanched and cold, perspire, and feel numb and prickly.

**d.** Group of small dilated blood vessels treated with scleropathy

**Activity B** *Match the diagnostic tests for cardiovascular disorders in Column A with their related descriptions in Column B.*

**Column A**

____ **1.** Echocardiogram

____ **2.** Nuclear scan

____ **3.** Electrocardiogram

____ **4.** Cardiac catheterization

**Column B**

**a.** Generally performed to detect ischemic patterns and to assess for viable myocardium

**b.** Performed to obtain information about congenital or acquired heart defects, to measure oxygen concentration, to determine cardiac output, or to assess the status of the heart's structure and chambers

**c.** Uses sound waves to produce a three-dimensional view of the heart and its blood flow. It is especially useful in the diagnosis and differentiation of heart murmurs.

**d.** Graphic record or tracing that represents the heart's electrical action. Provides essential information about the heart, including heart rate, rhythm, and the presence of certain disorders.

**Activity C** ***Mark each statement as either "T" (True) or "F" (False). Correct any false statements.***

1. T F A nuclear scan is generally performed to detect blood flow patterns and to assess for viable myocardium.
2. T F The nurse must ensure that the client is not allergic to thallium if he has to undergo thrombolytic therapy.
3. T F Hypertension can lead to myocardial infarction, kidney damage, congestive heart failure (CHF), and cerebrovascular accident (CVA).
4. T F Blood lipid studies are conducted to determine hyperlipidemia in clients with cardiovascular disorders.
5. T F Rubber gloves are recommended for the physician and the nurse during electrical defibrillation.
6. T F If sinus bradycardia occurs with digitalization, it is a symptom of heart block.
7. T F The first noticeable signs of a failing heart are numbness or tingling of fingers and sudden weight gain.
8. T F The first signs of chronic rheumatic heart disease are difficulty breathing, a cough, and sometimes cyanosis and expectoration of blood.

**Activity D** ***Fill in the blanks.***

1. A ___________ test is used to assess the severity of symptomatic and asymptomatic cardiac disease.
2. ___________ edema is a type of edema formed when a finger pressed on a swollen area leaves an indention that lasts longer than normal.
3. ___________, one of the symptoms of CHF, refers to the presence of albumin in the urine.
4. ___________ monitoring is a special kind of monitoring used when the heart pressures are increased.
5. ___________ refers to an inflammation of the sac surrounding the heart, which may be caused by infection, allergy, malignancy, trauma, or some other nonspecific problem.
6. ___________ angina is a type of angina pain that does not respond to therapy and is so persistent that the client cannot work.

**Activity E** ***Consider the following figure.***

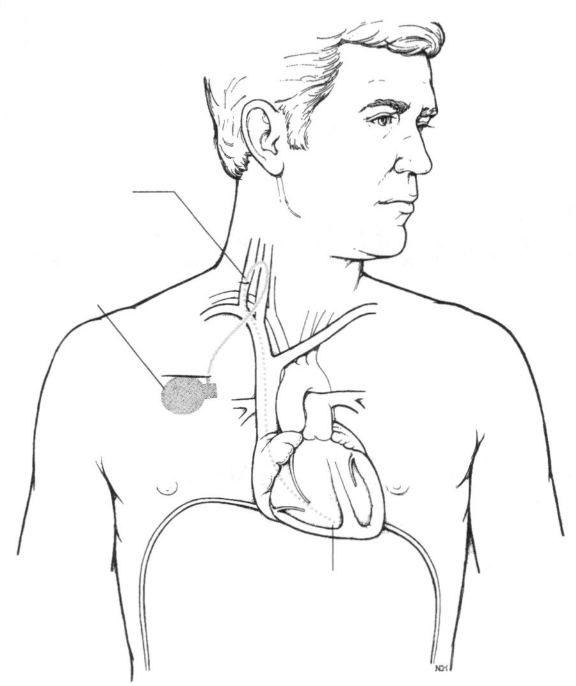

1. Identify the therapy depicted in the above figure. How does the therapy help?

___________________________________________

___________________________________________

2. List the nursing interventions involved when caring for the client who has undergone this therapy.

___________________________________________

___________________________________________

3. What precautions should a nurse take when caring for this client?

___________________________________________

___________________________________________

**Activity F** ***Briefly answer the following questions.***

1. Why should the nurse take the client's apical pulse before administering any digitalis preparation to the client?

___________________________________________

___________________________________________

2. Why should a nurse ask a client if he or she is allergic to shellfish or iodine before performing any test using radiopaque dye?

______________________________________

______________________________________

3. What are the nursing interventions when caring for a client who is scheduled to undergo cardiac catheterization?

______________________________________

______________________________________

4. What are the criteria for selection of clients for thrombolytic therapy?

______________________________________

______________________________________

5. What are the important preoperative considerations required for a client who is scheduled for cardiac surgery?

______________________________________

______________________________________

6. What do neck vein distention and muffled heart sounds indicate in a client with an implanted pacemaker?

______________________________________

______________________________________

7. Why is it important not to touch the client or the client's bed during electrical defibrillation?

______________________________________

______________________________________

## SECTION II: APPLYING WHAT YOU KNOW

**Activity G** ***Answer the following questions which involve the nurse's role in managing cardiac disorders.***

Nurses' role when caring for a client with a cardiovascular disorder includes data collection, nursing diagnosis, planning and implementation, teaching and prevention, and evaluation.

1. A client arrives at the healthcare facility complaining of a recurring chest pain. The initial interview reveals that the client has a positive family history of cardiovascular disorders. Diagnosis indicates hyperlipidemia. The physician suggests that an angiocardiogram be performed on the client.
   a. What nursing interventions should the nurse perform when caring for a client undergoing an angiocardiogram?
   b. What assessment findings are important in determining cardiovascular disorders?
   c. What instructions should the nurse include in the client teaching plan for the prevention of cardiovascular disorders?
2. A client arrives at a healthcare facility complaining of pain in the left arm. The initial interview reveals that the client has a recurring feeling of paleness and feels faint. Further assessment reveals that the client is dyspneic and experiences a tightening, vise-like, choking sensation in the chest along with indigestion.
   a. What condition do these symptoms indicate?
   b. What instructions should the nurse include in the client teaching plan for the prevention of client's disorder?
3. A client arrives at a healthcare facility complaining of difficulty in breathing and nausea. During the assessment, the nurse observes the following in the client: cold and clammy skin; cyanosis; rapid, thready, and irregular pulse; drop in blood pressure and body temperature.
   a. What condition do these symptoms indicate?
   b. What nursing interventions should the nurse perform when caring for this client?
   c. What instructions should the nurse include in the client and family teaching plan?
   d. What points should the nurse include in the rehabilitation plan for this client?
4. A client arrives at a healthcare facility complaining of chills and loss of appetite. During the assessment, the nurse observes that the client has a low-grade fever. The diagnosis indicates bacterial endocarditis.
   a. What assessment findings are important in determining bacterial endocarditis in a client?
   b. Which groups of clients are most susceptible to bacterial endocarditis?
   c. What are the nursing interventions involved when caring for this client?

5. A nurse has been caring for a client with thrombophlebitis. The client complains of a sudden, sharp chest pain. The nurse reports the client's symptom to the physician. A diagnostic test reveals a blood clot traveling to the lungs, causing obstruction of a small vessel.
   a. What does the client's diagnosis indicate?
   b. What signs and symptoms should the nurse monitor for in this client?
   c. What nursing interventions should the nurse perform when caring for this client?
6. A 30-year old female client arrives at the health care facility complaining of numb and prickly hands. When assessing the client, the nurse understands that the client is undergoing emotional stress and observes that her hands are blanched and perspiring. The physician suspects that the client has developed Raynaud's phenomenon.
   a. What symptoms should the nurse monitor for to assess Raynaud's phenomenon in this client?
   b. What instructions should a nurse give this client when caring for her?

## SECTION III: GETTING READY FOR NCLEX

**Activity H** *Answer the following questions.*

1. A client who has undergone treatment for a kidney failure arrives at a healthcare facility for a routine checkup. When assessing the client, the nurse observes a rise in the client's blood pressure and reports to the physician, who suspects hypertension. Which of the following instructions should the nurse offer the client to prevent the development of the hypertension?
   a. Refrain from caffeine intake
   b. Refrain from exercising
   c. Consume foods rich in carbohydrates
   d. Avoid consuming sugary snacks
2. A nurse is caring for a client who has had a CVA. As a result of the CVA, the client is experiencing hemianopsia. Which of the following nursing interventions should the nurse practice when caring for a client with hemianopsia?
   a. Teach the client to scan to see things.
   b. Reinforce the client's speech therapy.
   c. Encourage the client to read.
   d. Talk to the client even if the client does not respond.
3. A 35-year old client who is receiving treatment for a cardiovascular disorder is scheduled to undergo thrombolytic therapy. The nurse must monitor for which of the following complications that might occur due to the thrombolytic therapy? (Select all that apply.)
   a. Dyspareunia
   b. Fever
   c. Insomnia
   d. Bleeding
   e. Dysrhythmias
4. A nurse is caring for a client with a cardiovascular disorder who is scheduled to undergo an angiocardiogram. Which of the following signs should a nurse monitor for after the client has undergone an angiocardiogram?
   a. Clammy skin
   b. Shakiness
   c. High blood pressure
   d. Sleepiness
5. A client who has had a pacemaker implanted arrives at the healthcare facility complaining of dizziness. Which of the following instructions should the nurse offer the client to prevent the dizziness or light-headedness from occurring again?
   a. Get an adequate amount of sleep every night.
   b. Practice light exercises along with good nutrition.
   c. Move 6 feet away from source of electrical interference.
   d. Do not allow chilling of the hands or feet.
6. A nurse is required to care for a client with thrombophlebitis. Which of the following nursing interventions should the nurse perform when caring for this client?
   a. Use cold packs on the client.
   b. Stretch the client's knees.
   c. Mobilize the affected part.
   d. Maintain the client on bed rest.

**7.** A nurse is caring for a client who has just undergone a cardiac surgery. Which of the following postoperative nursing interventions should the nurse perform when caring for this client? (Select all that apply.)

**a.** Monitor the client's body temperature.
**b.** Control chest drainage with suction.
**c.** Monitor the client's sleep patterns.
**d.** Help relieve the client's pain.
**e.** Elevate the foot of the bed.

**8.** A nurse is caring for a client with CVA, who is in an unresponsive state. What are the important nursing activities to implement during this phase? (Select all that apply.)

**a.** Minimize talking with the client.
**b.** Encourage coughing and deep breathing.
**c.** Ensure that the client is positioned on the back.
**d.** Turn the client often, at least once every 2 hours.
**e.** Provide passive range-of-motion (PROM) exercises as ordered.

**9.** Which of the following symptoms should a nurse monitor for when assessing a client with CHF? (Select all that apply.)

**a.** Cold and clammy skin
**b.** Numbness or tingling in the fingers
**c.** Sudden weight gain
**d.** Visible pulsation of neck veins
**e.** Chills and perspiration

**10.** A nurse is required to administer a digitalis preparation to a client with CHF. Which of the following factors should a nurse keep in mind when doing so? (Select all that apply.)

**a.** Be aware of the various names used for digitalis preparations.
**b.** Ensure that the dosage does not differ if digitoxin is used instead of digoxin.
**c.** When setting up a digitalis derivative, keep it in its sealed package.
**d.** Identify the digitalis preparation in a separate medication cup.
**e.** Ensure that the digitalis preparation or derivative is diluted as required.

CHAPTER 82

# Blood and Lymph Disorders

## SECTION I: TESTING WHAT YOU KNOW

**Activity A** *Match the diagnostic test in Column A with its function in Column B.*

| Column A | Column B |
|---|---|
| ____ 1. Hematocrit | a. To monitor the clot formation pathway |
| ____ 2. Indirect Coombs' test | b. To detect antibodies already attached to RBC |
| ____ 3. Partial thromboplastin time | c. To screen for circulating Rh antibodies |
| ____ 4. Direct Coombs' test | d. To identify the percentage of RBCs in the blood |

**Activity B** *Match the disease in Column A with its features in Column B.*

| Column A | Column B |
|---|---|
| ____ 1. Leukemia | a. Increase in RBCs |
| ____ 2. Thalassemia | b. Increase in abnormal WBCs |
| ____ 3. Polycythemia | c. Decrease in RBCs, WBCs, and platelets |
| ____ 4. Pancytopenia | d. Deficiency and presence of damaged chains of hemoglobin |

**Activity C** *Mark each statement as either "T" (True) or "F" (False). Correct any false statements.*

1. T F The antidote for heparin therapy is warfarin sodium.
2. T F Neutropenia is a common side effect of antineoplastic drugs.
3. T F Non-Hodgkin's lymphoma initially affects only one lymphatic area.
4. T F The number of lymphocytes increases in bacterial infection, and the number of neutrophils increases in viral infection.
5. T F Bleeding time is a screening test that can be used to detect platelet disorders.

**Activity D** *Fill in the blank.*

1. The ____________ sedimentation rate measures the speed at which RBCs settle in 1 hour to the bottom of a tube of unclotted blood.
2. Hemolytic anemia is characterized by the presence of immature RBCs called ____________.
3. Removal of blood and simultaneous infusion of other solutions to maintain intravascular volume is known as acute normovolemic ____________.

4. If the donor in bone marrow transplantation is the recipient's identical twin, it is known as ____________ bone marrow transplantation.
5. Pernicious anemia is caused by a lack of ____________ factor.

**Activity E** *Consider the following figure.*

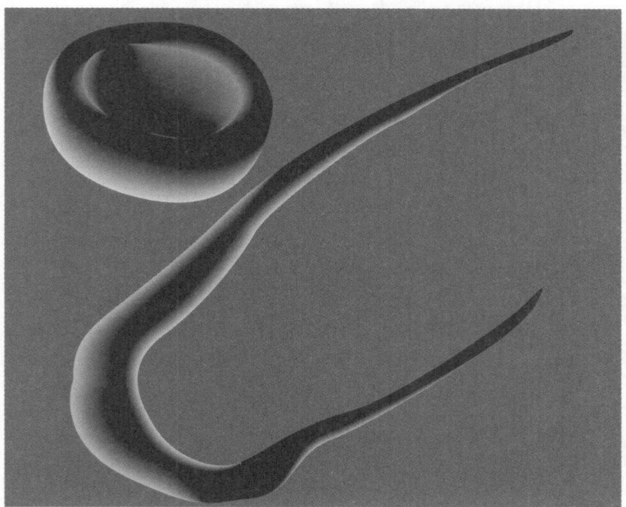

1. Identify the figure.

______________________________________

______________________________________

2. What disease is associated with this condition?

______________________________________

______________________________________

3. Explain the complications associated with this disorder.

______________________________________

______________________________________

**Activity F** ***Hodgkin's disease is the most common cancer occurring in young adults. The stage of the disease influences the client's treatment decisions. Various stages of Hodgkin's disease are given below in random order. Write the correct sequence in the boxes provided.***

1. The disease is present both above and below the diaphragm.
2. The disease is limited to a single node or a single extralymphatic site.
3. The disease is spread to one or more extralymphatic organs or tissues.
4. The disease is present on one side of the diaphragm and involves more than one lymph node.

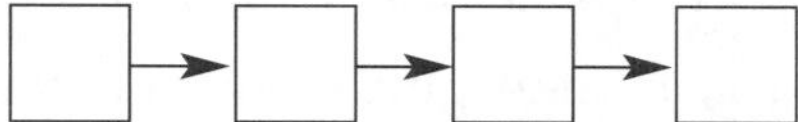

**Activity G** ***Briefly answer the following questions.***

1. Why is a blood type and crossmatch test done?

______________________________________

______________________________________

2. What is meant by a differential WBC count?

______________________________________

______________________________________

3. What is meant by the term plasmapheresis?

______________________________________

______________________________________

4. What are the signs and symptoms of Cooley's anemia?

______________________________________

______________________________________

5. What is the major cause of pernicious anemia?

______________________________________

______________________________________

6. What are the two types of acute leukemia?

______________________________________

______________________________________

7. What are petechiae?

______________________________________

______________________________________

## SECTION II: APPLYING WHAT YOU KNOW

**Activity H** *Answer the following questions, which involve the nurse's role in the management of blood and lymph disorders.*

A nurse's role in managing blood and lymph disorders involves monitoring the symptoms of the disorder and providing proper nursing care. The nurse also helps the clients with activities of daily living (ADL).

1. A nurse is caring for a client with late-stage pernicious anemia.
   a. What symptoms should the nurse monitor in the client?
   b. What nursing care measures should be employed when caring for the client?
2. A nurse is assessing a client who has been admitted to the healthcare facility for bone marrow transplantation.
   a. What data should the nurse collect from the client?
   b. What are the various nursing diagnoses that can be established based on the data collection?

## SECTION III: GETTING READY FOR NCLEX

**Activity I** *Answer the following questions.*

1. What should the nurse assess for in a client with multiple myeloma?
   a. Increased volume of urine
   b. Excessive sweating
   c. Watery, loose bowel movements
   d. Increase in body temperature
2. A client is diagnosed with granulocytopenia. A decrease in which of the following blood components is the nurse likely to notice in the client's hematology report?
   a. Neutrophils
   b. Platelets
   c. Immunoglobulin
   d. Hemoglobin
3. A nurse is caring for a client who is receiving a blood transfusion. The nurse notices a transfusion reaction in the client. Which of the following measures should the nurse take to manage the transfusion reaction? (Select all that apply.)
   a. Stop the blood transfusion procedure.
   b. Close the intravenous infusion line immediately.
   c. Discard the blood bag with attached administration set.
   d. Collect blood and urine samples and send to the laboratory.
   e. Report the reaction to the transfusion service.
4. A nurse is caring for a client with non-Hodgkin's lymphoma. When assessing the client, what signs and symptoms should the nurse look for?
   a. Excessive thirst and dehydration
   b. Enlargement of the liver
   c. Petechiae and ecchymosis
   d. Tenderness over the sternum
5. Which of the following nursing care measures should be employed when caring for a client with relative polycythemia?
   a. Take preventive measures against constipation.
   b. Instruct the client to use a soft toothbrush.
   c. Encourage the client to drink plenty of fluids, especially water.
   d. Monitor for symptoms of infection and bleeding.
6. A nurse is caring for a client with secondary polycythemia. Which of the following would show an increase in the laboratory report for this client?
   a. Thrombocytes
   b. Erythropoietin
   c. Plasma cells
   d. Serum albumin

**7.** A female client has chronic myeloid leukemia. What signs and symptoms should the nurse monitor in such a client? (Select all that apply.)

**a.** Night sweats

**b.** Excessive menses

**c.** Shortness of breath

**d.** Enlarged spleen

**e.** Weight gain

**8.** A client is admitted to a healthcare facility in a stage of hemorrhagic shock. What should be the primary concern of the nurse?

**a.** Clear the airway by providing suction.

**b.** Sustain the blood pressure by providing fluids.

**c.** Provide intravenous iron to make up for the blood loss.

**d.** Start blood transfusion immediately.

**9.** Which of the following should the nurse keep in mind when caring for the client who is receiving warfarin therapy? (Select all that apply.)

**a.** Avoid monitoring the rectal temperature of the client.

**b.** Avoid the administration of intramuscular injections.

**c.** Administer the anticoagulant before drawing a blood sample to check the prothrombin time (PT).

**d.** Administer vitamin K to enhance the action of warfarin.

**e.** Monitor the PT twice a week after stabilization of the blood anticoagulant level.

**10.** A nurse is caring for a client with a peptic ulcer. The client shows symptoms of anemia. Which of the following terms should the nurse use to describe the anemic condition of the client?

**a.** Chronic hemorrhagic anemia

**b.** Idiopathic aplastic anemia

**c.** Pernicious anemia

**d.** Hemolytic anemia

CHAPTER 83

# Cancer

## SECTION I: TESTING WHAT YOU KNOW

**Activity A** *Match the tumor marker in Column A with the corresponding tumor in Column B.*

| Column A | Column B |
|---|---|
| ____ 1. Beta$_2$-microglobulin | a. Thyroid carcinoma |
| ____ 2. Philadelphia chromosome | b. Breast carcinoma |
| ____ 3. Serum ferritin | c. Chronic myeloid leukemia |
| ____ 4. CA 15-3 tumor marker | d. Multiple myeloma |
| ____ 5. Thyrocalcitonin | e. Hepatocellular carcinoma |

**Activity B** *Match the type of tumor in Column A with its causative viral agent in Column B.*

| Column A | Column B |
|---|---|
| ____ 1. Kaposi's sarcoma | a. Human papillomavirus |
| ____ 2. Burkitt's lymphoma | b. Retrovirus of HIV |
| ____ 3. Cervical cancer | c. Epstein-Barr virus |

**Activity C** *Mark each statement as either "T" (True) or "F" (False). Correct any false statements.*

1. T F Carcinomas develop from connective tissues.
2. T F Biotherapy uses biologic response modifiers to enhance the immune system.
3. T F Benign tumors are composed of anaplastic cells.
4. T F Insecticides are chemical carcinogens.
5. T F Ovarian teratoma is a mixed-tissue tumor.

**Activity D** *Fill in the blanks.*

1. RNA viruses are known as ____________.
2. Brachytherapy is the placement of ____________ substances directly into a tumor site.
3. Viruses that can cause tumors are called ____________viruses.
4. Wilms' tumor is a tumor of the ____________.
5. ____________ swallow is a radiologic technique used to detect abnormalities of the gastrointestinal system.

**Activity E** *Consider the following figure.*

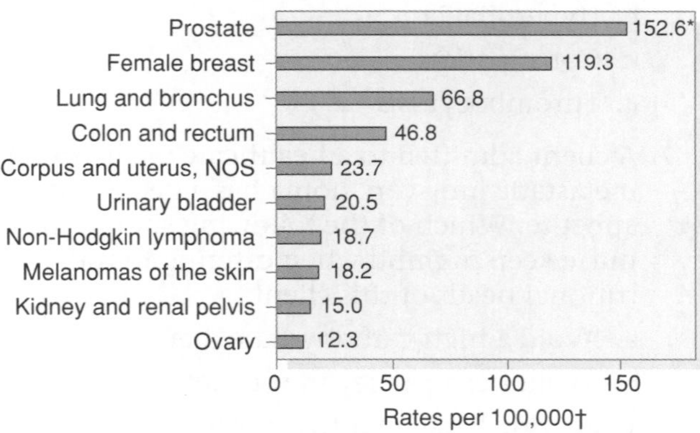


1. What is the leading cause of cancer deaths?

______________________________________________

______________________________________________

2. List some of the risk factors for developing cancer.

______________________________________________

______________________________________________

**Activity F** ***The nurse must follow safe handling procedures during the administration of chemotherapeutic agents, because they are extremely toxic. Some of the nursing steps performed when administering parenteral chemotherapy are given below in random order. Write the correct sequence in the boxes provided.***

1. Administer the chemotherapeutic agent such that it does not come in contact with eyes or mucous membranes.
2. Carefully review administration guidelines and side effects of the chemotherapeutic agent.
3. In case of contact, rinse the affected part with clear water for at least 5 minutes.
4. Wear gloves, gown, and protective eyewear during preparation and administration.

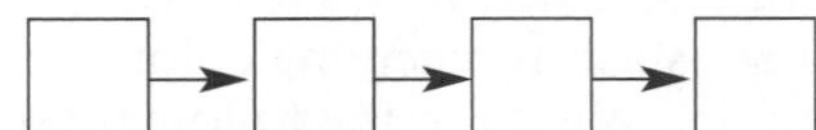

**Activity G** ***Briefly answer the following questions.***

1. What is carcinogenesis?

______________________________________________

______________________________________________

2. What measures should be emphasized to the public to prevent cancer?

______________________________________________

______________________________________________

3. What is the purpose of a biopsy examination?

______________________________________________

______________________________________________

4. What is photodynamic therapy?

______________________________________________

______________________________________________

5. What are the uses of monoclonal antibodies?

______________________________________________

______________________________________________

## SECTION II: APPLYING WHAT YOU KNOW

**Activity H** ***Answer the following questions, which involve the nurse's role in the management of cancer therapy.***

Cancer therapy is associated with unpleasant side effects. The nurse assists the client with strategies for managing side effects.

1. A client with acute leukemia develops stomatitis after chemotherapy.
   a. What instructions should the nurse provide to this client?
   b. What solution should the nurse recommend as an alternative to commercial mouthwash?
   c. What instructions should the nurse provide if the client is advised to use a swish-and-swallow solution?
2. A client with breast cancer who is undergoing radiotherapy frequently complains of excessive fatigue.
   a. What could be the cause of this fatigue?
   b. List a few recommendations that the nurse should make to help decrease the distress.

## SECTION III: GETTING READY FOR NCLEX

**Activity I** *Answer the following questions.*

1. A client undergoing chemotherapy for small cell carcinoma of the lung has a decreased white blood cell count. What precautions should the nurse take to avoid any secondary infection when caring for this client?
   a. Measure the client's temperature through the rectal route.
   b. Avoid multiple intravenous access attempts.
   c. Keep the client in an isolation ward.
   d. Shave the client with a blade razor.
2. A client diagnosed with medullary carcinoma of the thyroid is prescribed radiotherapy by the treating oncologist. The nurse is required to give information about the therapy to the client. Which of the following should the nurse tell the client?
   a. There is an increased risk of developing anemia.
   b. The procedure will be slightly painful.
   c. The procedure will last for half an hour.
   d. The area being treated will feel hot.
3. A client with metastatic renal cancer is receiving interleukin therapy. Which of the following side effects should the nurse monitor for in this client?
   a. Hypertension
   b. Bradycardia
   c. Hot flashes
   d. Dyspnea
4. A nurse is documenting the laboratory reports of a client with pancreatic carcinoma. Which of the following tumor markers is most likely to be found in this client?
   a. Neuron-specific enolase
   b. Alpha-fetoprotein
   c. CA 19-9 tumor marker
   d. Carcinoembryonic antigen
5. A nurse is administering 5-fluorouracil to a client with acute leukemia. To which category of chemotherapeutic agents does 5-fluorouracil belong?
   a. Antimetabolites
   b. Alkylating agents
   c. Hormonal agents
   d. Antitumor antibiotics
6. Which of the following side effects should the nurse look for in a client receiving radiotherapy?
   a. Skin irritation
   b. Hyperphagia
   c. Constipation
   d. Thrombocytosis
7. A client admitted to a healthcare facility with metastatic lung carcinoma has a decreased appetite. Which of the following should the nurse keep in mind when catering to the nutritional needs of this client?
   a. Avoid a high-carbohydrate diet.
   b. Avoid fresh parsley in the diet.
   c. Provide large-quantity meals.
   d. Provide a high-protein diet.
8. A client receiving chemotherapy for acute leukemia complains of nausea. The client refuses to take any antiemetic medication. Which of the following nonpharmacologic therapies can the nurse offer this client? (Select all that apply.)
   a. Diet modification
   b. Relaxation techniques
   c. Guided imagery
   d. Distraction techniques
   e. Herbal remedies
9. A client with promyelocytic leukemia is receiving retinoids. When monitoring the client for retinoic acid syndrome, which of the following should the nurse look for? (Select all that apply.)
   a. Respiratory distress
   b. Weight loss
   c. Pleuritic chest pain
   d. Unexplained fever
   e. Hypertension
10. A client diagnosed with breast cancer with liver metastasis is receiving colony-stimulating factors. Which of the following side effects should the nurse monitor this client for? (Select all that apply.)
    a. Bulimia
    b. Bone pain
    c. Fatigue
    d. Alopecia
    e. Fever

CHAPTER 84

# Allergic, Immune, and Autoimmune Disorders

## SECTION I: TESTING WHAT YOU KNOW

**Activity A** *Match the allergic reaction in Column A with the corresponding stimulating factor in Column B.*

| Column A | Column B |
|---|---|
| ____ 1. Urticaria | a. Exercise |
| ____ 2. Contact dermatitis | b. Pollen grains |
| ____ 3. Bronchial asthma | c. Poison ivy |
| ____ 4. Allergic rhinitis | d. Parasitic infections |

**Activity B** *Match the terms in Column A with their descriptions in Column B.*

| Column A | Column B |
|---|---|
| ____ 1. Antigen | a. A specific substance that produces a tissue reaction in the body |
| ____ 2. Histamine | b. A foreign protein substance to which the body reacts by producing antibodies |
| ____ 3. Allergen | c. An agent used to reduce congestion of bronchial mucosa |
| ____ 4. Epinephrine | d. A major chemical mediator involved in the allergic response |

**Activity C** *Mark each statement as either "T" (True) or "F" (False). Correct any false statements.*

1. T F Men are more likely to develop autoimmune disorders than women.
2. T F Allergic reactions to medications will occur rapidly and more severely if the medication is administered parenterally.
3. T F Clients should remain in the healthcare facility for at least 1 day after injections for desensitization.
4. T F Any medication allergies should be noted in large letters on the front of the medical record.
5. T F Narcotics are contraindicated in clients with bronchial asthma because they cause migraine headaches.

**Activity D** *Fill in the blanks.*

1. ____________ are antigens that cause an immune response in the body.
2. The physician who specifically treats allergies is called a/an ____________.
3. Leukotrienes are chemical mediators that are released by ____________ cells.
4. During anaphylaxis, the cardiac ____________ falls, and the heart cannot pump enough blood and oxygen to the tissues.

5. Autoimmunity is the process in which the body produces __________ against its own healthy cells.

**Activity E** *Consider the following figure.*

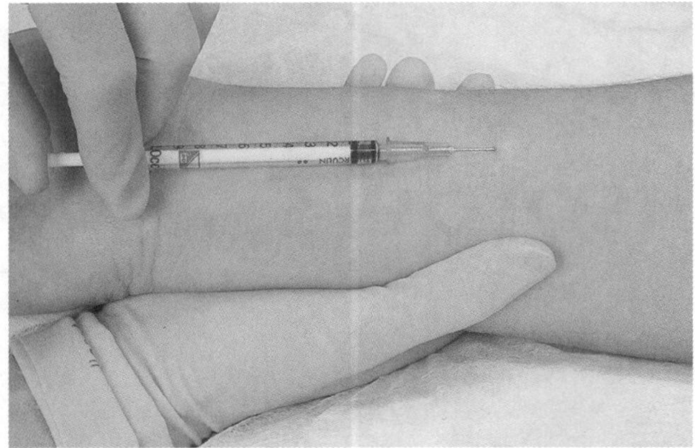

1. Identify the procedure shown in the figure.

______________________________

______________________________

2. How is this procedure performed?

______________________________

______________________________

3. How long does it take for signs of positive reaction to appear?

______________________________

______________________________

**Activity F** *Symptoms that are manifested in a client with latex sensitivity are given below in random order. Write the correct sequence in the boxes provided.*

1. Exhibits vesicles, papules, and crusting of the skin.
2. Exhibits warning signs and symptoms of cardiac arrest.
3. Demonstrates pruritus, erythema, and edema.
4. Develops wheezing, dyspnea, and bronchial spasm.

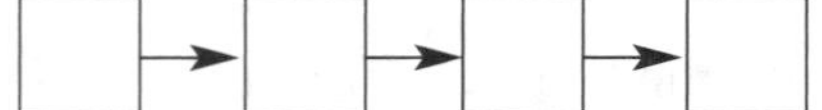

**Activity G** *Briefly answer the following questions.*

1. Describe antigen–antibody reaction.

______________________________

______________________________

2. Name the laboratory tests included in the detection of allergic disorders.

______________________________

______________________________

3. Explain the mechanism of autoimmune disorders.

______________________________

______________________________

4. How is bronchial asthma classified?

______________________________

______________________________

5. Name some of the common food allergens.

______________________________

______________________________

6. What is meant by an adverse drug reaction?

______________________________

______________________________

7. What are leukotriene antagonists?

______________________________

______________________________

## SECTION II: APPLYING WHAT YOU KNOW

**Activity H** *Answer the following questions, which involve the nurse's role in the management of allergic, immune, and autoimmune disorders.*

Nursing considerations for clients with allergic or immune disorders include careful observation and assessment of the client's symptoms, vigilant documentation and communication of the symptoms, and careful planning and implementation of the care plan, as well as client and family teaching.

**1.** A client is diagnosed with contact dermatitis after complaints of itching, redness, burning sensation, and rashes on his trunk.

**a.** What goals should the nurse include in the plan of care for this client?

**b.** What important client teaching should the nurse provide?

**c.** What information should the nurse provide about using the prescribed topical medications?

**2.** A client comes to the healthcare facility with complaints of recurring episodes of itching, excessive tearing, and sneezing. The client reports that these symptoms occur more often during the day and are exacerbated in cold weather.

**a.** What medical history should the nurse ask the client for during the nursing assessment?

**b.** What should the nurse assess the client's skin for?

**c.** What observations should the nurse make regarding the client's respiration?

## SECTION III: GETTING READY FOR NCLEX

**Activity I** *Answer the following questions.*

**1.** A nurse is required to assist a physician to perform an intradermal skin test in a client. What information should the nurse provide the client about skin testing?

**a.** Intradermal skin injections are extremely painful.

**b.** The degree of edema indicates the severity of the reaction.

**c.** Only a single antigen can be tested at one time.

**d.** Signs of positive reaction will appear in 1 week.

**2.** A nurse is assisting a healthcare provider to perform a skin test in a client. Which of the following suggests the appearance of induration on the client's skin? (Select all that apply.)

**a.** Lump

**b.** Redness

**c.** Wheal

**d.** Edema

**e.** Crust

**3.** A nurse is caring for a client with multiple sclerosis (MS). Which of the following should the nurse include in the nursing care plan for this client?

**a.** Airway clearance

**b.** Level of consciousness

**c.** Physical mobility

**d.** Aid in hearing

**4.** A female client is confirmed to have a penicillin allergy. What measures should the nurse employ to ensure the client's protection?

**a.** Prepare the client to deal with anaphylaxis as the first point in client teaching.

**b.** Ask the client to carry her medical records with her always.

**c.** Encourage dietary modifications.

**d.** Encourage the client to wear a MedicAlert tag.

**5.** A nurse is caring for a client who experienced an anaphylactic reaction after a bee sting. Which of the following measures should the nurse employ to open the client's airway?

**a.** Initiate cardiopulmonary resuscitation.

**b.** Make use of an endotracheal tube.

**c.** Administer antihistamines as ordered.

**d.** Place the client in the Trendelenburg position.

**6.** A nurse is required to assist a physician performing an intradermal skin test on a client. What information does the skin test provide?

**a.** Risk of anaphylactic reaction

**b.** Rate of antigen absorption

**c.** Cause of allergic reactions

**d.** Response to antiallergic therapy

**7.** Which of the following allergens can be a cause of contact dermatitis?

**a.** Poison ivy

**b.** Insect stings

**c.** Animal dander

**d.** Chocolate

8. What should the nurse look for in a client with atopic dermatitis?
   a. Bluish lips and fingernails
   b. Yellow mucous membranes
   c. Heavily pigmented skin
   d. Scaly, thickened skin

9. A nurse has been ordered to administer epinephrine to a client with an allergic disorder. When providing client education, what should the nurse say is the purpose of this injection?
   a. To reduce itching sensation
   b. To reduce bronchospasms
   c. To provide antiseptic effects
   d. To control spread of infection

10. A nurse is required to observe a client with a suspected immune disorder. What should the nurse look for? (Select all that apply.)
    a. Impaired gas exchange
    b. Recurrent infections
    c. Visual disturbances
    d. Impaired hearing
    e. Slow wound healing

CHAPTER 85

# HIV and AIDS

## SECTION I: TESTING WHAT YOU KNOW

**Activity A** *Match the important terminologies of HIV/AIDS in Column A with the correct definition in Column B.*

| Column A | Column B |
|---|---|
| ____ 1. Antiretroviral therapy | a. HIV is an example that invades a healthy normal cell |
| ____ 2. Opportunistic infections | b. Consists of a combination of five classes of medications |
| ____ 3. Retrovirus | c. Lymphocytes that mature in the thymus |
| ____ 4. T cells | d. Can occur when HIV positive person's T cell falls between 200 and 400/mm$^3$ |

**Activity B** *Match the most common opportunistic infections in Column A with the correct definition in Column B.*

| Column A | Column B |
|---|---|
| ____ 1. Candidiasis | a. One celled parasitic infection of the gastrointestinal tract causing diarrhea, fever, and weight loss |
| ____ 2. Cryptococcus | b. Yeast like fungus that overgrows, causing infections of the mouth (thrush), respiratory tract, and skin |
| ____ 3. Cytomegalovirus | c. Yeast like fungus causing infections of the lung, brain, and blood |

**Activity C** *Mark each statement as either "T" (True) or "F" (False). Correct any false statements.*

1. T F HIV infection is transmitted through coughing and sneezing.
2. T F The enzyme immunoassay (EIA) test is specifically done to confirm the presence of antibodies to HIV proteins.
3. T F HIV infection can be prevented through the use of antiretroviral medications.
4. T F A decrease in the number of CD4 cells below 500/mm$^3$ indicates an abnormality.
5. T F The OraQuick Rapid HIV-1 Antibody Test can determine HIV infection with 99% accuracy.

**Activity D** *Fill in the blanks.*

1. Persistent enlargement of lymph nodes is called ____________.
2. The antiretroviral zidovudine is a ____________ reverse transcriptase inhibitor.

3. A virus that overtakes the biosynthetic mechanism of living cells to duplicate itself is called a/an ____________.
4. T lymphocytes are the lymphocytes that mature in the ____________ gland of the human body.
5. Producing ____________ to elicit specific immune responses is one of the functions of T and B cells.

**Activity E** *Consider the following figures.*

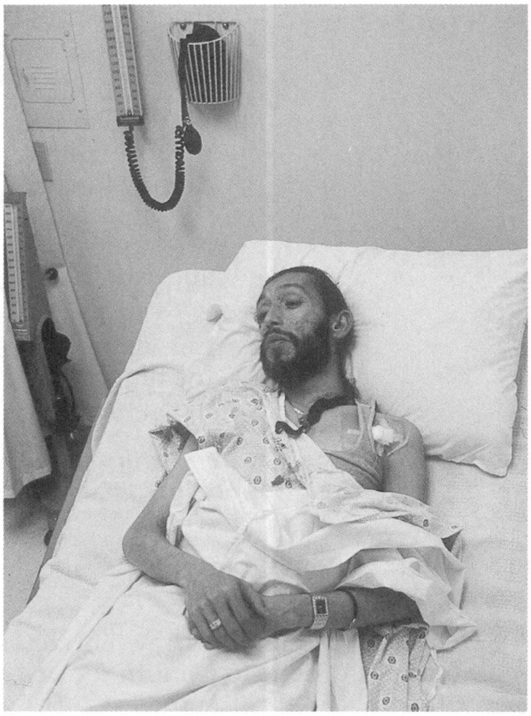

1. What is wasting syndrome of AIDS?

_______________________________________________

_______________________________________________

2. What is meant by opportunistic infection?

_______________________________________________

_______________________________________________

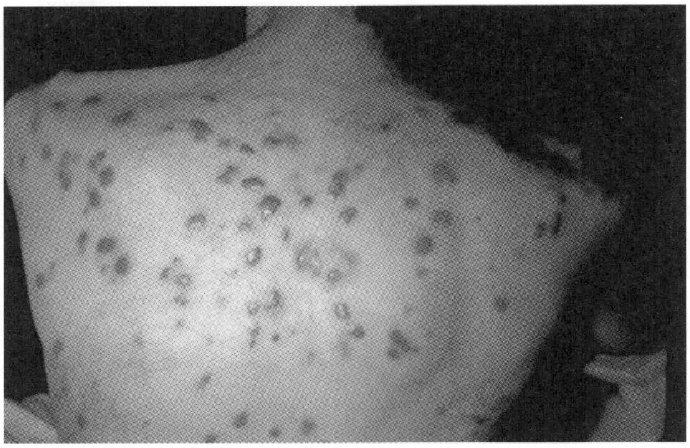

3. Identify the figure.

_______________________________________________

_______________________________________________

4. What is the major symptom of this disease?

_______________________________________________

_______________________________________________

**Activity F** *Briefly answer the following questions.*

1. What are the nursing implications for clients with HIV?

_______________________________________________

_______________________________________________

2. Explain the action of HIV virus.

_______________________________________________

_______________________________________________

3. What is meant by antiretroviral therapy?

_______________________________________________

_______________________________________________

4. What are the legal implications associated with HIV testing?

_______________________________________________

_______________________________________________

5. State the gastrointestinal manifestations associated with untreated HIV or AIDS infection.

_______________________________________

_______________________________________

6. Name the various HIV antibody tests.

_______________________________________

_______________________________________

7. What is meant by viral load?

_______________________________________

_______________________________________

8. Name the classes of antiviral medications used against HIV infection.

_______________________________________

_______________________________________

## SECTION II: APPLYING WHAT YOU KNOW

**Activity G** *Answer the following questions, which involve the nurse's role in the management of HIV and AIDS.*

A nurse's role in managing HIV and AIDS involves monitoring the symptoms and assisting the client to perform activities of daily living (ADL).

1. A nurse is caring for a client infected with HIV.
   a. What data should the nurse collect from the client?
   b. What are the various nursing diagnoses that can be established based on the data collection?
2. A nurse is required to care for a pregnant client who is at high risk for HIV infection.
   a. What information should the nurse provide to the client regarding signs and symptoms of HIV infection?
   b. What information should the nurse provide to the client regarding the routes of transmission of HIV?

## SECTION III: GETTING READY FOR NCLEX

**Activity H** *Answer the following questions.*

1. A 30-year-old client comes to the healthcare facility for HIV testing. Which of the following guidelines should be followed for HIV testing? (Select all that apply.)
   a. The nurse should obtain informed consent from the client before testing.
   b. The nurse should make arrangements for posttest counseling if the test is positive.
   c. If the client asks for results over the telephone, the results should be provided after verification of identity.
   d. The laboratory for HIV or AIDS testing must be approved by the state.
   e. The nurse should make arrangements for pretest counseling regardless of the test results.
2. A nurse is educating a family caregiver about the precautions to be taken when helping an HIV-infected client. Which of the following should the nurse tell the caregiver? (Select all that apply.)
   a. Avoid physical contact with an HIV-infected client.
   b. Disinfect the hands before recapping needles for disposal.
   c. Put on gloves before contact with blood or other body fluids.
   d. Cover cuts, sores, or breaks on the client's skin with bandages.
   e. Discourage the client from sharing razors or toothbrushes.
3. A nurse is educating an HIV-positive pregnant client about the precautions to be taken to reduce the risk of mother-to-child transmission. Which of the following can reduce the risk of HIV transmission from mother to child?
   a. Breast feeding the baby
   b. Avoiding kissing the baby
   c. Prophylactic antiretroviral treatment
   d. Administering HIV vaccines

4. A nurse is caring for an HIV-positive client. The nurse observes blisters on the lips, nose, and genitalia of the client and identifies this as an opportunistic infection. What is the cause of this condition?
   a. Toxoplasmosis
   b. Histoplasmosis
   c. Candidiasis
   d. Cryptococcosis

5. A nurse is educating a client about the routes of transmission of HIV infection. Which of the following should the nurse tell the client regarding the routes of transmission?
   a. HIV is transmitted through sharing of utensils.
   b. HIV is transmitted through hugging and kissing.
   c. HIV is transmitted through insect bites.
   d. HIV is transmitted through tattooing needles.

6. A client with HIV infection has been prescribed antiretroviral therapy. Which of the following statements is true regarding antiretroviral therapy? (Select all that apply.)
   a. Antiretroviral therapy helps to prevent the transmission of disease from one person to another.
   b. Antiretroviral drugs also lower blood cholesterol levels.
   c. Antiretroviral therapy helps to restore the immune function of the body.
   d. Antiretroviral therapy helps to lower the viral load to nondetectable levels.
   e. Peripheral neuropathy is one of the adverse effects of this therapy.

7. A pregnant client comes to the healthcare facility for a regular antenatal checkup. The client asks the nurse about HIV, AIDS, and related tests. Which of the following should the nurse tell the client?
   a. A person who is not infected with HIV will show an undetectable viral load.
   b. AIDS occurs in the initial stages of HIV infection.
   c. Constipation is a common gastrointestinal manifestation of the disease.
   d. The ELISA test is used to confirm the presence of HIV antibodies.

8. A nurse is required to monitor the clinical manifestations in an HIV positive client. What type of cells does HIV invade and deplete that reduces the function of the immune system?
   a. A
   b. B
   c. T
   d. X

9. A client asks the nurse about the various HIV antibody tests. Which test is done by testing saliva and blood?
   a. ELA
   b. Eastern blot
   c. Western blot
   d. OraQuick Rapid HIV-1 Antibody test

10. A client is diagnosed with AIDS-related toxoplasmosis. What kind of infection causes this condition?
   a. Fungal infection
   b. Viral infection
   c. Bacterial infection
   d. Protozoan infection

CHAPTER 86

# Respiratory Disorders

## SECTION I: TESTING WHAT YOU KNOW

**Activity A** *Match the diagnostic tests in Column A with their corresponding features in Column B.*

**Column A**

____ 1. Magnetic resonance imaging

____ 2. Bronchoscopy

____ 3. Throat culture

____ 4. Lung perfusion scan

**Column B**

a. Helps to observe lung tissue or to remove mucous plugs or foreign objects

b. Helps to determine which medication is most effective against an infecting organism

c. Illustrates different views through which lesions, pneumonia, and other disorders can be located

d. Noninvasive nuclear procedure used to diagnose disorders in the lungs and bronchi

**Activity B** *Match the respiratory disorders in Column A with their characteristic features in Column B.*

**Column A**

____ 1. Syncope

____ 2. Empyema

____ 3. Pneumothorax

____ 4. Hypoxemic hypoxia

**Column B**

a. Collection of pus-containing exudate in the pleural cavity

b. Temporary loss of consciousness and fainting

c. Decrease in blood oxygen level causing a decreased amount of oxygen in the tissues

d. Collection of air in the pleural cavity, causing collapse of all or part of the lung

**Activity C** *Mark each statement as either "T" (True) or "F" (False). Correct any false statements.*

1. T F Withdrawing a large amount of fluid during paracentesis can cause vasoconstriction.

2. T F The purpose of chest suction is to restore the negative pressure within the chest cavity.

3. T F Closed water-seal drainage uses position and gravity to drain secretions and mucus from the individual's lungs.

4. T F Tidal volume is the volume of air in an average breath.

5. T F Influenza is an active, contagious respiratory disease caused by one of several strains of fungi.

**Activity D** *Fill in the blanks.*

1. Collapse of a lung due to obstruction by mucus or a foreign object is called ___________.
2. The incentive ___________ helps the client to perform respiratory exercises and to maintain lung function.
3. An inflammation of the double membrane covering of the lungs is called ___________.
4. ___________ tuberculosis is a form of tuberculosis that is characterized by widespread dissemination into the body.
5. Profuse sweating at night is called nocturnal ___________.

**Activity E** *Consider the following figures.*

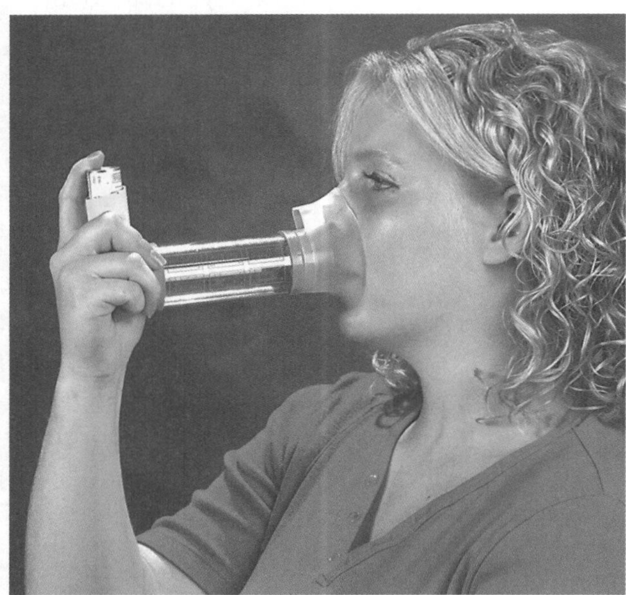

1. Identify the equipment in the figure.

_______________________________________

_______________________________________

2. Which health condition is this equipment used for?

_______________________________________

_______________________________________

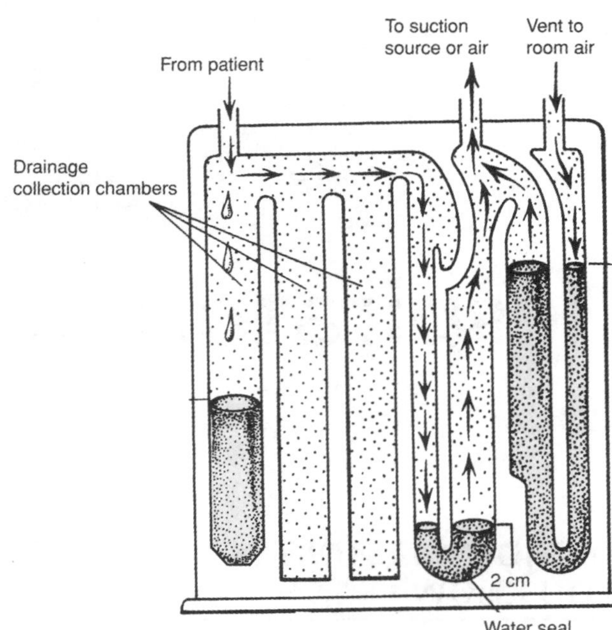


3. Identify the equipment shown in the figure.

_______________________________________

_______________________________________

4. What is the purpose of this equipment?

_______________________________________

_______________________________________

5. What are the different components of this system?

_______________________________________

_______________________________________

6. What are the nursing implications during this procedure?

_______________________________________

_______________________________________

**Activity F** ***Suctioning is a procedure done to remove excess secretions and mucus from the airway. Some of the steps used in preparing for suction are given below in random order. Write the correct sequence in the boxes provided.***

1. Open the sterile suction package.
2. Place the conscious client in a semi-Fowler's position.
3. Moisten the catheter with sterile saline.
4. Pick up the sterile catheter and connect it to the suction tubing.

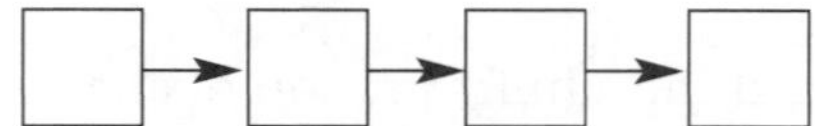

**Activity G** ***Briefly answer the following questions.***

1. What are the preventive measures against tuberculosis?

_______________________________________

_______________________________________

2. What are the signs and symptoms of influenza?

_______________________________________

_______________________________________

3. What are the major causes of epistaxis?

_______________________________________

_______________________________________

4. List a few structural disorders of the nose.

_______________________________________

_______________________________________

5. What are the symptoms of chronic sinusitis?

_______________________________________

_______________________________________

## SECTION II: APPLYING WHAT YOU KNOW

**Activity H** ***Answer the following questions, which involve the nurse's role in the management of respiratory disorders.***

A nurse's role in managing respiratory disorders involves monitoring the symptoms of the disorder and providing proper nursing care. The nurse also helps the clients with activities of daily living (ADL).

1. A nurse is assessing a client with respiratory difficulties.
   a. What data should the nurse collect from a client with respiratory disorders?
   b. What are the nursing diagnoses that can be established based on the data collection?
2. A nurse is caring for a client who has been admitted to the healthcare facility with pneumonia.
   a. What symptoms should the nurse monitor for in the client?
   b. How should the nurse care for the client?

## SECTION III: GETTING READY FOR NCLEX

**Activity I** Answer the following questions.

1. A nurse is caring for a client after a laryngectomy. Which of the following postoperative nursing care measures should be employed when caring for the client? (Select all that apply.)
   a. Reestablish oral feeding of the client.
   b. Remove secretions through the tracheostomy tube.
   c. Administer oxygen using a mask or T-piece.
   d. Instruct the client to wear a thin, filmy scarf over the opening.
   e. Teach the client how to use the tracheoesophageal puncture for speech.
2. A nurse is caring for a client with tuberculosis (TB). Which of the following information should the nurse provide to the client? (Select all that apply.)
   a. TB spreads by inhalation of infected droplets.
   b. Persons with latent TB show a negative skin test reaction.
   c. Pulmonary TB is characterized by high fever.
   d. Diabetic clients have an increased risk for TB infection.
   e. TB spreads to other parts of the body through the blood.

3. A nurse is caring for a client with bronchiectasis. Which of the following nursing care measures should be employed when caring for the client? (Select all that apply.)
   a. Monitor the client for the occurrence of hemoptysis.
   b. Take measures to reduce the humidity of the air.
   c. Discourage the client from breathing deeply.
   d. Provide special mouth care to the client.
   e. Perform a postural drainage procedure.

4. A nurse is preparing a client for bronchoscopy. Which of the following are possible complications of the procedure?
   a. Bleeding
   b. Pneumothorax
   c. Hemothorax
   d. Delirium

5. A nurse is caring for a client admitted to the pulmonary care unit. Which of the following is an early symptom of hypoxia that the nurse should assess for?
   a. Hypertension
   b. Bradycardia
   c. Dyspnea
   d. Stupor and coma

6. A client has been diagnosed with acute rhinitis. Which of the following information should the nurse provide to the client?
   a. The physician should be consulted if fever continues beyond 5 days.
   b. It is not transmitted through coughing or sneezing.
   c. Drinking plenty of fluid helps to reduce the fever.
   d. Antibiotics are effective against the disease.

7. A nurse is caring for a client with influenza. Which of the following nursing care measures should be followed when caring for the client?
   a. Monitor for the presence of purulent or rose-colored sputum.
   b. Instruct the client not to drink fresh fruit juice.
   c. Avoid the administration of analgesics to the client.
   d. Encourage the client to drink milk to improve the nutritional status.

8. A 60-year-old client complains of snoring when sleeping. Which of the following should the nurse suggest to the client as a remedy?
   a. Avoid using sleeping pills.
   b. Eat a heavy evening meal.
   c. Avoid using pillows for sleep.
   d. Sleep in the supine position.

9. A nurse is caring for a female client with asbestosis. Which of the following cancerous conditions is associated with asbestosis?
   a. Cervical carcinoma
   b. Mesothelioma
   c. Melanoma
   d. Kaposi's sarcoma

10. A nurse is caring for a client with chronic sinusitis. Which of the following symptoms of chronic sinusitis should the nurse assess for? (Select all that apply.)
    a. Cough
    b. Facial pain
    c. Nasal stuffiness
    d. Acute headaches
    e. Fatigue

CHAPTER 87

# Oxygen Therapy and Respiratory Care

## SECTION I: TESTING WHAT YOU KNOW

**Activity A** *Match the source of oxygen in Column A with the corresponding indication in Column B.*

| Column A | Column B |
|---|---|
| ____ 1. Oxygen cylinders | a. Home and extended care settings |
| ____ 2. Hyperbaric chambers | b. Administering portable liquid oxygen |
| ____ 3. Oxygen concentrators | c. Carbon monoxide poisoning |
| ____ 4. Oxygen strollers | d. Short-term emergencies |

**Activity B** *Match the oxygen delivery system in Column A with its distinguishing features in Column B.*

| Column A | Column B |
|---|---|
| ____ 1. Simple mask | a. Presence of valves on the outside of the mask |
| ____ 2. Partial-rebreathing mask | b. Transparent mask with a nipple adapter |
| ____ 3. Non-rebreathing mask | c. Presence of a hard plastic adapter with large windows |
| ____ 4. Venturi mask | d. Presence of a bag and the absence of valves |

**Activity C** *Mark each statement as either "T" (True) or "F" (False). Correct any false statements.*

1. T F An oxygen tank is much safer and more convenient to use than an oxygen concentrator.
2. T F Non-rebreathing masks are used only in one-on-one client care situations.
3. T F Oxygen concentrations can be more easily controlled with manual resuscitators.
4. T F A Venturi mask supplies the most reliable and consistent low levels of supplemental oxygen.
5. T F Low-flow oxygen delivery devices aid in supplying precise oxygen concentrations.

**Activity D** *Fill in the blanks.*

1. The pressure in the oxygen cylinder is measured in terms of pounds per square ____________.
2. The percentage of oxygen that reaches the lungs depends on the ____________ and depth of respirations.
3. ____________ mist treatment refers to the suspension of microscopic liquid particles in the air.
4. The ____________ pressure ventilator causes the chest to expand and air to flow into the lungs by lowering the pressure around the chest.

5. ____________ positive airway pressure helps to keep the client's lungs inflated and tends to improve lung function, even though breathing is spontaneous.

**Activity E** *Consider the following figures.*

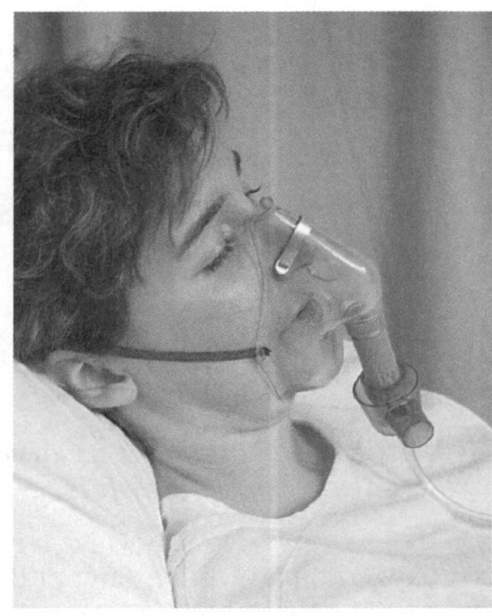

1. Identify the equipment shown in the figure.

______________________________

______________________________

2. Name the features of this equipment.

______________________________

______________________________

3. What is this equipment used for?

______________________________

______________________________

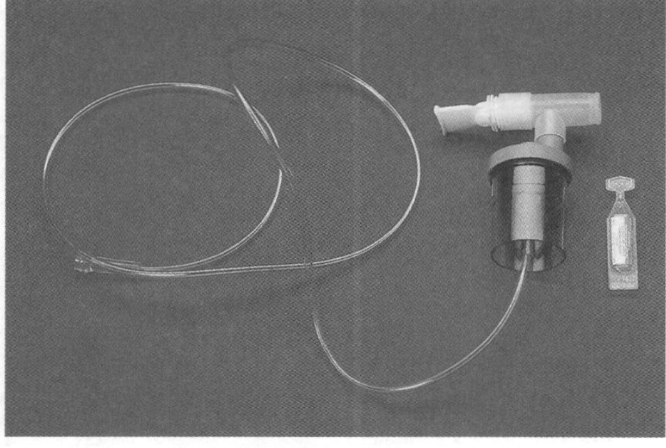

4. Identify the device shown in the figure.

______________________________

______________________________

5. Describe the device setup.

______________________________

______________________________

6. What are the common indications for this device?

______________________________

______________________________

**Activity F** ***The nursing steps involved in the application of the Venturi mask for a client with chronic obstructive pulmonary disease (COPD) are given below in random order. Write the correct sequence of steps in the boxes provided.***

1. Connect the tubing from the Venturi mask to the tailpiece.
2. Place the mask over the bridge of the client's nose and down onto the chin.
3. Attach the wing nut and tailpiece to the flow meter's threaded outlet.
4. Set the flow meter to the manufacturer's recommended flow rate.

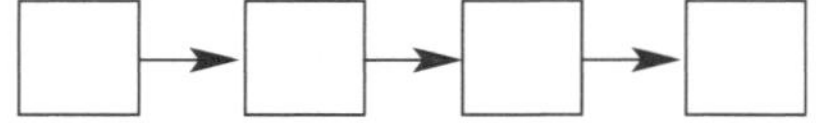

**Activity G** ***Briefly answer the following questions.***

1. What are the goals of oxygen therapy?

______________________________

______________________________

2. Why do clients with severe anemia show unreliable pulse oximeter readings?

______________________________

______________________________

3. What precautions must be taken with oxygen cylinders?

______________________________

______________________________

4. At what maximum rate should the nurse ensure flow of oxygen through a nasal cannula?

______________________________

______________________________

5. What is the goal of intermittent positive-pressure breathing (IPPB)? What steps should the nurse perform when providing an IPPB treatment?

______________________________

______________________________

## SECTION II: APPLYING WHAT YOU KNOW

**Activity H** ***Answer the following questions, which involve the nurse's role in the management of clients with breathing difficulties.***

Oxygen is a gas that is essential to life. When it is prescribed as a medication, it is administered under controlled conditions. Nursing considerations for clients with breathing difficulties include careful determination of the client's respiratory status, safe administration of oxygen therapy, and effective respiratory care.

1. A nurse is caring for a client with chronic obstructive pulmonary disease. The client is receiving supplemental oxygen via a high-flow Venturi mask.
   a. What observations should the nurse make in a client who is receiving oxygen?
   b. What precautions should the nurse take when caring for this client?
   c. What steps should the nurse follow when the physician has recommended discontinuing oxygen?
2. A nurse is caring for a client who underwent tracheostomy after a motor vehicle accident. The nurse is instructed to perform suctioning and provide tracheostomy care to the client.
   a. What steps should the nurse perform when preparing the suction equipment?
   b. How should the nurse change the tracheostomy tube tape?
   c. How should the nurse clean around the tracheostomy stoma and under the tracheostomy tube faceplate?

## SECTION III: GETTING READY FOR NCLEX

**Activity I** ***Answer the following questions.***

1. A nurse is performing pulse oximetry on a client in order to measure the oxygen saturation in the blood. Which of the following interventions should the nurse perform?
   a. Explain that there might be slight pain from the needle prick.
   b. Attach the pulse oximetry probe to the client's fingertip.
   c. Document the oximetry reading as liters per minute.
   d. Avoid using the pulse oximeter continuously.
2. A nurse is caring for a client who is receiving IPPB. What should the nurse assess for in this client? (Select all that apply.)
   a. Dizziness
   b. Bradycardia
   c. Headache
   d. Nausea
   e. Pressure ulcers
3. A nurse is caring for an asthmatic client who is receiving oxygen via a nasal cannula. What is the first step the nurse should take before administering oxygen?
   a. Adjust the flow meter to the recommended flow rate.
   b. Insert the prongs of the nasal cannula into the client's nostrils.
   c. Encourage the client to breathe through the nose rather than the mouth.
   d. Attach the cannula with the connecting tube to the adapter on the humidifier.
4. A nurse is caring for a client who is receiving oxygen with a simple mask. Which of the following measures should the nurse undertake when caring for this client?
   a. Turn the oxygen on after applying the mask.
   b. Ask the client not to move out of bed.
   c. Encourage the client to breathe through the mouth.
   d. Connect the mask tubing to the humidifier outlet.

5. A nurse is caring for a client who is receiving IPPB treatment. Which of the following measures should the nurse employ to ensure that mucus is removed?
   a. Encourage forceful exhalation.
   b. Perform airway suctioning.
   c. Provide IPPB for 2 to 4 minutes.
   d. Assist the client to lie supine on the bed.
6. A nurse is suctioning the airways in a client who recently underwent tracheostomy. Which of the following measures should the nurse employ when inserting the suction catheter?
   a. Apply suction while inserting the catheter.
   b. Assist the client to lie in a supine position.
   c. Insert the catheter until the client coughs.
   d. Suction for no longer than 20-second intervals.
7. A nurse who is new to the healthcare facility is becoming familiar with the wall outlet system used in the facility. Which of the following measures should the nurse employ?
   a. Practice inserting the adapter into the outlet.
   b. Reduce the outlet pressure to a safe level.
   c. Push gently to ensure the adapter is locked in place.
   d. Keep the wall outlets upright at all times.
8. A nurse is caring for a client who is receiving oxygen via a Venturi mask. Which of the following measures should the nurse employ to change oxygen concentrations?
   a. Change the humidifier.
   b. Change the mask regulator.
   c. Change the settings on the adapter.
   d. Change the window openings.
9. A nurse has been providing suctioning and tracheostomy care in a client receiving mechanical ventilation. What should be the maximum duration for each interval of suctioning?
   a. 10 seconds
   b. 20 seconds
   c. 30 seconds
   d. 40 seconds
10. A nurse is caring for a client who is receiving mechanical ventilation. Which of the following supplies are necessary at the client's bedside? (Select all that apply.)
    a. Mini-nebulizer with mask
    b. Manual breathing bag
    c. Extra tracheostomy tube
    d. Aerosolized medications
    e. A 10-mL syringe

CHAPTER 88

# Digestive Disorders

## SECTION I: TESTING WHAT YOU KNOW

**Activity A** *Match the terms related to digestive disorders in Column A with their descriptions in Column B.*

| Column A | Column B |
|---|---|
| ____ 1. Hyperalimentation | a. Inflammation of the gums and teeth |
| ____ 2. Ascites | b. Excessive intravenous administration of nutrients |
| ____ 3. Pyorrhea alveolaris | c. Difficulty in swallowing |
| ____ 4. Dysphagia | d. Accumulation of fluid in the peritoneal cavity |

**Activity B** *Match the tests and procedures in Column A with their purposes in Column B.*

| Column A | Column B |
|---|---|
| ____ 1. Hematest | a. Check for the presence of gallbladder stones |
| ____ 2. Cholecystogram | b. Remove stomach contents and wash out the stomach |
| ____ 3. Colonoscopy | c. Detect occult blood in the feces |
| ____ 4. Gastric lavage | d. Provide direct visualization of the large intestine |

**Activity C** *Mark each statement as either "T" (True) or "F" (False). Correct any false statements.*

1. T F A nurse who educates people to care for ostomies of the stomach, intestine, or colon is known as an enterostomal therapist.
2. T F A nurse inserts a nasogastric tube into a client before gastric lavage.
3. T F The solutions normally used when irrigating nasogastric tubes are tap water or sterile normal saline.
4. T F Periodic heparinization is a necessary process when using a Hickman catheter for parenteral nutrition.
5. T F Clients with bowel surgery can return to their normal diet after the surgery.

**Activity D** *Fill in the blanks.*

1. Serum aminotransferase was formerly known as serum glutamic ____________ transaminase.
2. The procedure that allows the removal and examination of polyps is termed ____________.
3. Leukoplakia buccalis is also known as ____________ patch.
4. ____________ is an endoscopic procedure for injecting caustic agents into the tissues near the varices.
5. The presence of more fat than normal in the stool is a condition known as ____________.

**Activity E** *Consider the following figure.*

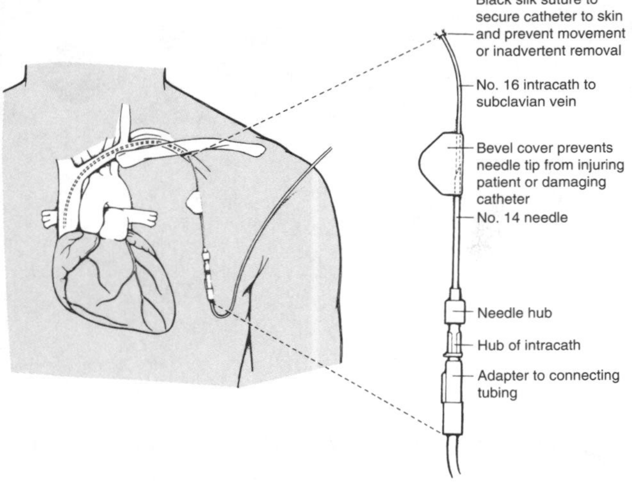


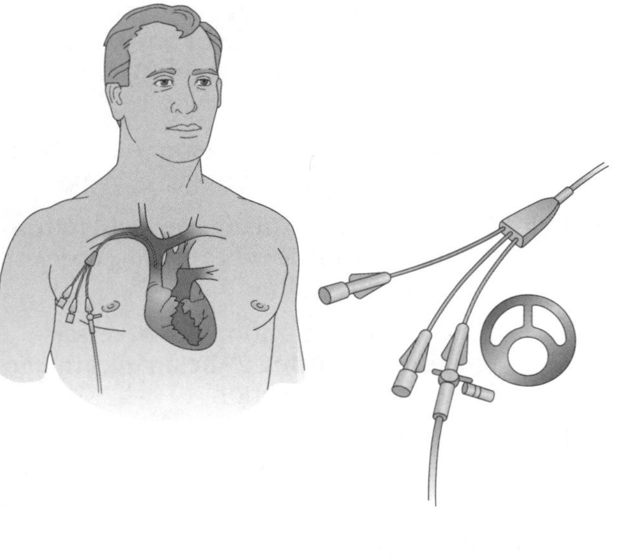

1. Identify the devices in the figure.

______________________________

______________________________

2. State the difference between these devices.

______________________________

______________________________

3. List three nursing considerations pertaining to the use of these devices.

______________________________

______________________________

**Activity F** *A nurse should follow certain guidelines when assisting a physician in removing the nasogastric tubes inserted into a client. Steps that are followed when removing a nasogastric tube are given below in random order. Write the correct sequence in the boxes provided.*

1. Instruct the client to hold his or her breath.
2. Crimp the tube to prevent leakage of its contents.
3. Temporarily clamp the tube, and make sure the client can tolerate its absence.
4. Pull the tube out slowly and then rapidly when the client begins to cough.

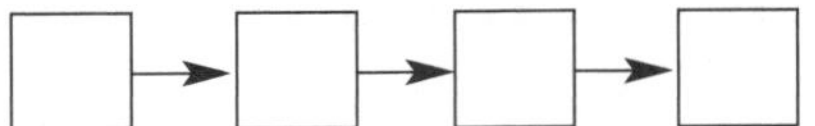

**Activity G** *Briefly answer the following questions.*

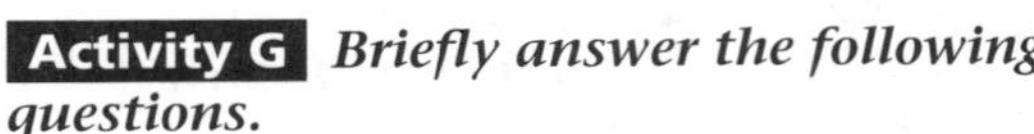

1. What are the causes of gingivitis?

______________________________

______________________________

2. What are the nursing considerations to be followed when preparing a client for a cholecystogram?

______________________________

______________________________

3. What are the nursing considerations to be followed when caring for a client after liver biopsy?

______________________________

______________________________

4. Why is it necessary for a client with gastroesophageal reflux disease (GERD) to follow a strict diet?

______________________________

______________________________

5. What nursing considerations should be kept in mind when antacids are given to a client with ulcers?

______________________________

______________________________

## SECTION II: APPLYING WHAT YOU KNOW

**Activity H** ***Answer the following questions, which involve the nurse's role in educating clients with various digestive disorders.***

A nurse's role in managing disorders of the digestive system involves assisting the clients in their diet and medication. The nurse also helps clients by educating them regarding causes, treatment, symptoms, and preventive measures.

1. A 60-year-old female client has lost two of her teeth and has been prescribed the use of dentures. She is anxious to know if she is losing her teeth due to advancing age.
   a. What should the nurse explain to the client?
   b. What preventive measures should the nurse recommend to the client to prevent further tooth loss?
   c. What client education should the nurse provide on the use of dentures?
2. A nurse is caring for a client with achalasia.
   a. How should the nurse teach the client to improve dietary and eating habits?
   b. What are the other points of care that a client with achalasia must be educated about?

## SECTION III: GETTING READY FOR NCLEX

**Activity I** ***Answer the following questions.***

1. A nurse is caring for a client who has undergone endoscopic retrograde cholangiopancreatography (ERCP). What should the nurse monitor for when assessing this client?
   a. Constipation
   b. Frequent urination
   c. Dysphagia
   d. Diaphoresis
2. A client with Crohn's disease is being weaned off steroid therapy. What withdrawal symptoms should the nurse monitor for in this client? (Select all that apply.)
   a. Body pain
   b. Yawning
   c. Dry mouth
   d. Blurred vision
   e. Goosebumps
3. A client with lactose intolerance has frequent diarrhea. Which of the following must the nurse ask the client to eliminate from the diet?
   a. Tomatoes
   b. Cheese
   c. Corn
   d. Grapes
4. A nurse is caring for a client who has undergone subtotal gastrectomy. What should the nurse monitor to assess dumping syndrome, which may occur as a postoperative complication in such a case? (Select all that apply.)
   a. Palpitation
   b. Steatorrhea
   c. Diaphoresis
   d. Diarrhea
   e. Gingivitis
5. A client who underwent gastric suction to relieve intestinal obstruction vomits during the procedure. What is the nursing consideration to be taken immediately?
   a. Apply K-Y jelly to the tube where it touches the nostril.
   b. Decrease the suction pressure to improve the client's comfort level.
   c. Change the tube and use a medium-length Dobbhoff tube instead.
   d. Note the incident on the client's chart and report it to the physician.
6. A client complains of discomfort in the lower abdomen after a colonoscopy. What should the nurse instruct the client to do to allow passage of air into the colon?
   a. Take a warm bath.
   b. Walk around the room.
   c. Lie on the right side.
   d. Take deep breaths.

7. A nurse is caring for a client who has been admitted to the healthcare center with chest pain. Which of the following distinguishes a heart attack from heartburn?
   a. Pain below the breastbone
   b. Pain immediately after meals
   c. Pain responds to antacids
   d. Pain responds to nitroglycerin

8. A nurse is assessing a client for cholecystitis. Which of the following should the nurse monitor the client for?
   a. Abdominal pain a few hours after food intake
   b. Dark, tarry stools that stick to the pan
   c. Cold and clammy extremities
   d. Intractable pain in the epigastric area

9. A nurse is assisting a physician in conducting a liver biopsy test. What is the first thing the nurse should do?
   a. Instruct the client to hold his or her breath.
   b. Insert the cannula.
   c. Anesthetize the skin.
   d. Withdraw the stylet.

10. A client with inflammatory bowel disease is prescribed steroid therapy. The nurse cautions the client against abruptly discontinuing steroid medication, because doing so could result in which of the following consequences?
    a. It could cause weight gain.
    b. It could reduce sleep.
    c. It could be life-threatening.
    d. It could cause puffiness of the eyelids.

CHAPTER 89

# Urinary Disorders

## SECTION I: TESTING WHAT YOU KNOW

**Activity A** *Match the type of urinary incontinence in Column A with the corresponding causative factor in Column B.*

**Column A**

____ **1.** True incontinence

____ **2.** Stress incontinence

____ **3.** Urge incontinence

____ **4.** Reflex incontinence

**Column B**

**a.** Irritation of the bladder wall by urine components

**b.** Bladder instability as a result of upper motor lesions

**c.** A sudden increase in intra-abdominal pressure

**d.** Almost continuous; commonly caused by prostatectomy

**Activity B** *Match the urinary disorder in Column A with its description in Column B.*

**Column A**

____ **1.** Cylindruria

____ **2.** Oliguria

____ **3.** Dysuria

____ **4.** Anuria

**Column B**

**a.** Painful or difficult urination

**b.** Presence of casts in the urine

**c.** Absence of urine formation

**d.** Production of less urine than normal

**Activity C** *Mark each statement as either "T" (True) or "F" (False). Correct any false statements.*

**1.** T F Extracorporeal shock wave lithotripsy (ESWL) is used when renal stones are present in the lower ureter.

**2.** T F Kidney transplantation is less complex than most other types of transplantation.

**3.** T F There is a significant elevation of serum creatinine when the glomerular filtration rate increases by at least 50%.

**4.** T F A pessary can be left in the vagina for about 4 to 8 weeks without the need for removal for cleaning or maintenance.

**5.** T F Uric acid stones are the most common form of kidney stones.

**Activity D** *Fill in the blanks.*

**1.** ____________ refers to the procedure of crushing the kidney stones.

**2.** ____________ are epithelial, fatty, or waxy tissue abnormally forced out of the renal tubules.

**3.** A ____________ is performed to measure bladder pressure during filling.

**4.** A primary cancer of the kidney is referred to as a/an ____________

**5.** A ____________ pouch is a type of continent diversion in which the middle portion of the ileum is folded and opened onto itself to create a pouch.

**Activity E** *Consider the following figures.*

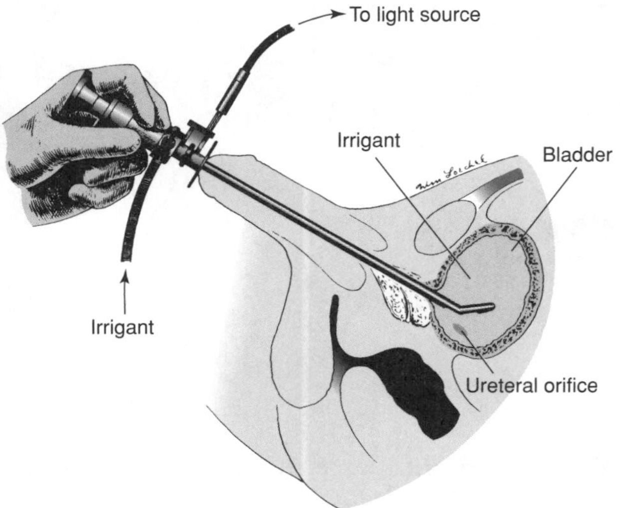


1. Identify the figure.

2. Describe the instrument shown in the figure.

3. What are the applications of this procedure?

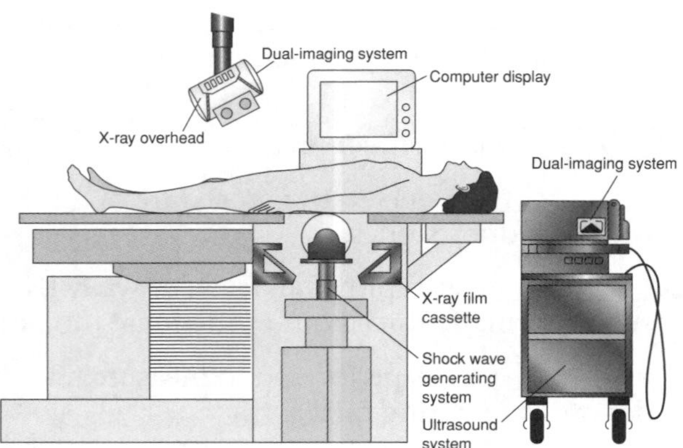


4. Identify the treatment shown in the figure.

5. How is this treatment performed?

6. Who performs this treatment?

**Activity F** ***The steps performed during a cystoscopy examination are given below in random order. Write the correct sequence of the steps in the boxes provided.***

1. Instill Xylocaine jelly into the urethra.
2. Encourage the client to drink fluids.
3. Obtain a urinalysis and a urine culture.
4. Pass the cystoscope into the client's bladder.

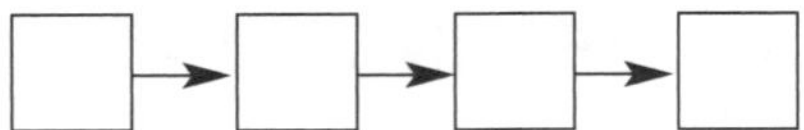

**Activity G** ***Briefly answer the following questions.***

1. What are the specialized imaging studies used to study the urinary tract?

2. What are urodynamic tests?

3. What are the factors that cause transient incontinence?

4. What factors make a person more susceptible to urinary tract infection (UTI)?

5. What is glomerulonephritis?

6. Who is considered a good candidate for kidney donation?

## SECTION II: APPLYING WHAT YOU KNOW

**Activity H** *Answer the following questions, which involve the nurse's role in the management of urinary disorders.*

Nursing care for urinary disorders focuses on maintaining and preserving renal function, decreasing discomfort, preventing infection, promoting skin integrity, maintaining fluid balance, restoring and maintaining the client's self-esteem, and client and family teaching.

1. A client comes to the healthcare facility with complaints of increased urinary frequency, especially during the night, for about the past week. The client also reports a painful, burning sensation felt when passing urine.
   a. What nursing diagnoses may be established for a client with a urinary disorder?
   b. What are the general nursing considerations undertaken when caring for clients with urinary disorders?
2. A client complains of urinary leakage when coughing or sneezing. The client has been experiencing these incidences since childbirth 6 months ago. The client is diagnosed with stress incontinence.
   a. What tips should the nurse provide the client to help empty the bladder completely?
   b. What client education is provided for the management of stress incontinence?

## SECTION III: GETTING READY FOR NCLEX

**Activity I** *Answer the following questions.*

1. A nurse is caring for a client who is experiencing a flare-up of chronic glomerulonephritis. Which of the following measures should the nurse employ when caring for this client?
   a. Encourage the client to drink plenty of fluids.
   b. Place the client in the orthopneic position.
   c. Provide the client with a protein-rich diet.
   d. Encourage the client to remain ambulatory.
2. A nurse is caring for a client who is receiving peritoneal dialysis. What measures should the nurse take after the procedure?
   a. Ask the client to avoid breathing deeply.
   b. Place the client flat for 24 hours.
   c. Assess the client for constipation.
   d. Encourage increased fluid intake for 24 hours.
3. A female client is required to provide a urine sample for a culture and sensitivity test. Which of the following interventions should the nurse perform?
   a. Ask the client to insert a container and start voiding.
   b. Send the urine sample to the laboratory within 24 hours.
   c. Instruct the client to clean the perineal area before voiding.
   d. Give the client nothing by mouth (NPO) for 8 to 10 hours before the test.
4. A nurse is preparing a client for a cystoscopy procedure. What information should the nurse provide the client?
   a. Voiding may be uncomfortable for 1 to 2 weeks.
   b. Salt and fluid intake should be restricted after the procedure.
   c. Urine is sent for culture immediately after cystoscopy.
   d. Urine may be reddish immediately after cystoscopy.
5. A nurse is assisting a healthcare provider perform a needle biopsy of a client's kidney. What is the first step the nurse should perform?
   a. Place a sandbag under the client's abdomen.
   b. Apply pressure to the biopsy site.
   c. Keep the client lying flat for 24 hours.
   d. Give the client a sedative as ordered.
6. A nurse is caring for a client with end-stage renal disease (ESRD). What measures should the nurse employ when caring for this client?
   a. Encourage fluid intake.
   b. Provide a sodium-rich diet.
   c. Weigh the client daily.
   d. Keep the room cool and breezy.

7. A nurse is caring for a client with renal calculi. Which of the following objectives should the nurse include in the short-term goals?
   a. Pain that is of tolerable level
   b. Urination without difficulty or pain
   c. Evidence of passage of stone
   d. Reduced urine output each time

8. A nurse is caring for a client with ESRD. What should the nurse monitor this client for? (Select all that apply.)
   a. Increased appetite
   b. Anasarca
   c. Uremic frost
   d. Hypotension
   e. Bleeding disorders

9. When educating the client who is a heavy smoker about his increased risk of developing various kinds of cancer, what should the nurse instruct the client to watch out for as the first sign of bladder cancer?
   a. Loss of body weight
   b. Pain in the flanks
   c. Sensation of a mass in the flanks
   d. Blood in the urine without any pain

10. A nurse is caring for a client with prerenal failure. The nurse is required to record the client's fluid intake and output. Which of these measures of 24-hour urine output would the nurse document as oliguria?
   a. 75 mL/day
   b. 250 mL/day
   c. 2.5 L/day
   d. 7.5 L/day

CHAPTER 90

# Male Reproductive Disorders

## SECTION I: TESTING WHAT YOU KNOW

**Activity A** *Match the surgical procedures in Column A with their features in Column B.*

**Column A**

____ 1. Plication

____ 2. Orchiopexy

____ 3. Orchiectomy

____ 4. Cavernostomy

**Column B**

a. Fixation of the testes to the scrotal sac

b. Stitching the folds in the hydrocele wall to reduce its size

c. Opening and drainage of a cavity

d. Removal of the testicle

**Activity B** *Match the type of prostatectomy in Column A with its description in Column B.*

**Column A**

____ 1. Radical

____ 2. Retropubic

____ 3. Suprapubic

**Column B**

a. Removal of the prostate through a low abdominal incision working behind the pubic bone

b. Removal of the prostate gland, seminal vesicles, and part of the urethra

c. Removal of the prostate through an incision below the umbilicus and above the symphysis pubis

**Activity C** *Mark each statement as either "T" (True) or "F" (False). Correct any false statements.*

1. T F In case of a varicocele, scrotal temperature is lower than normal body temperature.
2. T F The plaque or scar tissue formation in Peyronie's disease is idiopathic and benign.
3. T F Urinary difficulties are the initial symptoms of benign prostatic hyperplasia.
4. T F Radioactive seed implantation is a common method of treating erectile dysfunction.
5. T F Cancer of the penis is relatively rare in circumcised men.

**Activity D** *Fill in the blanks.*

1. The twisting of the ____________ cord is the actual cause of torsion of the testicle.
2. Inflammation of the epididymis is called ____________.
3. The condition of enlargement of the prostate gland is called benign prostatic ____________.
4. The condition of painful voiding is called ____________.
5. Inflammation of the rectum and anus is called ____________.

**Activity E** *Consider the following figures.*

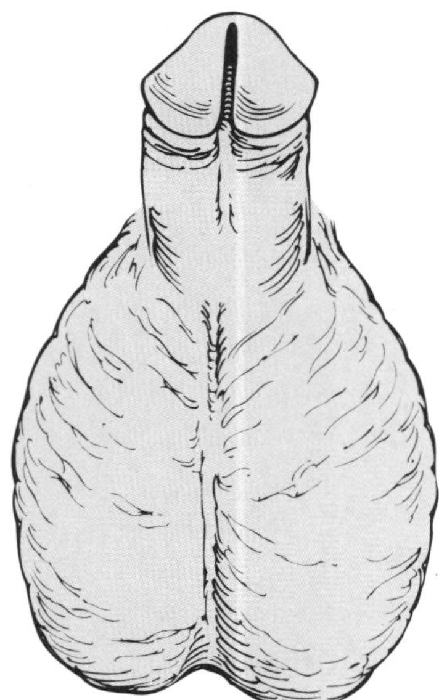

1. Identify the figure.

___

___

2. What is the major cause of this clinical condition?

___

___

3. What is the treatment available for this condition?

___

___

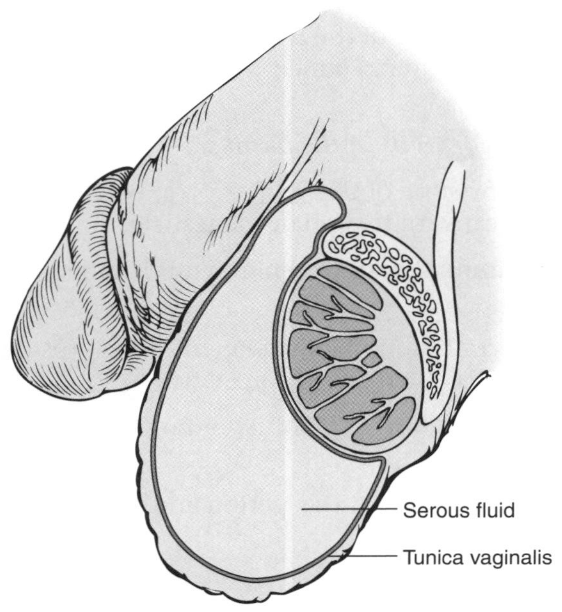


4. Identify the figure.

___

___

5. What is the major cause of this clinical condition?

___

___

6. Explain the treatment methods available for this condition.

___

___

**Activity F** ***Suprapubic prostatectomy is performed to remove the enlarged prostate gland. Some of the steps that occur during suprapubic prostatectomy are given below in random order. Write the correct sequence in the boxes provided.***

1. The enlarged prostate gland is removed.
2. A cystostomy is performed to relieve urinary retention.
3. The catheters are attached to two separate drainage containers.
4. One catheter is placed in the urethra and the other in the suprapubic wound.

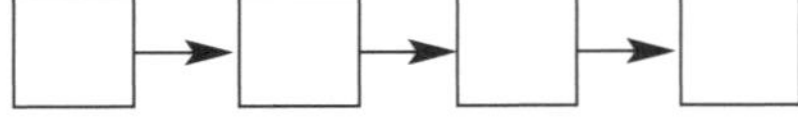

**Activity G** ***Briefly answer the following questions.***

1. What are the various nursing diagnoses that can be established for a male client with a reproductive disorder?

___

___

2. What is the purpose of giving a prostate-specific antigen (PSA) test?

___

___

3. What are intraurethral suppositories?

___

___

4. What are the causes of priapism?

______________________________

______________________________

5. What are the symptoms of epididymitis?

______________________________

______________________________

## SECTION II: APPLYING WHAT YOU KNOW

**Activity H** ***Answer the following questions, which involve the nurse's role in the management of male reproductive disorders.***

A nurse's role in managing male reproductive disorders involves monitoring the symptoms of the disorder and providing proper nursing care.

1. A nurse is assessing a client with erectile dysfunction.
   a. What data should the nurse collect from the client?
   b. How should the nurse care for the client?
2. A nurse is assessing a client with possible testicular cancer.
   a. What information should the nurse provide to the client regarding the risk factors for developing testicular cancer?
   b. How should the nurse instruct the client to perform testicular self-examination?

## SECTION III: GETTING READY FOR NCLEX

**Activity I** ***Answer the following questions.***

1. What interventions should the nurse adopt when caring for the client with epididymitis? (Select all that apply.)
   a. Avoid the administration of antibiotics to the client.
   b. Inform the client that the disease can affect fertility.
   c. Provide scrotal support to the client.
   d. Monitor if the condition is interfering with the client's ambulation.
   e. Discourage the client from applying cold packs to the scrotum.
2. A nurse is caring for a 25-year-old client who has been admitted for a prostatectomy. Which of the following preoperative nursing care measures should be employed when caring for this client? (Select all that apply.)
   a. Alert the client about postoperative erectile dysfunction.
   b. Restrict the fluid intake of the client before the procedure.
   c. Encourage the client to consider sperm banking before the surgery.
   d. Avoid catheterization of the client before the procedure.
   e. Administer the prescribed dose of antibiotics.
3. A client has to undergo a nocturnal penile tumescence (NPT) test. Which of the following measures should the nurse perform with regard to the procedure?
   a. Explain that it helps to determine the degree and duration of the erection.
   b. Inject a vasodilator into the corpora cavernosa of the penis before the test.
   c. Explain that the procedure can cause mild discomfort and pressure.
   d. Assist the physician during the procedure by providing a sterile endoscope.
4. A client has to undergo a suprapubic prostatectomy. Which of the following measures should the nurse perform with regard to the procedure?
   a. Inform the client that it is necessary because the prostate is enlarged to more than 50 g.
   b. Assist the surgeon by providing a sterile suprapubic Cystocath.
   c. Monitor the urethral catheter attached to the irrigation apparatus.
   d. Avoid fecal contamination of the surgical incision.
5. A nurse is preparing a postoperative plan of care for a client who has undergone a radical prostatectomy. Which of the following measures should be included in the client's plan of care? (Select all that apply.)
   a. Avoid using antiembolism stockings.
   b. Teach how to use an incentive spirometer.
   c. Administer the prescribed dose of stool softeners.
   d. Remove the urethral catheter after 1 week.
   e. Monitor the intake and output of the client.

6. Which of the following measures should be adopted when caring for a client after a suprapubic prostatectomy?
   a. Assure the client that urinary urgency during bladder irrigation should not cause concern.
   b. Perform continuous irrigation to wash out clots that plug the catheter.
   c. Monitor the client for overdistention of the bladder due to clogging of the catheter.
   d. Instruct the client to avoid all exercises for 2 days after catheter removal.

7. A client has to undergo a nerve-sparing radical prostatectomy. Which of the following measures should the nurse adopt when caring for this client?
   a. Explain that the prostate is removed through the urethra.
   b. Care for the incision area by frequently changing the dressing.
   c. Provide the prescribed dose of aspirin to relieve the pain of the incision.
   d. Avoid the administration of antispasmodics to the client.

8. During assessment, the client informs the nurse of abnormal and persistent penile erection without any sexual stimulation. Which of the following terms should the nurse use to document the condition?
   a. Orchitis
   b. Phimosis
   c. Epispadias
   d. Priapism

9. A nurse is caring for a 20-year-old client with orchitis. Which of the following nursing care measures should be employed when caring for the client?
   a. Assure the client that the disease does not affect fertility.
   b. Apply heat to relieve the pain associated with the disease.
   c. Provide scrotal support to the client.
   d. Teach the client Kegel exercises for sphincter retraining.

10. A nurse is educating a client with erectile dysfunction about Viagra. Which of the following side effects should the nurse tell the client about?
   a. Priapism
   b. Hydrocele
   c. Phimosis
   d. Varicocele

CHAPTER 91

# Female Reproductive Disorders

## SECTION I: TESTING WHAT YOU KNOW

**Activity A** *Match the disorders related to the menstrual cycle in Column A with their characteristics in Column B.*

| Column A | Column B |
|---|---|
| ____ 1. Menorrhagia | a. Bleeding between menstrual periods |
| ____ 2. Amenorrhea | b. Painful menstruation |
| ____ 3. Dysmenorrhea | c. Absence or abnormal stoppage of menses |
| ____ 4. Metrorrhagia | d. Excessive bleeding in amount or duration during menstruation |

**Activity B** *Match the surgical procedure in Column A with its description in Column B.*

| Column A | Column B |
|---|---|
| ____ 1. Oophorectomy | a. Removal of an oviduct |
| ____ 2. Mastectomy | b. Removal of an ovary |
| ____ 3. Salpingectomy | c. Removal of the entire uterus including the cervix |
| ____ 4. Panhysterectomy | d. Removal of a breast |

**Activity C** *Mark each statement as either "T" (True) or "F" (False). Correct any false statements.*

1. T F Tubal ligation increases the chances of developing ovarian cancer.
2. T F The first symptom of a fibroid tumor is abnormal vaginal bleeding.
3. T F Cystic disease is the most common breast disorder in postmenopausal women.
4. T F Following a high-oxalate diet helps in the treatment of vulvodynia.
5. T F Untreated trichomoniasis can lead to a fragile cervix.

**Activity D** *Fill in the blanks.*

1. Infection of the oviducts is called ____________.
2. Accumulation of lymphatic fluid in the tissues after the removal of a lymph node is called ____________.
3. The surgical procedure removing the entire contents of the pelvis is called pelvic ____________.
4. Inflammation of the cervix is called ____________.
5. Thick, whitish vaginal discharge is called ____________.

**Activity E** *Consider the following figure.*

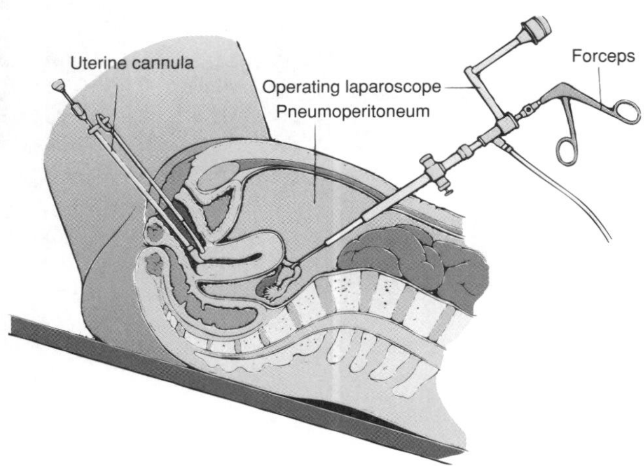


1. Identify the equipment shown in the figure.

______________________________

______________________________

2. What is the purpose of this equipment?

______________________________

______________________________

3. Explain how this equipment works.

______________________________

______________________________

**Activity F** ***Vaginal irrigation helps to remove excess discharge from the vaginal canal and to relieve pain and inflammation. Some of the steps that occur during the vaginal irrigation procedure are given below in random order. Write the correct sequence in the boxes provided.***

1. Carefully inspect the douche tip to make sure that it is not cracked or rough.
2. Release the clamp to let air out of the tubing before inserting the nozzle.
3. Place the irrigating bag slightly above the client's hip level.
4. Have the client lie back and place her on the bedpan.

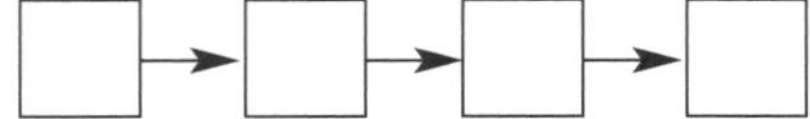

**Activity G** ***Briefly answer the following questions.***

1. What are the risk factors for developing cervical cancer?

______________________________

______________________________

2. What are the signs and symptoms of breast cancer?

______________________________

______________________________

3. What are the stages of cervical cancer?

______________________________

______________________________

4. What are the signs and symptoms of rectocele?

______________________________

______________________________

5. What are the discomforts associated with menopause?

______________________________

______________________________

## SECTION II: APPLYING WHAT YOU KNOW

**Activity H** ***Answer the following questions, which involve the nurse's role in the management of female reproductive disorders.***

A nurse's role in managing reproductive disorders in female clients involves monitoring the symptoms of the disorder and providing proper nursing care.

1. A nurse is caring for a client who has undergone a mastectomy. The surgeon has asked the client to do rope-turning exercises.
   a. How should the nurse instruct the client to do the rope-turning exercise?
   b. What are the postoperative nursing care measures to be employed when caring for this client?

2. A nurse is assessing a client for possible vaginal candidiasis.
   a. What data should the nurse collect from this client?
   b. What self-care tips should the nurse provide to the client?

## SECTION III: GETTING READY FOR NCLEX

**Activity I** *Answer the following questions.*

1. A nurse is preparing a client for mammography. Which of the following instructions should be given to the client? (Select all that apply.)
   a. Wear a gown that opens in the front.
   b. Remove any neck jewelry before the procedure.
   c. Avoid the use of deodorant or powder containing zinc.
   d. Maintain a knee-chest position during the procedure.
   e. Take an analgesic as needed (PRN) to relieve postprocedure pain.
2. A nurse is assisting the physician during a pelvic examination. Which of the following nursing care measures should be employed? (Select all that apply.)
   a. Place the client in Fowler's position.
   b. Place drapes around the client to provide privacy.
   c. Instruct the client to void before the procedure.
   d. Discourage the client from breathing deeply.
   e. Assist the physician by providing a vaginal speculum.
3. A nurse is preparing a postoperative nursing care plan for a mastectomy client. Which of the following nursing care measures should be included in the nursing care plan? (Select all that apply.)
   a. Avoid obtaining blood pressure on the operative side.
   b. Provide a sodium-rich diet to the client.
   c. Monitor drains that are placed in the surgical wound.
   d. Discourage the client from walking and moving around.
   e. Place the affected arm in an elevated position for several days.
4. A nurse is caring for a client affected with chronic cystic mastitis. Which of the following food items may aggravate the formation of cysts?
   a. Coffee
   b. Spinach
   c. Celery
   d. Green beans
5. A 40-year-old client with a family history of breast cancer has come for a routine health checkup. When educating the client, which of the following groups should the nurse say is at a risk for developing breast cancer?
   a. Women who attain menopause before the age of 40 years
   b. Women who have had more than three children
   c. Women who eat a low-fat diet
   d. Women with an irregular menstrual cycle
6. A nurse is preparing a client for culdoscopy. In which of the following positions should the nurse place the client?
   a. Fowler's position
   b. Supine position
   c. Knee-chest position
   d. Lithotomy position
7. A nurse is caring for a client with toxic shock syndrome. Which of the following may have caused this condition?
   a. Using Astroglide during sexual intercourse
   b. Using tampons during menstruation
   c. Using soap to disinfect the perineal area
   d. Using intrauterine devices for contraception

8. A nurse is caring for a client with toxic shock syndrome. What should the nurse monitor in the client during nursing assessment?
   a. Increase in body temperature
   b. Increase in urinary output
   c. Hypertension
   d. Constipation

9. A nurse is educating a 45-year-old client about measures to be taken to relieve menopausal symptoms. Which of the following information should be provided to the client?
   a. Drink a cup of coffee early every morning.
   b. Take vitamin C supplements daily.
   c. Avoid using K-Y jelly during intercourse.
   d. Include ginseng root in the diet.

10. A nurse is caring for a client with pelvic inflammatory disease. Which of the following instructions should the nurse provide to the client?
    a. Maintain the lithotomy position for drainage.
    b. Avoid sexual intercourse.
    c. Perform frequent vaginal douching.
    d. Avoid taking sitz baths.

CHAPTER 92

# Gerontology: The Aging Adult

## SECTION I: TESTING WHAT YOU KNOW

**Activity A** *Match the disorder in Column A with its description in Column B.*

| Column A | Column B |
|---|---|
| ____ 1. Presbycusis | a. Impaired vision due to normal aging |
| ____ 2. Presbyopia | b. Inability to use or understand speech |
| ____ 3. Aphasia | c. Curvature of the spine |
| ____ 4. Kyphosis | d. Sensorineural hearing problem |

**Activity B** *Match the systemic changes due to aging in Column A with their manifestations in Column B.*

| Column A | Column B |
|---|---|
| ____ 1. Receding capillaries | a. Decreased ability to maintain hydration |
| ____ 2. Erratic pigment production | b. Sallow skin and thick nails |
| ____ 3. Loss of subcutaneous fat | c. Increased incidence of trauma |
| ____ 4. Loss of elasticity | d. Senile lentigines and keratoses |

**Activity C** *Mark each statement as either "T" (True) or "F" (False). Correct any false statements.*

1. T F Retirement communities are nursing homes exclusively for the care of older adults.
2. T F A nurse should not "trick" an older adult into taking medication by hiding it in food.
3. T F Older adults should have a restricted fluid intake because of the risk of incontinence.
4. T F A client with aphasia often has clear thinking processes.
5. T F A nurse should discourage excessive use of laxatives by older adults.

**Activity D** *Fill in the blanks.*

1. The study of the effects of normal aging and age-related diseases is called ___________.
2. Awareness of posture, movement, and changes in equilibrium in relation to objects is called ___________.
3. The single most highly recommended exercise for adults is ___________.

4. The branch of medicine concerned with the disorders of aging and their treatment is ___________.

5. The toes or fingernails of older diabetic adults are cut by ___________.

**Activity E** *Consider the following figures.*

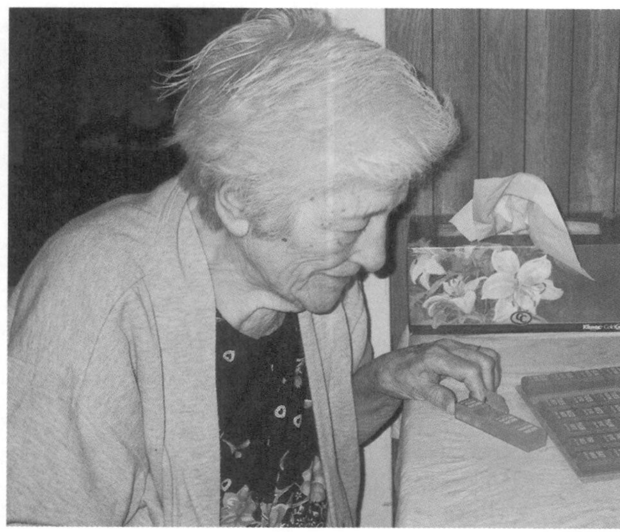

1. Identify the figure.

_______________________________________________

_______________________________________________

2. What are the advantages of such measures?

_______________________________________________

_______________________________________________

3. List at least three changes in the use of medications that are related to the process of aging.

_______________________________________________

_______________________________________________

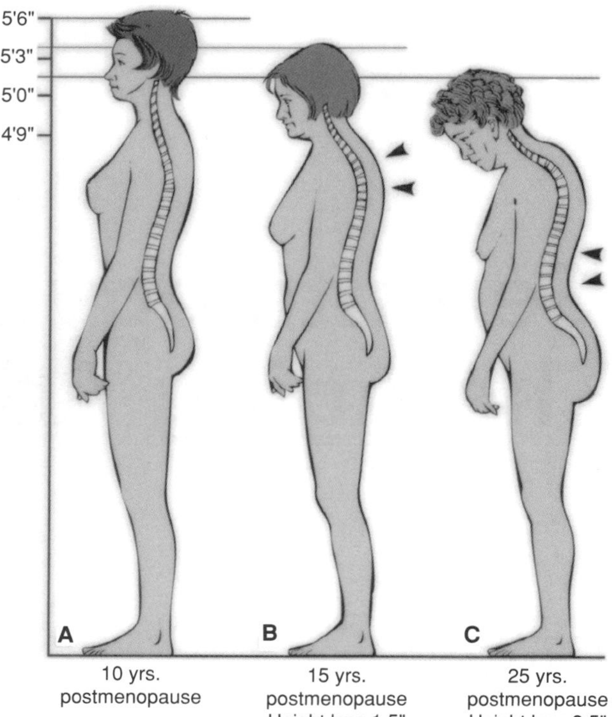


4. Identify the figure.

_______________________________________________

_______________________________________________

5. How does exercise help in reducing the disorder?

_______________________________________________

_______________________________________________

**Activity F** *Briefly answer the following questions.*

1. Why is it important for an older adult to maintain proper weight?

_______________________________________________

_______________________________________________

2. What is caregiver stress, and why is it an important consideration?

_______________________________________________

_______________________________________________

3. What are the nursing considerations to be followed when caring for a client with incontinence?

_______________________________________________

_______________________________________________

4. Why are family members usually unable to detect an older adult's alcohol abuse?

______________________________________

______________________________________

5. What are the nursing considerations to be followed when caring for an elderly adult with visual impairment?

______________________________________

______________________________________

6. Why do elderly clients usually have difficulties with elimination?

______________________________________

______________________________________

7. Why do elderly clients face difficulty in voiding urine?

______________________________________

______________________________________

## SECTION II: APPLYING WHAT YOU KNOW

**Activity G** *Answer the following questions, which involve a nurse's role in caring for older adults.*

A nurse's role when caring for older adults involves assisting the clients in their basic needs, such as nutrition, elimination, and hygiene. The nurse also helps clients by providing emotional and psychological assistance, encouraging them in self-care, and educating them to maintain good health.

1. A nurse is caring for an elderly client with presbycusis.
   a. What nursing considerations should be kept in mind when caring for this client?
   b. How can communication be improved in aging adults?
2. A nurse is caring for an elderly client who is obese.
   a. When providing client education, what should the nurse explain about the benefits of physical activity?
   b. What dangers of immobility should the nurse caution the client about?

## SECTION III: GETTING READY FOR NCLEX

**Activity H** *Answer the following questions.*

1. Which of the following indicates the presence of hirsutism in a client?
   a. Impaired vision due to aging
   b. Altered sense of equilibrium
   c. Involuntary voiding of urine
   d. Presence of facial hair
2. An elderly client has difficulty swallowing food. How can a nurse help in such a condition? (Select all that apply.)
   a. Place the client in a lateral recumbent position.
   b. Elevate the head end of the client's bed.
   c. Encourage the client to bend his chin toward the chest.
   d. Cut the food into smaller bites.
   e. Provide less frequent meals to the client.
3. An elderly client's daughter wants to leave her mother at a senior care center when she goes out to work. What facilities are available at senior care centers? (Select all that apply.)
   a. Educational discussions
   b. Laundry services
   c. Recreational games
   d. Monitored healthcare
   e. Lunchtime meals
4. A nurse is caring for an older adult who is obese. What health risk should the nurse point out as associated with obesity?
   a. Hypotension
   b. Diabetes insipidus
   c. Tuberculosis
   d. Myocardial infarction
5. A client has been admitted to a healthcare facility due to elder abuse. What is the most common category of elder abusers?
   a. Siblings
   b. Children
   c. Friends
   d. Spouses

6. A nurse is providing assistance to a diabetic elderly client. Which of the following is a major nursing consideration when providing nail and foot care for the client?
   a. Wash the client's legs in cold water.
   b. Cut the overgrown nails of the foot.
   c. Document any injury to the client's foot.
   d. Encourage client to inspect the feet once a week.
7. An older adult decides to live away from his family, but wants to stay in a care center where he can be provided both care and privacy. Which of the following types of facilities should a nurse suggest?
   a. Senior care centers
   b. Assisted living facilities
   c. Retirement complexes
   d. Rehabilitative care facilities
8. An aging adult is being treated for constipation. Which of the following should the nurse include in the client's diet?
   a. Increased protein intake
   b. Increased fiber intake
   c. Increased vitamin intake
   d. Increased fat intake
9. A nurse is caring for an aging adult who has been prescribed an enteric-coated medication. The client is not agreeing to swallow the medication. Which of the following should the nurse do?
   a. Crush the tablet before administering it.
   b. Hide the tablet in the client's food.
   c. Tell the client that she must take the medicine.
   d. Ask the client to chew the tablet before swallowing it.
10. A nurse is providing care for an elderly client who has diabetes. What nursing measure is the nurse likely to undertake when caring for such a client?
   a. Provide bladder retraining.
   b. Provide a daily bath to the client.
   c. Cut the client's fingernails.
   d. Shave the client's facial hair.

CHAPTER 93

# Dementias and Related Disorders

## SECTION I: TESTING WHAT YOU KNOW

**Activity A** *Match the classification of dementia in Column A with its characteristic feature in Column B.*

**Column A**

____ **1.** Wernicke-Korsakoff syndrome

____ **2.** Pick's disease

____ **3.** Creutzfeldt-Jakob disease

____ **4.** Multi-infarct dementia

**Column B**

**a.** Caused by a slow virus, considered transmissible

**b.** Vascular; progresses in a stepwise fashion

**c.** Nerve cells are pale and swollen with globules of protein

**d.** Alcohol-related; short-term memory is most impaired

**Activity B** *Match the terms related to mental disorders in Column A with their corresponding descriptions in Column B.*

**Column A**

____ **1.** Dementia

____ **2.** Delirium

____ **3.** Aphagia

____ **4.** Akinesia

**Column B**

**a.** Inability to eat or swallow

**b.** Does not affect level of consciousness

**c.** Complete or partial loss of muscle control

**d.** Causes an altered level of consciousness

**Activity C** *Mark each statement as either "T" (True) or "F" (False). Correct any false statements.*

**1.** T F Confusion characterized by loss of cognitive function is a normal component of the aging process.

**2.** T F Delirium has a sudden onset and is often reversible.

**3.** T F Medications given in the early to middle stages of Alzheimer's disease (AD) will stop the progression of the disease.

**4.** T F Pick's disease has an earlier onset than AD.

**5.** T F Accidental or intentional suicide is a risk during the later stages of AD.

**Activity D** *Fill in the blanks.*

**1.** Inability to recognize objects or persons through auditory, visual, sensory, or tactile sensations is referred to as ____________.

**2.** Bayle's disease is a type of progressive dementia caused by tertiary ____________.

**3.** AD is characterized by a significant reduction in the brain's ability to make ____________, which is a vital neurotransmitter.

**4.** Definite diagnosis of AD can be made only via autopsy or ____________.

**5.** A/An ____________ directive indicates the client's preferences for caregiving procedures, treatments, and life-sustaining measures.

**Activity E** *Consider the following figures.*

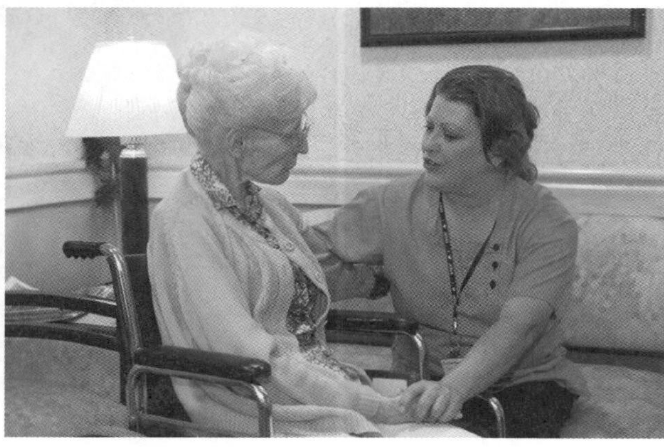

1. What does the figure show?

2. How should the nurse communicate with a client diagnosed with AD?

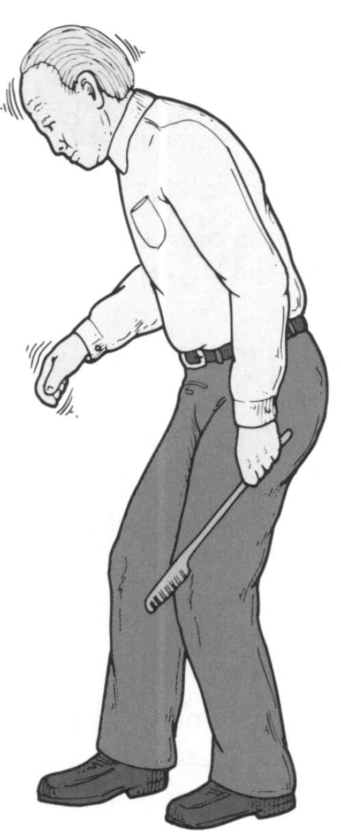

3. Identify the figure.

4. Describe the characteristic feature of the disorder.

**Activity F** ***The stages of AD are given below in random order. Write the correct sequence of progression of the disease in the boxes provided.***

1. The client may take longer than normal to complete routine chores.
2. The client loses the ability to speak and becomes incontinent.
3. The client may not be able to function normally in a work environment.
4. The client tends to wander and gets lost easily, even at home.

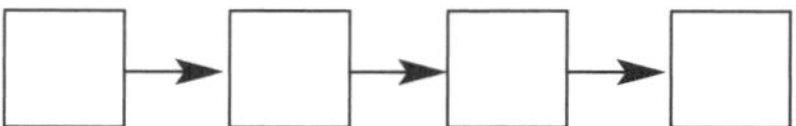

**Activity G** ***Briefly answer the following questions.***

1. What are the brain cell changes that occur in AD?

2. How should the nurse handle paranoia in clients with dementia?

3. What tests are performed in a neurologic examination for diagnosis of dementia?

4. What are the causes of delirium?

5. What measures should the nurse employ for bladder and bowel management in a client with dementia?

______________________________________

______________________________________

## SECTION II: APPLYING WHAT YOU KNOW

**Activity H** *Answer the following questions, which involve the nurse's role in the management of dementia and related disorders.*

Nursing actions when caring for the demented client include assisting with activities of daily living (ADL), using communication skills, managing difficult behaviors, and providing education and support to caregivers.

1. A nurse is caring for an elderly client with AD. The client is completely edentulous and wears dentures. The client exhibits aggressive behavior, making verbal threats and lashing out at the nurse.
   a. What evaluation should the nurse make regarding oral care in an AD client with dentures?
   b. What measures should the nurse take to maintain the client's nutrition and hydration?
   c. How should the nurse handle aggressiveness in this client?
2. A client with dementia is brought to the healthcare facility. The client resides with her daughter, who accompanies her to the visit. The client's daughter works as a high school teacher and finds it difficult to care for the client during the day.
   a. What measures should the nurse take when communicating with a client who has dementia?
   b. What assistance should the nurse provide the client's caregivers?
   c. What information should the nurse provide the client's daughter regarding respite care?

## SECTION III: GETTING READY FOR NCLEX

**Activity I** *Answer the following questions.*

1. A nurse is caring for a client with AD who needs assistance with dressing. Which of the following measures should the nurse employ for this client?
   a. Allow the client to choose clean clothes.
   b. Provide clothing with Velcro and elastic waistbands.
   c. Provide all instructions before the client starts to dress.
   d. Encourage the client to wear pullovers instead of buttoned clothes.
2. A nurse is assessing a client for progressive dementia. Which of the following should the nurse assess for in this client? (Select all that apply.)
   a. Difficulty with functional skills
   b. Signs of hyperactivity
   c. Impaired arithmetic calculations
   d. Loss of language skills
   e. Altered level of consciousness
3. A nurse is required to assess a client with dementia for signs of paranoid behavior. Which of the following demonstrates paranoia?
   a. Client accuses others of stealing her belongings.
   b. Client has false perception of hearing voices.
   c. Client believes that her spouse is trying to kill her.
   d. Client uses hostile language and makes verbal threats.
4. A nurse is caring for a client with dementia who is agitated and refuses to take directions. What measures should the nurse employ in this client?
   a. Touch the client gently when talking.
   b. Try to reason with the client.
   c. Try to talk with a pleasant tone.
   d. Go away briefly and come back later.

5. A nurse is caring for a client with dementia who needs assistance with daily care. What measures should the nurse employ?
   a. Keep ready all the clothes to be worn.
   b. Give pain medication before bathing the client.
   c. Provide clothes with buttons and zippers.
   d. Give the client a cup of coffee immediately after the bath.

6. A nurse is caring for a client with Wernicke-Korsakoff syndrome. The nurse might find it difficult to care for the client for which of the following reasons?
   a. Language problems
   b. Impaired long-term memory
   c. Belligerent behavior patterns
   d. Perceptual problems

7. A nurse is assisting the physician in assessing a client for dementia. Which of the following is part of the assessment during psychometric testing?
   a. Identifying behavioral problems in the client
   b. Determining judgment and planning abilities
   c. Assessing for sleep pattern disturbances
   d. Testing the client for the ability to communicate

8. A nurse is employed at a long-term facility caring for clients with dementia. Which of the following nursing diagnoses should be included on nursing care plans for these clients?
   a. Age when changes began
   b. Association with medical events
   c. Deteriorating mental status
   d. Ineffective family coping

9. The nurse is asked to test a client's skin turgor. What should the nurse assess for by performing this test?
   a. Signs of dehydration
   b. Pressure areas
   c. Peripheral edema
   d. Tactile sensation

10. A nurse is caring for a paranoid client with dementia. The nurse should remove which of the following items from the client's environment? (Select all that apply.)
   a. Electric razors
   b. Mirrors
   c. Intercoms
   d. Door buzzers
   e. Lamps

CHAPTER 94

# Psychiatric Nursing

## SECTION I: TESTING WHAT YOU KNOW

**Activity A** *Match the defense mechanisms in Column A with their corresponding definitions in Column B.*

**Column A**

____ 1. Suppression

____ 2. Displacement

____ 3. Reaction-formation

____ 4. Projection

**Column B**

a. Displaying a feeling opposite to that which one would normally exhibit in the same situation

b. Attributing to another person one's unacceptable thoughts and feelings

c. Unconsciously transferring feelings onto another person or object

d. Inhibiting consciously an emotion that is unacceptable

**Activity B** *Match the personality disorders in Column A with their deviation patterns in Column B.*

**Column A**

____ 1. Histrionic

____ 2. Narcissistic

____ 3. Schizotypal

____ 4. Paranoid

**Column B**

a. Pervasive distrust and suspiciousness of others, with marked hypervigilance

b. Excessive emotionality marked by severe attention-seeking behavior

c. Social and interpersonal deficits; showing acute discomfort with close relationships

d. Grandiosity, need for admiration, lack of empathy, and sense of entitlement

**Activity C** *Mark each statement as either "T" (True) or "F" (False). Correct any false statements.*

1. T F Major depressive disorder tends to last longer than dysthymia.
2. T F Negative reinforcement in behavior modification is usually ineffective because it does not promote and teach positive behavior.
3. T F All antidepressants take 1 to 6 months from initiation of administration for symptom relief to occur.
4. T F The nurse cannot have any contact with a mentally ill client outside the health-care setting under any circumstances.
5. T F The new classes of antipsychotics are commonly used to treat the positive symptoms of psychosis.
6. T F Intellectualization is a defense mechanism in which the client uses reasoning as a means of avoiding confrontation with objectionable impulses.

**Activity D** *Fill in the blanks.*

1. ___________ are sensory perceptions, not based in reality, wherein a client can hear, see, and feel things that are not there.
2. The sense of markedly diminished interest or loss of interest or pleasure in all or most activities is termed ___________.
3. The clients should sign a pass ___________ in which they promise to return and release the facility from liability when they are going for outings.
4. ___________ adult legislation protects intellectually impaired and mentally ill clients who are unable to protect themselves.
5. Difficulty falling or staying asleep is referred to as ___________.
6. ___________ is a defense mechanism in which the client disavows the existence of unpleasant realities.

**Activity E** *Consider the following figure.*

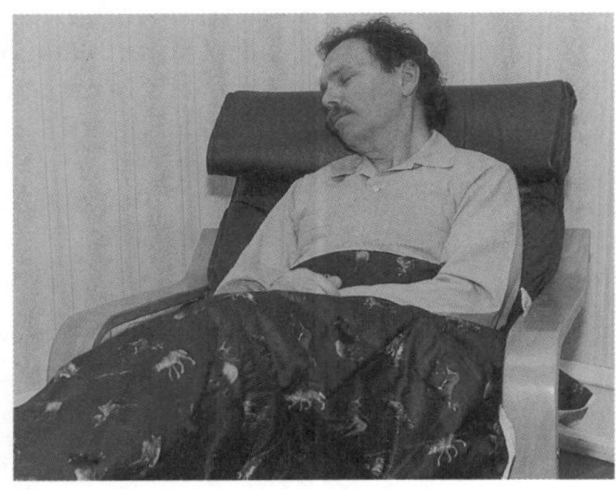

1. Identify the type of schizophrenia experienced by the client shown in the figure.

___________________________________________

___________________________________________

2. What are the symptoms noticed in this condition?

___________________________________________

___________________________________________

3. How are clients with this condition managed?

___________________________________________

___________________________________________

**Activity F** *The nurse needs to assist the physician during the administration of electroconvulsive therapy (ECT). The nursing steps followed during ECT are given below in random order. Write the correct sequence in the boxes provided.*

1. Achieve paralysis by use of short-acting anesthetic agents.
2. Start an IV line to administer routine medications.
3. Assist the client to put on hospital garb and remove contact lenses or jewelry.
4. Apply a tourniquet to obstruct the entry of anesthetics into the limb.

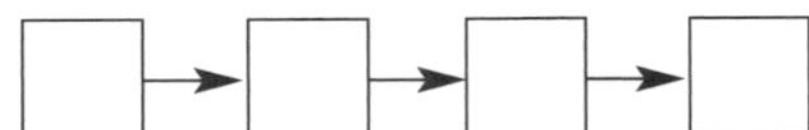

**Activity G** *Briefly answer the following questions.*

1. What is the *Diagnostic and Statistical Manual of Mental Disorders?*

___________________________________________

___________________________________________

2. State the method and purpose of performing lumbar puncture.

___________________________________________

___________________________________________

3. What is post-traumatic stress disorder (PTSD)?

___________________________________________

___________________________________________

4. Who pays the cost of mental healthcare?

___________________________________________

___________________________________________

5. What is seclusion?

___________________________________________

___________________________________________

## SECTION II: APPLYING WHAT YOU KNOW

**Activity H** *Answer the following questions, which involve the nurse's role in the care of clients with mental illness.*

Basic principles of mental health apply to the care of all clients, no matter what the setting. Primary prevention and counseling can help to avoid later problems. The primary goal of a psychiatric nurse practitioner is to use concepts learned in psychiatry or mental health classes in all interactions with mentally ill clients.

1. An 18-year-old client is brought to the healthcare facility with complaints of depression. The client's grandmother reports that the client has been experiencing crying spells, irritability, anxiety, poor concentration, and isolation since the death of her parents in an accident. The client is also noticed to have poor eating and sleeping habits. The healthcare provider instructs the nurse to observe the client for depression.
   a. What assessment should be done by the nurse regarding the client's speech?
   b. What observations should the nurse make regarding the client's sleep patterns?
   c. What goals should the nurse include in the plan of care for this client?
2. A 32-year-old client is brought to the healthcare facility, accompanied by her husband, with complaints of severe behavior changes. The client's husband reports that the client has become irritable, frustrated, and assaultive in nature. The client also seems to be making unreasonable demands, such as demanding that he move out of their apartment. The healthcare provider confirms the diagnosis of mania and advises hospitalization.
   a. What measures should the nurse employ when caring for a client with mania?
   b. What safety devices should the nurse use for these clients?

## SECTION III: GETTING READY FOR NCLEX

**Activity I** *Answer the following questions.*

1. The healthcare provider informs the nurse that a client is extremely agoraphobic. Which of the following is fearful for this client?
   a. Enclosed places
   b. Open spaces
   c. Heights
   d. Public speaking
2. A 31-year-old client is hospitalized and kept under observation for severe behavioral changes. The physician confirms the diagnosis of obsessive-compulsive disorder and starts the client on buspirone (BuSpar). Which of the following side effects should the nurse watch for in clients receiving BuSpar?
   a. Headache
   b. Hypertension
   c. Peripheral edema
   d. Pain in calves
3. The healthcare provider prescribes monamine oxidase inhibitors (MAOI) to a client to treat major depression. The nurse is asked to provide client teaching regarding the medication. Which of the following instructions should the nurse give to this client?
   a. Encourage the client to eat ripe fruits, bananas, and yogurt.
   b. Instruct the client to drink large amounts of water to avoid dryness of the mouth.
   c. Tell client not to take over-the-counter (OTC) drugs containing sympathomimetic amines.
   d. Advise the client to restrict salt consumption as much as possible.
4. A client accused of a serious crime is admitted to the healthcare facility for an extended period. The client is reported to exhibit aggressive behavior and has twice escaped from the facility. Which of the following steps should the nurse employ to prevent the client from escaping?
   a. Use a whiplash collar
   b. Use leather restraints
   c. Lock the nursing unit
   d. Use sally-port doors

5. A psychiatric nurse is caring for a client with severe psychosis who is being treated with neuroleptics. The nurse is instructed to administer anticholinergic medication to the client. For which of the following reasons should the client take this medication?
   a. To prevent the side effects of neuroleptics
   b. To increase the absorption of neuroleptics
   c. To reduce the elimination of neuroleptics
   d. To increase nutrient absorption capacity

6. A nurse is caring for a client with a mental disorder who was diagnosed with neuroleptic malignant syndrome (NMS) soon after the first administration of a neuroleptic medication. Which of the following is considered the most frequent cause of death from NMS?
   a. Congestive heart failure
   b. Respiratory failure
   c. Severe infections
   d. Myocardial infarction

7. A nurse is caring for a client who is diagnosed with schizophrenia. Which of the following negative symptoms should the nurse expect to find in this client?
   a. Hallucinations
   b. Delusions
   c. Withdrawal
   d. Muscle rigidity

8. A nurse is caring for a client who was recently admitted to the healthcare facility with severe bipolar disorder. Which of the following measures should the nurse employ when assisting the client to fall asleep? (Select all that apply.)
   a. Encourage use of relaxation tapes.
   b. Encourage watching television at bedtime.
   c. Provide a snack before bedtime.
   d. Administer sleeping pills as needed (PRN).
   e. Encourage increased fluid intake.

9. A nurse is caring for mentally ill clients in the psychiatric unit. In what capacity should the nurse act to support mentally disordered clients? (Select all that apply.)
   a. Socializing agent
   b. Support person
   c. Dietitian
   d. Chaplain
   e. Counselor

10. A mentally disordered client is receiving therapeutic recreation as a part of his psychotherapy regimen. What are the roles of a recreational therapist? (Select all that apply.)
    a. To offer spiritual counseling and support
    b. To encourage the client to engage in games
    c. To help clients find a safe place to live
    d. To take clients on outings
    e. To assist clients in cooking a meal or dessert

CHAPTER 95

# Substance Abuse

## SECTION I: TESTING WHAT YOU KNOW

**Activity A** *Match the terms in Column A with the symptoms they represent in Column B.*

| Column A | Column B |
|---|---|
| ____ 1. Diaphoresis | a. Runny nose |
| ____ 2. Rhinorrhea | b. Excessive sweating |
| ____ 3. Bradypnea | c. Drooping eyelids |
| ____ 4. Ptosis | d. Respiratory depression |

**Activity B** *Match the terms in Column A with the clinical conditions they indicate in Column B.*

| Column A | Column B |
|---|---|
| ____ 1. Laennec's cirrhosis | a. Extreme sleepiness and drowsiness |
| ____ 2. Delirium tremens | b. Rapid eyeball movement from side to side |
| ____ 3. Somnolence | c. Vivid and terrifying auditory, visual, and tactile hallucinations |
| ____ 4. Horizontal nystagmus | d. Chronic interstitial inflammation of the liver |

**Activity C** *Mark each statement as either "T" (True) or "F" (False). Correct any false statements.*

1. T F Methamphetamine can be used as an adjunct treatment for alcoholism.
2. T F The abuse of gamma hydroxybutyrate can be detected by conducting routine U-tox screening tests.
3. T F Abuse of cocaine can cause organic brain syndrome.
4. T F Elevated vital signs are the first indicator of alcohol withdrawal.
5. T F The acute detoxification process from alcohol begins within 96 hours after the last ingestion.

**Activity D** *Fill in the blanks.*

1. Alcohol can cause ____________ alcohol syndrome when used by a pregnant woman.
2. When an alcoholic blames others for his or her problems, this defense mechanism is termed ____________.
3. Binding of carbon monoxide present in cigarette smoke with ____________ reduces the oxygen carrying capacity of the blood.
4. Fear or panic without any reason is called ____________.
5. Anabolic steroids are substances derived from ____________ the male hormone.

**Activity E** *Consider the following figure.*

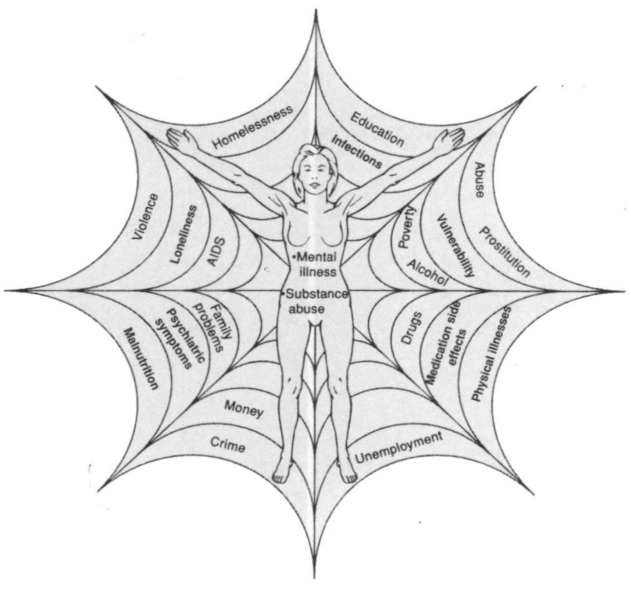


1. Explain the figure.

2. How can a nurse identify a chemically dependent client?

3. Why is a mentally ill person more prone to such a disorder?

**Activity F** ***Unmanaged alcohol withdrawal can lead to life-threatening complications. Symptoms seen during alcohol withdrawal are given below in random order. Write the correct sequence of occurrence of these symptoms in the boxes provided.***

1. A feeling that the person is being persecuted
2. Copious vomiting and dry heaves
3. Blackouts and cardiac arrest
4. Two to eight tonic-clonic seizures close together

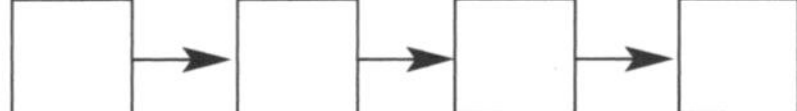

**Activity G** ***Briefly answer the following questions.***

1. What is meant by the term codependent?

2. What are the common characteristics of a substance abuser's personality?

3. What are the symptoms associated with amphetamine abuse?

4. What are the symptoms of abuse of cannabis-related drugs?

5. What are the side effects of anabolic steroid abuse?

## SECTION II: APPLYING WHAT YOU KNOW

**Activity H** ***Answer the following questions, which involve the nurse's role in substance abuse management.***

A nurse's role in managing substance abuse involves identifying a chemically dependent client and providing appropriate nursing care while monitoring the withdrawal symptoms during the time of detoxification.

1. A nurse is caring for a chain smoker during the detoxification process.
   a. What are the withdrawal symptoms the nurse should monitor in this client?
   b. What information should the nurse provide to the client regarding the adverse effects of smoking?

2. A nurse suspects alcohol abuse in a client who is 16 weeks pregnant and arrives at the health-care facility for a regular checkup.
   a. How can a nurse identify whether the client is an alcoholic?
   b. What information should the nurse provide to the client regarding the adverse effects of consuming alcohol during pregnancy?

## SECTION III: GETTING READY FOR NCLEX

**Activity I** *Answer the following questions.*

1. During the data gathering process, a 30-year-old methamphetamine abuser complains to the nurse that he has the sensation of insects or snakes crawling on the skin. Which of the following terms should the nurse use to document the condition?
   a. Formications
   b. Anhedonia
   c. Tweaking
   d. Huffing
2. A client has been prescribed Antabuse therapy for chronic alcohol abuse. Which of the following is true regarding Antabuse therapy?
   a. Antabuse can be started within 12 hours after alcohol ingestion.
   b. Therapy should be continued for a maximum of 6 months.
   c. Cough syrups should be avoided during Antabuse therapy.
   d. Antabuse drugs can be safely used in diabetic clients.
3. A nurse is caring for a client with Wernicke-Korsakoff syndrome. Which deficiency should the nurse monitor this client for?
   a. Vitamin A
   b. Vitamin B
   c. Vitamin C
   d. Vitamin D
4. A nurse is caring for a client with unmanaged alcohol withdrawal. Which of the following symptoms indicate that the client's condition is life-threatening?
   a. Delirium tremens
   b. Subjective internal tremors
   c. Somnolence
   d. Horizontal nystagmus
5. A nurse is teaching an elderly client about the adverse effects of over-the-counter (OTC) drug abuse. Which of the following drugs can be cited as an example of an OTC drug?
   a. Naltrexone (Depade, ReVia)
   b. Amphetamine (Dexadrine, DextroStat)
   c. Methadone (Dolophine)
   d. Caffeine (Vivarin)
6. A nurse is required to care for a cocaine abuser who is in the detoxification process. Which of the following withdrawal symptoms should the nurse monitor in the client? (Select all that apply.)
   a. Dilated pupils
   b. Increased urinary output
   c. Unreasonable fear and panic
   d. Increase in respiratory rate
   e. Sleep disturbances
7. A 30-year-old client with suspected chronic alcohol abuse is brought to the detoxification center. Which of the following symptoms should the nurse monitor to identify the abuse? (Select all that apply.)
   a. Palmar erythema
   b. Formication
   c. Tachypnea
   d. Spider angioma
   e. Dementia
8. A nurse is conducting a blood alcohol test for a motorist who is suspected of alcohol abuse. Which of the following statements are true regarding the rate of absorption of alcohol? (Select all that apply.)
   a. Aspirin decreases the absorption of alcohol.
   b. Carbonation decreases the rate of absorption.
   c. The absorption rate is faster in women than in men.
   d. Ranitidine enhances the absorption of alcohol.
   e. The ratio of muscle to fat affects the rate of absorption.

9. A 45-year-old drug abuser who is in the detoxification process has developed refeeding syndrome. The excess and rapid introduction of which of the following substances is the actual cause of the syndrome?
   a. Protein
   b. Carbohydrates
   c. Fat
   d. Vitamins

10. A nurse is required to care for a 40-year-old client who is receiving acamprosate therapy. Which of the following is true regarding the use of acamprosate?
    a. Extreme sleepiness is one of the side effects of this drug.
    b. Administration of the drug along with antidepressants causes weight loss.
    c. The drug should be administered before withdrawal is complete.
    d. The drug is used to reduce the craving for alcohol.

CHAPTER 96

# Extended Care

## SECTION I: TESTING WHAT YOU KNOW

**Activity A** *Match the type of extended-care facility in Column A with its distinguishing feature in Column B.*

| Column A | Column B |
|---|---|
| ____ 1. Continual care | a. Provide 24-hour care; always have a licensed nurse on duty |
| ____ 2. Medically complex care | b. Provide room, board, and some nursing care; involve licensed nurses on call |
| ____ 3. Skilled nursing | c. Provide care for clients who do not require hospitalization or care in subacute units |
| ____ 4. Intermediate care | d. Provide highly sophisticated care, but are less expensive than hospitals |

**Activity B** *Match the extended-care team members given in Column A with their functions given in Column B.*

| Column A | Column B |
|---|---|
| ____ 1. Ombudsperson | a. Organizes fund-raising for special programs and activities |
| ____ 2. Care manager | b. Ensures that the client's rights are not violated |
| ____ 3. Volunteer | c. Visits clients at regular intervals and draws blood for tests |
| ____ 4. Home care nurse | d. Local advocate who ensures appropriate client care |

**Activity C** *Mark each statement as either "T" (True) or "F" (False). Correct any false statements.*

1. T F A client must have a formal case manager irrespective of the duration of stay in the facility.
2. T F The client may need to pay a higher cost or a penalty if he does not sign up for a plan when becoming eligible for Medicare.
3. T F A person's treatment may be classified as "subacute" for 2 months under Medicare.
4. T F The client's case manager or a family member may be designated as the client's payee.
5. T F A skilled nursing facility stabilizes the person during the acute phase of illness.

**Activity D** *Fill in the blanks.*

1. The Long Term Care ____________ works to ensure that Americans will have access to much-needed long-term care services.
2. Specific ____________ certification in long-term care is available for licensed practical nurses.

3. Pay for ____________ is a program in which the facility's future reimbursement is based on the quality of care provided.
4. A stay in a/an ____________ care facility may occur between the skilled nursing facility and the client's home.
5. The ____________ is often the first step in the continuum of care for the injured or disabled person.

**Activity E** *Consider the following figure.*

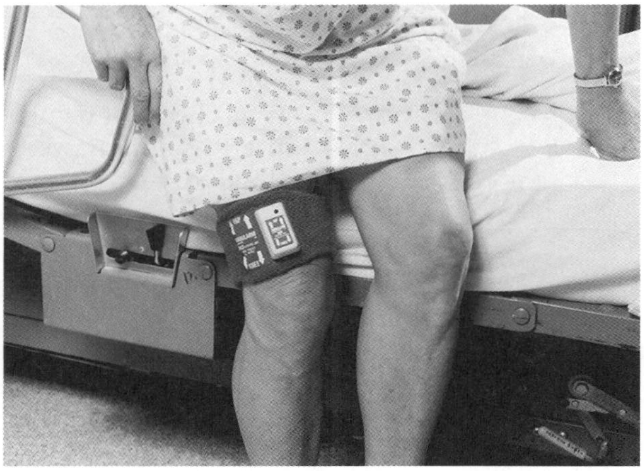

1. Identify the device shown in the figure.

________________________________________

________________________________________

2. What is the purpose of this device?

________________________________________

________________________________________

**Activity F** ***A client who has had a stroke may be admitted to various healthcare facilities in sequence. The types of facilities in which a client with a stroke is provided care are given below in random order. Write the correct sequence in the boxes provided.***

1. Cardiac monitoring in a skilled nursing facility
2. Management in an assisted living facility
3. Management in an intensive care unit
4. Treatment at an intermediate care facility

☐ → ☐ → ☐ → ☐

**Activity G** ***Briefly answer the following questions.***

1. What are the common nursing considerations provided at all extended care facilities?

________________________________________

________________________________________

2. What nursing functions are included in subacute-care facilities?

________________________________________

________________________________________

3. What is the role of short-term rehabilitation units?

________________________________________

________________________________________

4. What problem is faced by clients at extended-care facilities regarding elective meal programs?

________________________________________

________________________________________

5. What is the role of therapeutic swimming and aquatic exercises in extended-care facilities?

________________________________________

________________________________________

6. Briefly describe the function of the Long Term Care Community Coalition (LTCCC) program.

________________________________________

________________________________________

7. State the functions of a Quality Improvement Organization (QIO) and give two examples of QIOs.

________________________________________

________________________________________

8. What are supervised group homes?

________________________________________

________________________________________

9. What are senior apartment complexes?

________________________________________

________________________________________

## SECTION II: APPLYING WHAT YOU KNOW

**Activity H** *Answer the following questions, which involve the nurse's role in extended-care facilities.*

Extended-care facilities and assisted living facilities provide many lifestyle options and housing alternatives to clients outside hospitals. These facilities provide the nurses with an opportunity to work with clients and their family members over a longer period of time.

1. An elderly client with breast cancer is admitted to the skilled nursing facility. The client is a widow and has no children. The client is extremely depressed about her condition.
   a. What information should the nurse give the client regarding meal programs?
   b. What are the various recreational activities the nurse should involve this client in?
2. An elderly client with Alzheimer's disease (AD) is admitted to an extended-care facility. The client's daughter reports that she cannot afford the treatment for her father and cannot care for him herself.
   a. What measures should the nurse undertake to maintain the client's safety?
   b. What suggestions should the nurse provide the client's daughter regarding Medicare Part D?

## SECTION III: GETTING READY FOR NCLEX

**Activity I** *Answer the following questions.*

1. A client with a chronic illness is provided extended care in his own home. What role does a home care assistant play in providing care for this client?
   a. Draws blood for tests
   b. Helps in bathing and laundry
   c. Sets up client's medications
   d. Assists with finances
2. A client with AD is admitted to a long-term care facility. Which of the following services do volunteers provide? (Select all that apply.)
   a. Take residents on outings
   b. Oversee the client's dietary intake
   c. Organize fund-raising programs
   d. Help with the client's daily care
   e. Receive the client's monthly check
3. An elderly client with a chronic condition is being cared for by unlicensed assistive personnel (UAP) at an assisted living facility. Which of the following team members monitors the functions of the UAP?
   a. Care manager
   b. Ombudsperson
   c. Visiting nurse
   d. Physicians on call
4. Which of the following clients is a good candidate for an extended care facility?
   a. A client with a recent hip fracture
   b. A client admitted for joint surgery
   c. A client with head trauma after an accident
   d. An elderly client with AD
5. An elderly client with AD is admitted to the extended-care facility. Which of the following are part of an extended-care facility? (Select all that apply.)
   a. Intensive care unit
   b. Skilled nursing care unit
   c. Subacute-care unit
   d. Emergency department
   e. Nursing home beds
6. An elderly client with dementia is brought to the healthcare facility by her son, who is unable to care for her during the day because of his job. Which of the following programs should the client be involved in?
   a. Hospice care
   b. Nursing home
   c. Respite care
   d. Transitional care

7. An elderly client recovering from stroke was discharged from an extended-care facility after 20 days. Which of the following types of facilities was the client admitted to?
   a. Continual care facility
   b. Medically complex care
   c. Skilled nursing facility
   d. Intermediate care facility

8. A client living at a long-term care facility feels that the staff is neglecting him. What measures should he take?
   a. Contact the facility's nursing director.
   b. Use a buzzer to warn the staff members.
   c. Speak to the facility's social services director.
   d. Contact the facility's local administration.

9. An elderly client is being cared for at an assisted living facility. Which of the following services is available at an assisted living facility?
   a. 24-hour care by a licensed nurse
   b. Grocery and medication delivery
   c. Bowel and bladder retraining program
   d. Primary healthcare facilities

10. An elderly client is admitted to a skilled nursing facility two months after the death of her husband of 60 years. Which of the following recreational activities should the nurse involve the client in? (Select all that apply.)
   a. Crafts, cards, and other games
   b. Independent outings in the community
   c. Wii golf or bowling
   d. Monthly theme carnival with games and food for residents and family members
   e. Musical programs
   f. Cultural events such as a play

CHAPTER 97

# Rehabilitation Nursing

## SECTION I: TESTING WHAT YOU KNOW

**Activity A** *Match the terms in Column A with their disease conditions in Column B.*

| Column A | Column B |
|---|---|
| ____ 1. Aphasia | a. Difficulty in performing coordinated movements |
| ____ 2. Dyspraxia | b. Difficulty in speaking |
| ____ 3. Dysphagia | c. Paralysis of the four limbs and trunk |
| ____ 4. Quadriplegia | d. Difficulty in swallowing |

**Activity B** *Match the prostheses in Column A with their applications in Column B.*

| Column A | Column B |
|---|---|
| ____ 1. Inflatable trousers | a. Hold the body part stationary and prevent the contraction of the limb |
| ____ 2. Dynamic splints | b. Provide support during walking and allow hands to be freed when needed |
| ____ 3. Resting splints | c. Help to maintain an upright position and prevent vascular collapse |
| ____ 4. Lofstrand crutches | d. Enable movement and function of the whole body |

**Activity C** *Mark each statement as either "T" (True) or "F" (False). Correct any false statements.*

1. T F Paralysis of one side of the body is known as paraplegia.
2. T F Ability to communicate with others is an instrumental activity of daily living.
3. T F Braces or splints help the client to achieve greater mobility and support.
4. T F An occupational therapist is not a member of a rehabilitation team.
5. T F Vocational assessment of the client is done prior to the rehabilitation procedure.

**Activity D** *Fill in the blanks.*

1. The process of attending regular class in schools by physically or mentally challenged young people is known as ____________.
2. Constructing ramps for wheelchairs and elevators to make public buildings accessible and safe for all people is known as reduction of ____________ barriers.
3. The condition of swelling of the lymph nodes is known as ____________.
4. During the process of functional electrical stimulation, a stimulus is sent to the nerves to move ____________.
5. Ability to self-administer medications is a/an ____________ activity of daily living category.

**Activity E** *Consider the following figures.*

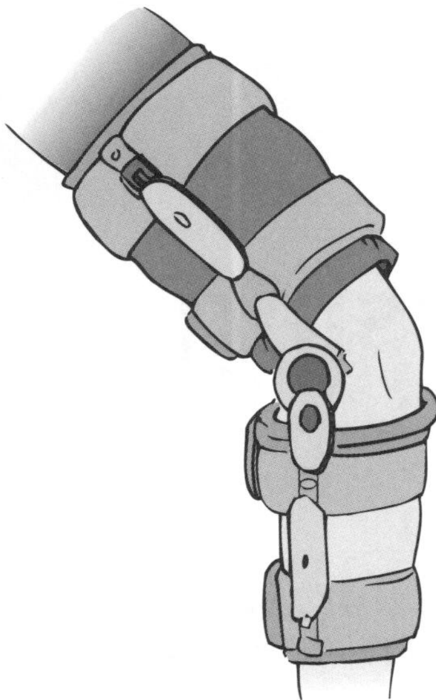

1. Identify the equipment in the figure.

______________________________

______________________________

2. Explain the use of this equipment.

______________________________

______________________________

3. Name the health conditions in which this equipment is used.

______________________________

______________________________

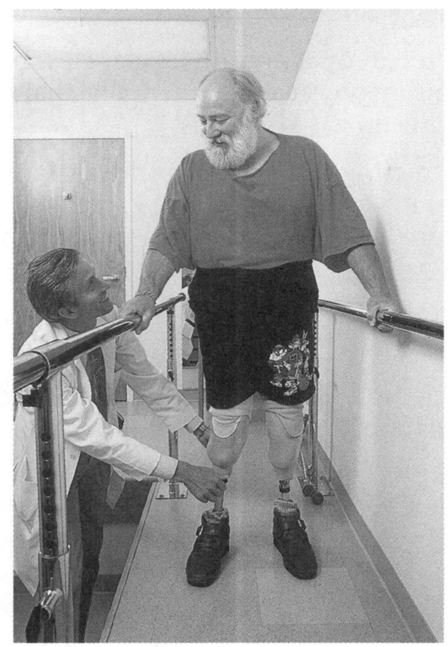

4. Identify the equipment in the figure.

______________________________

______________________________

5. Explain the use of this equipment.

______________________________

______________________________

6. What nursing care should the nurse provide to a client using this equipment?

______________________________

______________________________

**Activity F** ***Early recognition and individualized planning for each client are the main principles of rehabilitation. Maslow's hierarchy of needs is generally applied to the rehabilitation process. Steps involved during the rehabilitation of clients on the basis of Maslow's hierarchy of needs are given below in random order. Write the correct sequence in the boxes provided.***

1. Assist the client in self-actualization.
2. Assist in independent eating and dressing.
3. Ensure adequate oxygenation.
4. Assist the client to move about independently.

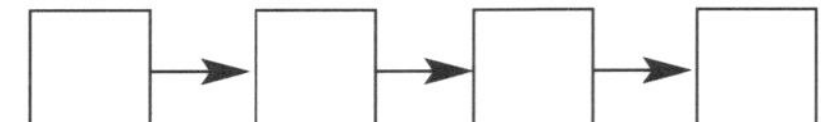

**Activity G** ***Briefly answer the following questions.***

1. Explain the legislative barriers of rehabilitation.

______________________________

______________________________

2. Explain the nursing care measures associated with cancer rehabilitation.

______________________________

______________________________

3. What are the different types of canes used to achieve mobility?

______________________________

______________________________

4. Explain the term "functional activity of daily living" with examples.

_______________________________________________

_______________________________________________

5. Explain about the kinds of adaptive equipment that are available for people with limited vision.

_______________________________________________

_______________________________________________

## SECTION II: APPLYING WHAT YOU KNOW

**Activity H** *Answer the following questions, which involve the nurse's role in rehabilitation.*

A nurse's role in rehabilitation involves providing suitable rehabilitation nursing care and assisting the client with mental and physical support.

1. A 20-year-old female client was brought to the healthcare facility with severe burns on her face and neck. The nurse notices that the client appears withdrawn and depressed all the time.
   a. How should the nurse comfort her?
   b. What rehabilitation nursing care should the nurse provide to the client?
2. An 80-year-old female client with complaints of upper back pain and pain in her middle back radiating to her sides is brought to the primary healthcare center. She also complains of numbness and lack of sensation in her right arm.
   a. List the nursing measures to be employed for the management of pain.
   b. What measures should the nurse take when providing skin care for this client?

## SECTION III: GETTING READY FOR NCLEX

**Activity I** *Answer the following questions.*

1. A 50-year-old client with paralysis of his lower limb is brought to the rehabilitation center. The client is apprehensive that he may not be able to participate in sexual activity. The nurse should tell the client which of the following regarding sexual activity? (Select all that apply.)
   a. The client may require a penile implant before sexual activity.
   b. The client should avoid participating in sexual activity.
   c. The client and his partner should be interviewed by a sex therapist.
   d. The client should be educated about comfortable positions.
   e. The client should take medication to increase sexual activity.
2. A nurse is caring for a 30-year-old female client with complaints of lack of lower limb movement and sensation. Which of the following instructions should be given to the client to prevent bladder infection? (Select all that apply.)
   a. Have frequent examinations by a physician
   b. Avoid drinking cranberry juice
   c. Consume an acidophilus-free diet
   d. Drink an adequate amount of fluid
   e. Clean the perineal area from front to back
3. A nurse is required to care for a 50-year-old client with lung cancer. Which of the following nursing care measures should be included in the client's rehabilitation care plan? (Select all that apply.)
   a. Assist the client in performing activities of daily living.
   b. Provide the client with electrical therapy.
   c. Carry out the client's gait analysis.
   d. Assist the client in doing physiotherapy.
   e. Provide the client with mental and emotional support.

4. A nurse is required to care for a 25-year-old male client in braces after paralysis of his lower limb. Which of the following specific nursing care measures should be included in the client's rehabilitation care plan?
   a. Provide the client with special tight gloves or body wraps.
   b. Assist the client with chest physiotherapy.
   c. Assist the client with range-of-motion exercises.
   d. Provide the client with assistance in taking medications.
5. A 35-year-old female client brought to the healthcare facility by her husband complains of disorientation, confusion, distractibility, and high blood pressure. Which of the following psychiatric rehabilitation care measures should be employed when caring for this client?
   a. Assist in managing physical problems.
   b. Assist in performing breathing exercises.
   c. Provide the client with compression appliances.
   d. Assist in doing range-of-motion exercises.
6. A nurse is caring for a 30-year-old female client with an acute spinal cord injury. Which of the following should the nurse tell the caregivers regarding homemaking adaptations for this client?
   a. Construct ramps instead of stairs.
   b. Provide lever-style doorknobs.
   c. Provide lever-style faucet handles.
   d. Use a combination washer and dryer.
7. A 50-year-old female client with 50% burns was admitted to the healthcare facility. Which of the following prostheses helps to provide tissue compression and vascular support to the client?
   a. Supportive braces
   b. Compression appliances
   c. Special tight gloves
   d. Dynamic splints
8. A nurse is caring for a client with quadriplegia. Which of the following prostheses helps the client maintain an upright position and prevents vascular collapse?
   a. Hook with adaptive splint
   b. Resting hand splint
   c. Lofstrand crutch
   d. Inflatable trousers
9. A psychiatric client is living at home with a service dog to help her with certain activities. She had been prescribed clozapine. Which of the following can the nurse do when paying a weekly visit?
   a. Encourage seeking full guidance.
   b. Pat and praise the service dog.
   c. Draw the client's blood for laboratory tests.
   d. Assist the client in spirometry exercises.
10. A 30-year-old woman was brought to the healthcare facility three months after a double mastectomy and vaginal hysterectomy. The client was unable to have any children. The nurse notices that the client is depressed and withdrawn all the time. How should the nurse comfort the client? (Select all that apply.)
   a. Make arrangements for individual counseling
   b. Make arrangements for group therapy
   c. Encourage the client to move on with her life
   d. Provide physical support to the client
   e. Provide emotional support to the client

CHAPTER 98

# Home Care Nursing

## SECTION I: TESTING WHAT YOU KNOW

**Activity A** *Match the community service organizations in Column A with the services they provide in Column B.*

| Column A | Column B |
|---|---|
| ____ 1. Lifeline | a. Housing assistance |
| ____ 2. Habitat for Humanity | b. Respite care for caregivers |
| ____ 3. YMCA | c. Electronic alert equipment |

**Activity B** *Match the personnel in Column A with the roles they play in Column B.*

| Column A | Column B |
|---|---|
| ____ 1. LPN | a. Provides spiritual support to the client to help in holistic healing |
| ____ 2. Case manager | b. Assists clients in learning appropriate self-care techniques |
| ____ 3. Parish nurse | c. Evaluates the safety of the home and the adequacy of available family caregivers |

**Activity C** *Mark each statement as either "T" (True) or "F" (False). Correct any false statements.*

1. T F A new nursing graduate may be employed for providing home care.
2. T F The Pay for Performance (P4P) rule applies when Medicare reimbursement is used for funding home care.
3. T F The Centers for Medicare and Medicaid Services (CMS) promote increased immunization of seniors for pneumonia.
4. T F A case manager visits the client's home to make an evaluation of the safety guidelines.
5. T F The Joint Commission certifies all agencies providing home care services.

**Activity D** *Fill in the blanks.*

1. A client is assigned to a Home ____________ Resource Group for 60 days of care during prospective payment system assessment.
2. The ____________ care hospitalization measure of the Outcome and Assessment Information Set (OASIS) aims to reduce the number of home care clients readmitted to hospitals.
3. The Centers for ____________ Nurses serve as consultants to the staff nurse from the local home care agency.
4. Centers for Medicare and Medicaid contracts ____________ Improvement Organizations to work with home care agencies.
5. A licensed practical nurse serves as a team member under the supervision of a ____________ manager.

**Activity E** *Consider the following figure.*

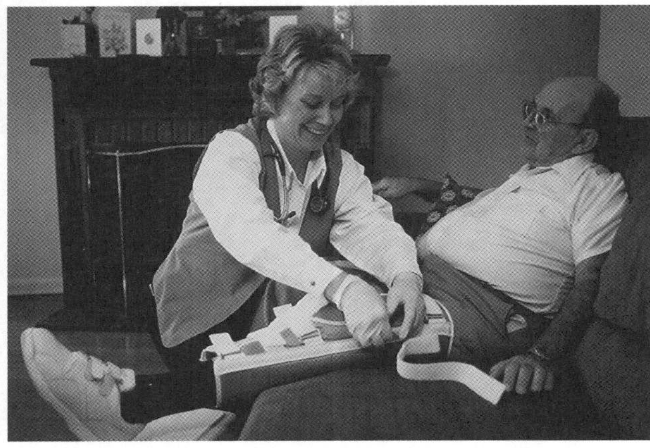

1. What does the figure show?

______________________________

______________________________

2. What are the qualities that a nurse must possess when providing home care?

______________________________

______________________________

3. What are the nursing duties to be followed when providing home care to a client?

______________________________

______________________________

**Activity F** *An elderly adult client is in need of home health care. Services provided by the client's case manager are given below in random order. Write the correct sequence in the boxes provided.*

1. Assistance to the family in home setup
2. Meeting with the home care team
3. Assessment of the client's needs
4. Assessment of the client's home

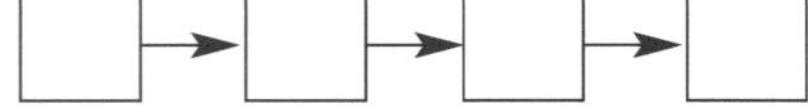

**Activity G** *Briefly answer the following questions.*

1. What are the characteristics of a long-term home care service?

______________________________

______________________________

2. What are the services provided by home care service agencies?

______________________________

______________________________

3. List the expertise of a Center of Excellence (COE) team.

______________________________

______________________________

4. What are the benefits of the prospective payment system (PPS)?

______________________________

______________________________

5. What are the advantages for a nurse working for home care services?

______________________________

______________________________

## SECTION II: APPLYING WHAT YOU KNOW

**Activity H** *Answer the following questions, which involve a nurse's role in providing home care to clients.*

A nurse's role when providing home care for clients with various diseases or disorders involves assisting the clients with a variety of needs and educating them about various measures to be implemented to improve health conditions.

1. A nurse is providing short-term care to a new mother.
   a. What are the nursing duties to be followed when providing care for the client?
   b. What does the new mother learn from home care visits?

2. A client who has undergone spinal surgery is being shifted from hospital care to home health care. The client is on a patient-controlled analgesia (PCA) pump to self-deliver analgesics as needed.
   a. What are the nursing guidelines to be implemented when providing care for the client?
   b. What outcome measures of the services of the home care agency does Medicare look for from the OASIS when deciding on the payments?

## SECTION III: GETTING READY FOR NCLEX

**Activity I** *Answer the following questions.*

1. A nurse is providing hospice home care for an older client with dementia. What is a nursing consideration when caring for this client?
   a. Decide on the combination of medications to be given.
   b. Encourage the client to interact and to recollect memories.
   c. Decide on the necessary dietary changes to be made.
   d. Comfort and assure the client of providing a cure for dementia.
2. A nurse is appointed to provide short-term care to a new mother. Which of the following is an important measure the nurse should implement?
   a. Avoid visiting the client's home too frequently.
   b. Set up prescribed medications in organizers.
   c. Educate the mother about the feeding procedures.
   d. Notify the care-providing agency before each visit.
3. A nurse is providing home care to a terminally ill child. A third-party payor is funding the treatment. Which of the following is an important nursing duty to be implemented?
   a. Call the client when visits are not scheduled.
   b. Provide curative treatment for the client.
   c. Instruct relatives to document all teachings.
   d. Complete and submit all records to a physician.
4. A nurse is assisting a family caregiver in providing home care to a client. Which of the following should the nurse do?
   a. Teach the family caregiver to prepare the home for the client.
   b. Report any emergencies to the family caregiver.
   c. Evaluate the relationship between the caregiver and the physician.
   d. Assess whether the family caregiver needs respite from caring.
5. A nurse is caring for an older adult in his home. Which of the following are the important nursing measures to be implemented? (Select all that apply.)
   a. Provide care for the client on weekdays or holidays.
   b. Provide transportation when going to a physician.
   c. Work in teams when caring for the client.
   d. Evaluate the client's home for safety issues.
   e. Restrict interactions with the client's family members.
6. A nurse is providing short-term home care to a client whose primary caregiver is a family member. Which of the following should the nurse implement when providing respite to the caregiver?
   a. Suggest that the caregiver increase his intake of food.
   b. Suggest that the caregiver drink more coffee.
   c. Suggest that the caregiver increase his intake of water.
   d. Suggest that the caregiver reduce salt intake.

**7.** A nurse is providing home care for a client who recently underwent surgery. Which of the following guidelines should the nurse follow?

   **a.** Change dressings once every 3 days for 2 weeks.

   **b.** Teach family members to monitor signs of infection.

   **c.** Transmit information on the wound to the physician via computer.

   **d.** Educate the family caregiver on administering intravenous antibiotics.

**8.** A nurse is providing home care to a client. Which of the following safety measures should the nurse implement when going on home visits?

   **a.** Get into the vehicle and ensure that the back seat is empty.

   **b.** Call and inform the client of the time of visit.

   **c.** Use a shortcut to reach the client's home.

   **d.** Knock on the door and enter the client's home.

**9.** A nurse is providing short-term home care to a mentally retarded child. Which of the following should the nurse do during her visit to the client's home?

   **a.** Evaluate medications given and suggest changes.

   **b.** Evaluate changes in the client's behavior.

   **c.** Evaluate the family's expenditures on the client.

   **d.** Evaluate the relationship between the parents.

**10.** A nurse is providing short-term home care to an elderly client. Which of the following actions should the nurse take?

   **a.** Instruct caregivers to take vitamin supplements.

   **b.** Place all medications close to the client's bed.

   **c.** Observe the client for signs of possible abuse.

   **d.** Decide on dietary changes necessary for the client.

CHAPTER 99

# Ambulatory Nursing

## SECTION I: TESTING WHAT YOU KNOW

**Activity A** *Match the types of surgical equipment in Column A with their functions in Column B.*

| Column A | Column B |
|---|---|
| ____ 1. Fiberoptics | a. Accurate visualization and location of internal structures |
| ____ 2. Ultrasound | b. Immobilization in clients with a fracture or neck injury |
| ____ 3. Laser | c. Light and magnification at a distance |
| ____ 4. Halo device | d. Cutting and vessel cauterization that can be controlled from a distance |

**Activity B** *Match the surgical procedures in Column A with their descriptions in Column B.*

| Column A | Column B |
|---|---|
| ____ 1. Lithotripsy | a. Surgical removal of a kidney or section of a kidney |
| ____ 2. Nephrectomy | b. Use of small scopes to visualize and manipulate internal structures |
| ____ 3. Endoscopy | c. Insertion of a device to hold a blood vessel open after a heart attack |
| ____ 4. Stent placement | d. Pulverization of kidney or bladder stones without open surgery |

**Activity C** *Mark each statement as either "T" (True) or "F" (False). Correct any false statements.*

1. T F Nursing responsibilities are greater in inpatient settings than in same-day surgery.
2. T F Crisis intervention centers handle all medical emergencies.
3. T F Vertical clients are clients with critical conditions.
4. T F Robotic equipment assists surgeons to perform procedures that were previously impossible.
5. T F Basic hearing and vision screening is performed by a school nurse.

**Activity D** *Fill in the blanks.*

1. ___________ anesthesia greatly reduces the risk of postoperative complications.
2. The nurse should call ambulatory surgery clients on the ___________ postoperative day.
3. ___________ personnel maintain the client receiving general anesthesia during the procedure.

4. The primary care provider gives permission for the client to receive emergency care if the client belongs to a/an __________ maintenance organization.
5. Safety, asepsis, and confidentiality are the underlying principles of __________ care.

**Activity E** *Consider the following figures.*

1. Explain the figure.
2. What are specialized clinics?
3. What are the services offered at these clinics?

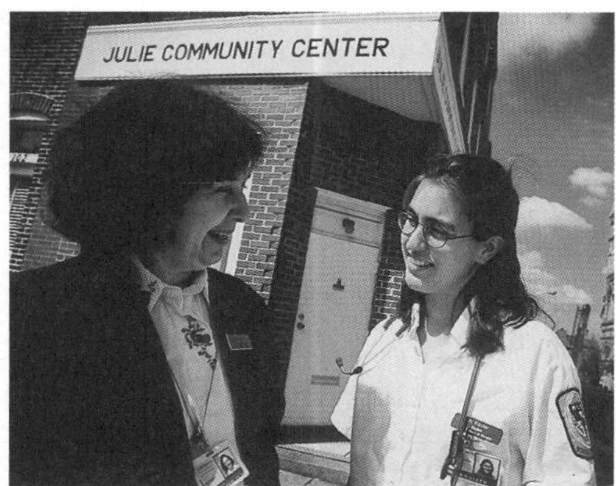


4. How is a community health center different from other healthcare providers?
5. Who provides most of the primary care in the community health center?
6. What is meant by "managed care protocols?"

**Activity F** ***One of the primary functions of the nurse in a day-surgery center is educating the client and the family. Steps that occur during of the instruction of the client and the family before surgery are listed below in random order. Write the correct sequence in the boxes provided.***

1. Give instructions in writing.
2. Teach the client about preoperative preparations.
3. Document all teaching accurately.
4. Refer to appropriate sources for supplies.

☐ → ☐ → ☐ → ☐

**Activity G** ***Briefly answer the following questions.***

1. What is a patient-controlled analgesia (PCA) pump?
2. What are the functions of the employee health service?
3. What is a mental health crisis center?

4. List some ambulatory care sensitive conditions.

______________________________

______________________________

5. What is telehealth service?

______________________________

______________________________

## SECTION II: APPLYING WHAT YOU KNOW

**Activity H** *Answer the following questions, which involve the nurse's role in ambulatory care.*

The nurse's role in an ambulatory setting is to deliver primary healthcare. The nurse also performs other duties not usually performed by nurses in acute-care settings.

1. A nurse is preparing a 25-year-old client admitted to an ambulatory surgery center for wound debridement.
   a. What factors are used to determine a client's appropriateness for ambulatory surgery?
   b. What should the nurse look for when following the preoperative checklist?
   c. What are the functions of the nurse in the recovery room?
2. A nurse is assessing a 35-year-old client who has come to an ambulatory healthcare facility with complaints of lower back pain.
   a. What baseline client data should the nurse gather?
   b. List the non-nursing procedures performed by the nurse in such a setting.
   c. What treatments can the nurse administer in an ambulatory setting?

## SECTION III: GETTING READY FOR NCLEX

**Activity I** *Answer the following questions.*

1. An obese 65-year-old client who is a known diabetic is admitted to an ambulatory surgery center for cataract removal. In which of the following groups will the nurse classify the client?
   a. Class I
   b. Class II
   c. Class III
   d. Class IV
2. A nurse is assuring a potential client for breast lumpectomy that ambulatory surgery is associated with fewer complications and faster recovery than inpatient surgery. Which of the following is responsible for the fastest recovery and fewer complications after same-day surgery?
   a. Small incision
   b. General anesthesia
   c. Heavy sedation
   d. Slow ambulation
3. A nurse is providing a client who is to undergo tonsillectomy at an ambulatory surgery center with information about the procedure. Which of the following precautions should the nurse emphasize when teaching this client?
   a. Perform preoperative preparation at hospital.
   b. Discontinue aspirin one day before surgery.
   c. Continue herbal medication.
   d. Avoid driving immediately after surgery.
4. After a multiple casualty event, a nurse at the emergency room is performing triage assessment of the clients. Which of the following clients should be seen first?
   a. Non-hemorrhaging wound
   b. Green-stick fracture
   c. Severe asthma attack
   d. Abdominal discomfort

**5.** A nurse is assessing a client admitted to the emergency department with complaints of chest pain. Which of the following procedures may the nurse in the emergency department perform?

**a.** Evaluate the electrocardiogram.

**b.** Perform defibrillation.

**c.** Monitor intravenous lines.

**d.** Stabilize the client.

**6.** A school nurse is performing a routine health checkup of all the students in an elementary school. The nurse notices that one of the students has multiple bruises and cigarette burn marks on her arms and appears frightened and depressed. The nurse suspects child abuse. What action should the nurse take?

**a.** Report her suspicions to child protection services.

**b.** Perform a forensic examination.

**c.** Report her suspicions to the child's parents.

**d.** Obtain custody of the child.

**7.** A 45-year-old client who sustained head trauma due to a vehicular injury is admitted to an emergency department. The client is found to be unresponsive and is declared dead after examination. His driving license indicates that he has designated himself as a donor. From whom should the nurse seek permission to proceed with the organ donation procedure?

**a.** Primary healthcare provider

**b.** Clinical nurse specialist

**c.** Advance practice nurse

**d.** Client's next of kin

**8.** A nurse is providing preoperative and postoperative information to a client who is scheduled for tubal ligation. Under which of the following conditions will surgery be cancelled? (Select all that apply.)

**a.** Client voids immediately before surgery.

**b.** Client has not made arrangements to get back home.

**c.** Client has a common cold or influenza.

**d.** Client is extremely fearful of the procedure.

**e.** Client is a known diabetic or hypertensive.

**9.** A visually impaired client, who has no perception of light, is scheduled for a corneal transplant. How should the nurse instruct this client? (Select all that apply.)

**a.** Provide written instructions in Braille.

**b.** Ask the client whether he or she has understood the instructions.

**c.** Provide taped instructions.

**d.** Make the client repeat the instructions to the nurse.

**e.** Instruct only the client's family members.

**10.** How is a community health center different from other healthcare providers? (Select all that apply.)

**a.** It charges uniform fees regardless of clients' financial status.

**b.** It provides comprehensive primary care services.

**c.** It is located in a "high-need" community.

**d.** It is available only to clients with insurance.

**e.** It targets medically underserved populations.

CHAPTER 100

# Hospice Nursing

## SECTION I: TESTING WHAT YOU KNOW

**Activity A** *Match the medications in Column A with their indications in Column B.*

| Column A | Column B |
|---|---|
| ____ 1. Cyclizine | a. Anxiety |
| ____ 2. Bisacodyl | b. Seizures |
| ____ 3. Furosemide | c. Constipation |
| ____ 4. Carbamazepine | d. Nausea |
| ____ 5. Alprazolam | e. Edema |

**Activity B** *Match the types of opioid medications in Column A with their examples in Column B.*

| Column A | Column B |
|---|---|
| ____ 1. Mild | a. Morphine sulfate |
| ____ 2. Mid-range | b. Hydrocodone |
| ____ 3. Strong | c. Oxycodone |

**Activity C** *Mark each statement as either "T" (True) or "F" (False). Correct any false statements.*

1. T F A temporary nerve block is applied under general anesthetic.
2. T F Transcutaneous electrical nerve stimulation interrupts transmission of pain sensations.
3. T F United States hospice programs advocate euthanasia.
4. T F A registered nurse does the initial evaluation of the client and the home.
5. T F Depressed clients often have hypersomnia.

**Activity D** *Fill in the blanks.*

1. ____________ is the surgical removal of the pituitary gland.
2. The ____________ electrical nerve stimulation (TENS) unit applies electrical stimulation directly to nerves and interrupts transmission of pain sensations.
3. The ____________ movement acknowledges that not all illnesses are curable and emphasizes the management of uncomfortable symptoms.
4. Permanent nerve block is achieved with a ____________ agent.
5. Belladonna suppositories are used to relieve bladder ____________.

**Activity E** *Consider the following figures.*

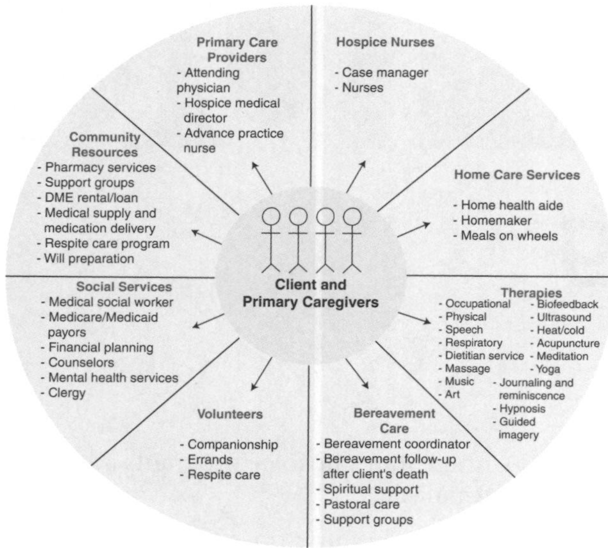


1. Identify what is shown in the figure.

_______________

2. List the staff involved in this type of care.

_______________

3. What is the role of the nurse in this setting?

_______________

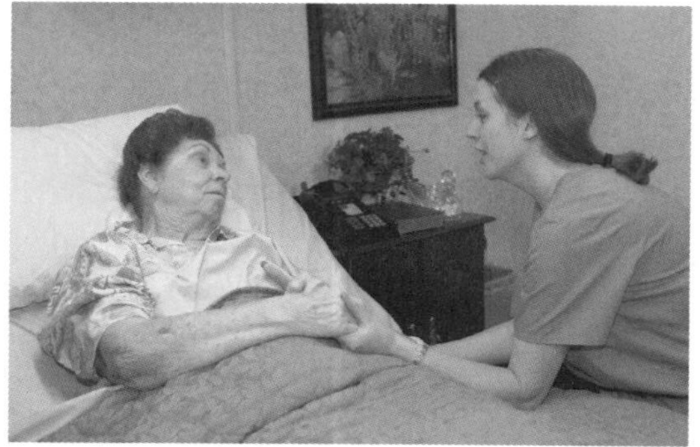

4. Identify what is shown in the figure.

_______________

5. What are the greatest fears of terminally ill clients?

_______________

6. How is emotional support offered to the family members of the client?

_______________

**Activity F** ***The nurse and family caregivers perform final care and make final preparations after the client dies. Nursing steps performed for a client who dies at home are given below in random order. Write the correct sequence in the boxes provided.***

1. Prepare the body for transportation to a funeral home.
2. Remove all the equipment that was used for the client.
3. Refer the client's family to a bereavement support group.
4. Allow the family time alone with the deceased client.

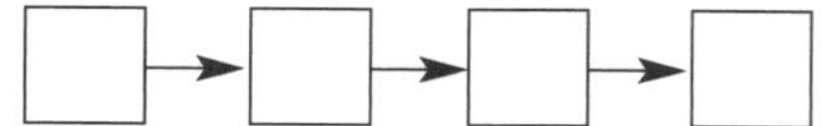

**Activity G** ***Briefly answer the following questions.***

1. What are the measures to manage odor in terminally ill clients?

_______________

2. Which areas of human needs does hospice care focus on?

_______________

3. What does durable medical equipment include?

_______________

4. Discuss the criteria an agency should meet to be called a hospice.

______________________________

______________________________

5. What is meant by the term bereavement?

______________________________

______________________________

## SECTION II: APPLYING WHAT YOU KNOW

**Activity H** *Answer the following questions, which involve the nurse's role in hospice care.*

Aggressive pain management is a primary goal of hospice nursing. The nurse, along with the client's family caregivers, performs final care and makes final preparations after the client dies.

1. A hospice nurse assists with postmortem care.
   a. What is the nursing responsibility when a client dies?
   b. How do hospice staff members give bereavement care?
   c. What support is available for hospice staff members?
2. A nurse is caring for a client with gastric carcinoma who is experiencing abdominal pain.
   a. How should the nurse evaluate the client's pain?
   b. What activities can the nurse suggest to divert the client's attention from the pain?
   c. What points should a nurse consider when administering pain relief medications to hospice clients?

## SECTION III: GETTING READY FOR NCLEX

**Activity I** *Answer the following questions.*

1. A client with a diagnosis of small cell carcinoma of the lung, who has been admitted to a home care hospice, complains to the home nurse that he has a bowel movement only once every 2 days. What action should the nurse take?
   a. Refer the client to a specialist.
   b. Reassure the client that it is normal.
   c. Increase the dietary fiber intake.
   d. Increase the client's fluid intake.
2. A client is admitted to a hospice program with carcinoma of the colon. The nurse observes a reddened area that does not return to its normal hue after pressure is removed on the client's lower back. What action should the nurse take?
   a. Change client's position frequently.
   b. Massage that area.
   c. Apply antifungal powder.
   d. Apply a moist cloth.
3. A client in home care hospice with terminal-stage cervical cancer complains of watery diarrhea. What action should the nurse take?
   a. Encourage a high-residue diet.
   b. Encourage the client to drink only water.
   c. Avoid any kind of food restrictions.
   d. Provide good skin care around the rectum.
4. A hospice nurse is caring for a client with a diagnosis of acute leukemia who has undergone chemotherapy and is complaining of nausea. What action should the nurse take?
   a. Assist the client to a supine position.
   b. Avoid carbonated beverages.
   c. Provide ice chips for a soothing effect.
   d. Avoid dry foods such as popcorn.

5. A nurse caring for a client with end-stage AIDS observes that the client has a dry mouth and is dehydrated. Which is a complication of dehydration?
   a. Nausea
   b. Choking
   c. Constipation
   d. Ascites

6. A client diagnosed with Ewing's sarcoma who is under hospice care complains of constipation. Which of the following should be evaluated before treating constipation with laxatives?
   a. Bowel obstruction
   b. Diabetes mellitus
   c. Hypertension
   d. Peptic ulceration

7. A client who has been admitted to a hospice program with a diagnosis of metastatic prostate carcinoma is unable to eat because of a decreased appetite. Which of the following will improve intake in this client?
   a. Providing low-calorie supplements
   b. Providing milk rather than clear fluids
   c. Providing large-quantity meals
   d. Providing soft foods that are easy to swallow

8. A client admitted to a hospice program for mesothelioma is constipated and is given a "colon cocktail" by the home nurse. What are the constituents of a "colon cocktail?" (Select all that apply.)
   a. Strawberries
   b. Applesauce
   c. Prune juice
   d. Miller's bran
   e. Pasteurized milk

9. A client with gastric carcinoma who is receiving morphine for pain management appears to be somnolent. What action should the nurse take? (Select all that apply.)
   a. Withhold the opioid medications.
   b. Make the client lie in a lateral position.
   c. Consult the healthcare provider.
   d. Provide naloxone after physician consultation.
   e. Provide relaxation techniques to the client.

10. A hospice nurse is ordered to give a client diagnosed with metastatic liver disease more than the usual dose of analgesic medication because of the considerable liver damage that has occurred. Which of the following can also necessitate a higher dose of pain-relieving medications? (Select all that apply.)
   a. Cognitive impairment
   b. Substance abuse
   c. Cigarette smoking
   d. Sedentary lifestyle
   e. Kidney damage

CHAPTER 101

# From Student to Graduate Nurse

## SECTION I: TESTING WHAT YOU KNOW

**Activity A** *Match the phase of the nursing process in Column A with its explanation in Column B.*

| Column A | Column B |
|---|---|
| ____ **1.** Data collection | **a.** Setting goals and designing strategies for meeting client needs |
| ____ **2.** Planning | **b.** Measurement of the effectiveness of nursing care |
| ____ **3.** Implementation | **c.** Setting up a database of client needs and clinical findings |
| ____ **4.** Evaluation | **d.** Provision of actual nursing care to achieve goals |

**Activity B** *Match the category of client need in Column A with its explanation in Column B.*

| Column A | Column B |
|---|---|
| ____ **1.** Safety and infection control | **a.** Nursing care that promotes and supports the emotional, mental, and social well-being of the client |
| ____ **2.** Psychosocial integrity | **b.** Reducing the likelihood of clients' developing complications related to existing conditions or treatments |
| ____ **3.** Reduction of risk potential | **c.** Managing and providing care for clients with acute, chronic, or life-threatening health conditions |
| ____ **4.** Physiologic adaptation | **d.** Protecting clients, family, and healthcare personnel from health and environmental hazards |

**Activity C** *Mark each statement as either "T" (True) or "F" (False). Correct any false statements.*

**1.** T F In most states, a specific score is given as the result for the NCLEX examination.

**2.** T F No telephone or verbal order is valid unless it is read back to the person issuing the order.

**3.** T F The case manager in home care is almost always a licensed practical nurse.

**4.** T F A nurse is required to complete an application and pay a fee to transfer licensure to another state.

**5.** T F Satisfactory completion of a test is necessary to obtain continuing education units.

**Activity D** ***Fill in the blanks.***

1. ___________ assistive personnel are members of the nursing team in community settings.
2. The NCLEX examination measures ___________-level competencies in nursing.
3. The ___________ license is usually not transferable to another state.
4. In a nursing home setting, the licensed practical nurse often works as a ___________ nurse.
5. ___________ overtime occurs when the nurses from the preceding shift must stay on or return to the facility and cover additional time.

**Activity E** ***Consider the following figures.***

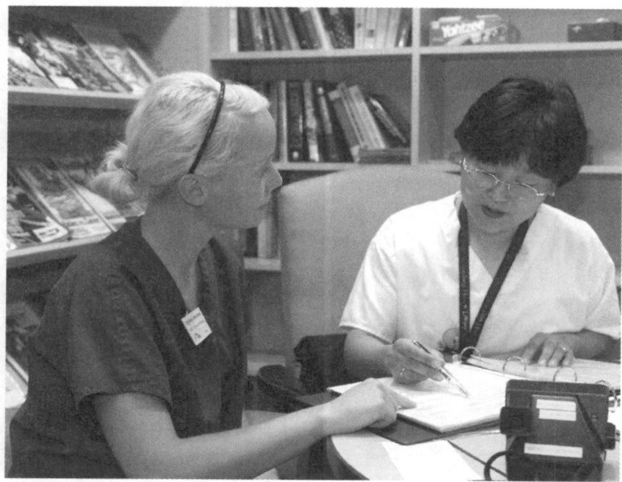

1. Identify what is shown in the figure.

_______________________________________

_______________________________________

2. What is the role of a mentor?

_______________________________________

_______________________________________

3. How long is the orientation period?

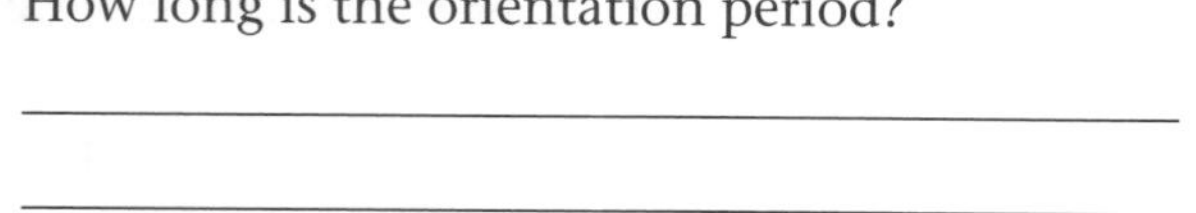

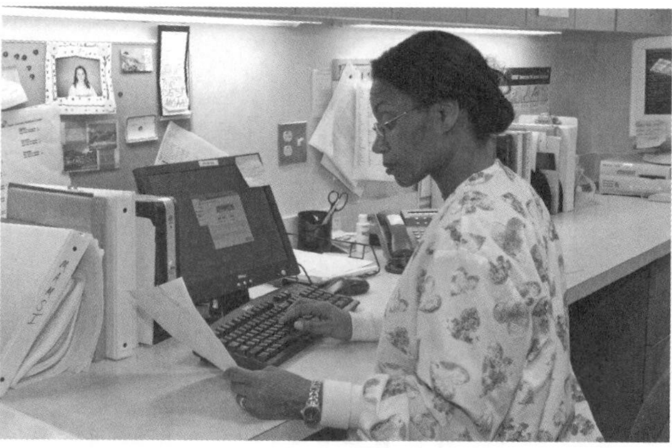

4. Identify what is shown in the figure.

_______________________________________

_______________________________________

5. List five uses of a computer in a healthcare facility.

_______________________________________

_______________________________________

6. What are the various aids available to familiarize nurses with computers?

_______________________________________

_______________________________________

**Activity F** ***To ensure client safety, the nurse must follow certain guidelines when discontinuing medication orders. Nursing steps that are performed when a medication is discontinued are given below in random order. Write the correct sequence in the boxes provided.***

1. Make out a drug credit and send leftover medications back to the pharmacy.
2. Cross out the item and write "discontinued" on the medical administration record.
3. Note completion of the order, indicating time and date, and sign the order.
4. Inform the nurse in charge of the client about the medication discontinued.

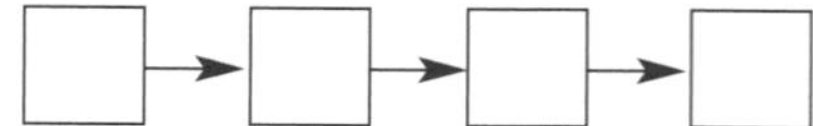

**Activity G** *Briefly answer the following questions.*

1. What is the responsibility of a nurse after receiving the license?

_______________________________________________

_______________________________________________

2. What actions can be taken in case of license revocation?

_______________________________________________

_______________________________________________

3. What is the primary role of a licensed practical nurse?

_______________________________________________

_______________________________________________

4. What is meant by the term "political activism?"

_______________________________________________

_______________________________________________

5. What precautions should the nurse take to maintain client confidentiality when using the computer charting system?

_______________________________________________

_______________________________________________

## SECTION II: APPLYING WHAT YOU KNOW

**Activity H** *Answer the following questions, which involve the nurse's role obtaining a nursing license and working as a licensed nurse.*

On completion of a nursing program, a graduate nurse is eligible to take the licensing examination and obtain a nursing license. The newly licensed nurse faces challenges of balancing work and personal responsibilities.

1. A new graduate nurse is learning organizational skills from her mentor.
   a. What are the guidelines to help organize the workload?
   b. What are the challenges that the new graduate faces with regard to work shifts?
   c. Name some factors that will contribute to the nurse's feelings of professional satisfaction.
2. A nurse is planning to take the NCLEX licensing examination.
   a. What are the eligibility criteria for taking the licensure examination?
   b. What aspects are assessed in the NCLEX examination?
   c. How should the nurse prepare before appearing for the NCLEX examination?

## SECTION III: GETTING READY FOR NCLEX

**Activity I** *Answer the following questions.*

1. The new nurse is working on the evening shift. Which of the following should the nurse keep in mind when on evening shifts?
   a. More staff are on duty during evening shifts.
   b. Clients experience fever more often in the evening.
   c. Most orders are written during evening shifts.
   d. Clients are usually discharged in the evening.
2. A new nurse receives a verbal order of medications to be given to a client scheduled for hip surgery. What action should the nurse take in case the order is not clear?
   a. Keep it pending until clarified by the person issuing it.
   b. Carry it out after clarifying with a colleague.
   c. Carry it out in the best way understood.
   d. Refer to the Internet or to a nursing book.
3. A new nurse is put on the night shift as part of the orientation to a healthcare facility. Which of the following should the nurse consider when on night shift?
   a. Avoid taking short naps during breaks.
   b. Avoid consuming too much fluid.
   c. Limit caffeine intake after about 6 AM.
   d. Eat a snack or meal during the shift.

4. A nurse is transcribing medication orders issued by a physician for a client admitted with acute gastroenteritis. Which of the following guidelines should the nurse follow when transcribing medication orders?
   a. Document "stat" orders toward the end of the day.
   b. Read written orders back to the physician so that they are valid.
   c. Check medications on arrival against the physician's orders.
   d. Discard any medication that is left over.

5. A nurse needs to obtain the signature of the primary care provider for a verbal order that was given for a client admitted with fever. Which of the following is the time frame for getting the verbal order signed by the primary care provider?
   a. Within 24 hours
   b. Within 36 hours
   c. Within 48 hours
   d. Within 72 hours

6. A new nurse is given probationary employment as an intern in a healthcare facility. Which of the following are the benefits of the probationary period?
   a. Cannot be terminated without cause
   b. One week vacation time
   c. Ample use of sick leave
   d. Orientation to appropriate job placement

7. The Board of Nursing has revoked a nurse's license due to negligent behavior. Which of the following is a just cause for revoking a license?
   a. Chemical dependency and addiction
   b. Accidental needlestick injury to self
   c. Recent detection of HIV infection
   d. Use of more sick leave time than permitted

8. A nurse working at a pediatric healthcare facility is exempted from working night shifts due to a health problem. Which of the following conditions exempt a nurse from night shifts? (Select all that apply.)
   a. Neurofibromatosis
   b. Heart disorders
   c. Seizure disorders
   d. Bipolar disorder
   e. Immature cataract

9. A nurse chooses a permanent night shift so as to suit her daily schedule. Which of the following are the advantages of night shifts over day shifts? (Select all that apply.)
   a. Less stressful
   b. Less work
   c. Higher pay
   d. Easier parking
   e. More staff

10. A new graduate nurse is compiling a personal nursing file for the purpose of seeking a job. The nurse should include copies of which of the following in his personal nursing file? (Select all that apply.)
   a. Driving license
   b. Resume
   c. Original nursing license
   d. Bank statement
   e. Immunization records

CHAPTER 102

# Career Opportunities and Job-Seeking Skills

## SECTION I: TESTING WHAT YOU KNOW

**Activity A** *Match the nursing area in Column A with nursing duties specific to that area in Column B.*

| Column A | Column B |
|---|---|
| ____ 1. Home care | a. Performing telephone follow-up after client returns home |
| ____ 2. Private duty and travel | b. Making an evaluation visit to client's home |
| ____ 3. Hospice | c. Caring for a client on a journey |
| ____ 4. Ambulatory | d. Providing end-of-life care to terminally ill clients |

**Activity B** *Match the document related to job seeking and employment in Column A with its content in Column B.*

| Column A | Column B |
|---|---|
| ____ 1. Letter of application | a. Source of information regarding the position applied for |
| ____ 2. Resume | b. Candidate's interest in the position and a note of thanks |
| ____ 3. Follow-up letter | c. Responsibilities of the employee and employer |
| ____ 4. Job contract | d. Special skills, training, honors, or volunteer positions held |

**Activity C** *Mark each statement as either "T" (True) or "F" (False). Correct any false statements.*

1. T F A licensed practical nurse (LPN) may work as a lead circulating nurse in operating rooms.
2. T F Special training should be given to nurses performing phlebotomy.
3. T F A private duty nurse may care for a client in his or her home.
4. T F It is better to submit a handwritten cover letter than a printed one when applying for a job.
5. T F An LPN may work as a certified public health nurse.

**Activity D** *Fill in the blanks.*

1. A nurse should pass an emergency ____________ technician course to work in air-rescue services.
2. ____________ oxygenation provides oxygen under pressure to clients with carbon monoxide poisoning.

3. The ___________ card is a work permit that is required to work in the United States.
4. Each state's employment service is affiliated with the local ___________.
5. A ___________ letter should accompany a resume.

**Activity E** ***Consider the following figures.***

1. Identify the figure shown.

_______________________________________

_______________________________________

2. What are the job opportunities for a nurse outside the hospital setting?

_______________________________________

_______________________________________

3. What are the duties of a registered home care nurse?

_______________________________________

_______________________________________

4. Identify the figure.

_______________________________________

_______________________________________

5. How should a man dress for a personal interview?

_______________________________________

_______________________________________

6. How should a woman dress for a personal interview?

_______________________________________

_______________________________________

**Activity F** ***As the time of graduation approaches, a nurse should look at future career plans. Recommended steps for securing the desired employment are given below in random order. Write the correct sequence in the boxes provided.***

1. Decide on the type of employment to seek.
2. Build networks to learn about positions as they become available.
3. Prepare a neatly printed and error-free resume and cover letter.
4. Evaluate personal and family requirements.

☐ → ☐ → ☐ → ☐

**Activity G** ***Briefly answer the following questions.***

1. What are the shift options available for a nurse working in a long-term healthcare facility?

_______________________________________

_______________________________________

2. What are the advantages of using a nurses' registry for employment?

_______________________________________

_______________________________________

3. What are the limitations of using a nurses' registry for employment?

_______________________________________

_______________________________________

4. How should a nurse resign from a position?

______________________________________

______________________________________

5. What are the responsibilities of a nurse as an employee?

______________________________________

______________________________________

6. What are the advantages of attending an informational interview?

______________________________________

______________________________________

7. What are the advantages of using the Internet for job searching?

______________________________________

______________________________________

8. What are the personal factors that should be considered by the nurse when looking for a place of employment?

______________________________________

______________________________________

9. What benefits should a nurse consider when choosing a place of employment?

______________________________________

______________________________________

## SECTION II: APPLYING WHAT YOU KNOW

**Activity H** ***Answer the following questions related to career opportunities for nurses.***

A nurse can apply for jobs in a hospital or a nonhospital setting.

1. A recently graduated nurse is preparing a resume to apply for a staff nurse position in a long term care facility.
   a. What items should the nurse include in a suitable resume?
   b. How should the nurse apply for the position?
2. An LPN is searching the Internet for job opportunities in ambulatory clinics.
   a. How should the nurse effectively use the Internet for conducting a job search?
   b. What are the duties of a nurse working in clinics?

## SECTION III: GETTING READY FOR NCLEX

**Activity I** ***Answer the following questions.***

1. An LPN is assigned to work as a parish nurse in a church. Which of the following duties should the nurse perform? (Select all that apply.)
   a. Providing hands-on nursing care
   b. Making an evaluation visit to the client's home
   c. Writing newsletter articles
   d. Visiting parishioners in nursing homes
   e. Assisting in training family caregivers
2. A registered nurse seeks employment at a rehabilitation center. Which of the following guidelines should be followed for writing a good resume? (Select all that apply.)
   a. State the career objective.
   b. Emphasize the past 5 years' experience.
   c. Keep the resume elaborate and detailed.
   d. List personal data at the beginning of the resume.
   e. Use white bond paper for the resume.
3. An LVN is assigned to work as a member of an employee health service team in a healthcare facility. Which of the following duties should the nurse perform? (Select all that apply.)
   a. Conduct physical examinations.
   b. Conduct yearly tuberculin testing.
   c. Renew the license of an LPN nurse.
   d. Work as an Emergency Medical Technician (EMT).
   e. Issue permits to return to work after an illness.

**4.** An LPN is assigned to work in a hyperbaric chamber. Which of the following duties does the nurse have to perform?

- **a.** Receive and preserve biopsied material.
- **b.** Monitor the administration of oxygen.
- **c.** Measure the skinfold thickness of the client.
- **d.** Teach the client how to operate the hyperbaric chamber.

**5.** A nurse is assigned to work in a health maintenance organization. Which of the following duties should the nurse perform?

- **a.** Review clients' records.
- **b.** Evaluate clients' progress.
- **c.** Update the clients' nursing plans.
- **d.** Supervise other health caregivers.

**6.** An LVN nurse is preparing to attend a personal interview. Which of the following guidelines should the nurse follow when attending the interview?

- **a.** Avoid asking the interviewer about notification about the position.
- **b.** Address the interviewer by first name only.
- **c.** Decline offers for coffee or food.
- **d.** Avoid keeping hands on the table.

**7.** A nurse is planning to work in a physician's office. Which of the following should the nurse be prepared to do?

- **a.** Work night shifts
- **b.** Work as a claims analyst
- **c.** Perform home visits
- **d.** Serve as a receptionist

**8.** A nurse is seeking employment in hospice care. What should the nurse know about the job profile of a hospice nurse?

- **a.** The nurse should provide emotional support to client and family.
- **b.** The nurse should have completed post-graduate surgical and technical training.
- **c.** The nurse should assist the surgeon in surgical procedures.
- **d.** The nurse must be familiar with high-tech equipment.

**9.** A nurse is looking for employment opportunities in a practical nursing program. What prerequisites do employers look for most when hiring a nurse in a practical nursing program?

- **a.** The nurse should be a certified public health nurse.
- **b.** The nurse should have previous teaching experience.
- **c.** The nurse should have patent auditory tubes.
- **d.** The nurse should be a registered nurse (RN).

**10.** A nurse is employed in a school summer camp program. Which of the following duties would the nurse need to perform?

- **a.** Teach flower essence therapy.
- **b.** Facilitate bereavement support groups.
- **c.** Teach about wilderness safety.
- **d.** Manage blood drives.

CHAPTER 103

# Advancement and Leadership in Nursing

## SECTION I: TESTING WHAT YOU KNOW

**Activity A** *Match the topics covered by questions on the NAPNES certification exam in Column A with the issues they relate to in Column B.*

**Column A**

____ 1. Cardiovascular status

____ 2. Potential for violence

____ 3. Communication

____ 4. Cost containment

**Column B**

a. Leadership and management

b. Physiologic integrity

c. Psychosocial integrity

d. Special practice issues

**Activity B** *Match the characteristic of a leader in Column A with the role it pertains to in Column B.*

**Column A**

____ 1. Accountability

____ 2. Advocacy

____ 3. Values clarification

**Column B**

a. Provide information and support to the team members

b. Choose from alternatives and act consistently on the choice

c. Be responsible for values and actions

**Activity C** *Mark each statement as either "T" (True) or "F" (False). Correct any false statements.*

1. T F To qualify for the NAPNES examination, the nurse needs to have practiced long-term care for 3,000 hours in the last 2 years.

2. T F Refresher courses are taught by practicing nurses.

3. T F A nurse must evaluate his or her own leadership abilities when working as a leader.

4. T F Health Care Financing Administration (HCFA) is the former name of the Omnibus Budget Reconciliation Act.

5. T F A nurse working as a manager should work without constant guidance from others.

**Activity D** *Fill in the blanks.*

1. The NAPNES certification for a licensed practical nurse is valid for ____________ years.

2. New nursing graduates feel comfortable with the ____________ style of leadership until they gain self-confidence.

3. A charge nurse is responsible for writing ____________ reviews of staff members.

4. An employer can terminate an employee as per process only after the ___________ period of employment.
5. A nurse is a leader in the healthcare facility and also in the ___________.

**Activity E** *Consider the following figure.*

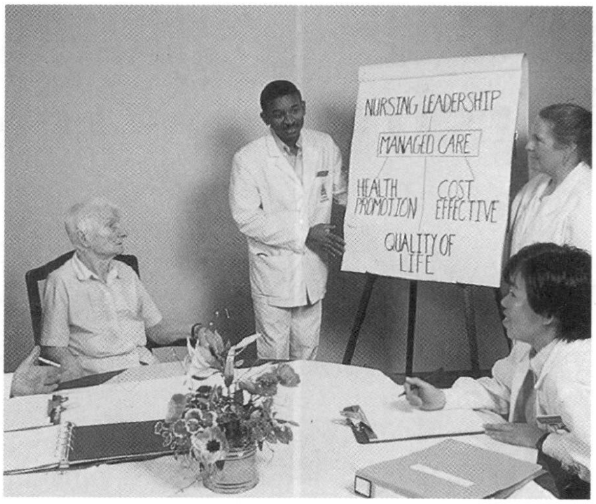

1. Identify the figure.

_______________________________________

_______________________________________

2. List at least four characteristics of an efficient manager.

_______________________________________

_______________________________________

3. How is a manager different from a leader?

_______________________________________

_______________________________________

4. List at least three characteristics of a manager that overlap with those of a leader.

_______________________________________

_______________________________________

**Activity F** ***A charge nurse is evaluating a staff nurse on the care provided to the clients. The steps of an evaluation process are given below in random order. Write the correct sequence in the boxes provided.***

1. Write the performance review.
2. Write a brief description of care provided.
3. Ask the member to write comments.
4. Inform the member on concerns noted.

☐ → ☐ → ☐ → ☐

**Activity G** ***Briefly answer the following questions.***

1. What are the reasons for which a nurse could be suspended or terminated from service?

_______________________________________

_______________________________________

2. What are the features of the NAPNES examination?

_______________________________________

_______________________________________

3. What is the advantage for a nurse opting for a one-plus-one program?

_______________________________________

_______________________________________

4. How can a nurse repay the tuition reimbursement provided by an employer?

_______________________________________

_______________________________________

5. How can a nurse with a bachelor's degree in a major other than nursing obtain a registered nurse (RN) license?

_______________________________________

_______________________________________

6. What information regarding legislation should a nurse in a leadership position have?

_______________________________________

_______________________________________

7. List the specialty care fields for which certification programs are available.

_______________________________________

_______________________________________

8. What are the areas in which a charge nurse should be experienced?

_______________________________________

_______________________________________

9. What are the requirements for an LPN/LVN to serve as a leader in specialty care?

_______________________________________

_______________________________________

## SECTION II: APPLYING WHAT YOU KNOW

**Activity H** ***Answer the following questions, which involve a nurse's role as a leader in a healthcare facility.***

A nurse in a leadership position should be mature, tactful, and responsible for providing quality care to a client. This involves not only leading a team but also reviewing the team and evaluating the care provided.

1. A team is providing care for an elderly client.
   a. What are the duties of the charge nurse with respect to implementing care for the client?
   b. Whom should a charge nurse approach if in need of assistance?
2. An LPN is working as a supervisor for unlicensed assistive personnel (UAP) in a healthcare facility.
   a. What are the other leadership roles available for LPN/LVNs?
   b. What are the higher education options available for LPN/LVNs?

## SECTION III: GETTING READY FOR NCLEX

**Activity I** ***Answer the following questions.***

1. What is the duty of a team leader?
   a. Instruct the staff to resolve a conflict among themselves.
   b. Assist authorities in hiring skilled nurses.
   c. Assist staff to update nursing procedures.
   d. Assist authorities to appoint a safety officer.
2. A team of nurses is assigned to care for an elderly diabetic client who has undergone surgery. Which of the following is the duty of a manager when providing care for the client?
   a. Monitor and suggest changes in the client's diet.
   b. Instruct staff members to determine the client's needs.
   c. Check the blood sugar testing equipment.
   d. Receive written reports on the client from the staff.
3. A charge nurse is assigned the task of providing care for elderly clients in a healthcare facility. Which of the following should the nurse do when assigning work to the staff?
   a. Assist a staff member to collect change-of-shift reports.
   b. Provide staff members with protocols for the procedures.
   c. Assist the staff members in planning their workloads.
   d. Assign staff members based on the needs of the clients.
4. A charge nurse has evaluated a staff member. Which of the following functions should the charge nurse perform after the evaluation?
   a. Call for a team meeting to discuss the results of the evaluation.
   b. Ask team members to write their comments on the evaluation.
   c. Sign and date a note containing the details of the meeting.
   d. Give a copy of the evaluation document to the evaluated member.
5. A nurse is working as a charge nurse in a healthcare facility. Which of the following is the duty of a charge nurse with respect to the shifts of the staff members?
   a. Converse with the staff members in all shifts.
   b. Plan on assigning staff members for the next shift.
   c. Check the primary care providers' orders after the shift.
   d. Instruct a staff member to collect the shift reports.

6. During evaluation of a staff member, a charge nurse observes life-threatening deficiencies in the staff member. What is the first step the charge nurse should follow when suspending the staff member?
   a. Suspend the staff member.
   b. Provide treatment to the staff member.
   c. Notify the Director of Nursing.
   d. Investigate the issue.
7. A nurse is preparing to appear for a "nurse refresher" course. Which of the following is the most likely reason for taking a "nurse refresher" course?
   a. The nurse plans to live and work in another state.
   b. The nurse plans to resume work after a gap of several years.
   c. The nurse intends to take the RN licensure examination.
   d. The nurse wants to obtain advanced training in emergency rescue.
8. A team leader in a healthcare facility is providing care to a child who has undergone surgery. Which among the following should the nurse perform when making a decision in the case of an infection?
   a. Gather relevant information on the symptoms.
   b. Decide on actions to be taken immediately.
   c. Follow personal intuition in providing care.
   d. Seek assistance from team members for caring.
9. A nurse is leading a team in a healthcare facility and wishes to use a laissez-faire leadership style. Which aspect of the team should the leader consider in using the desired style?
   a. The team members need to discuss before making a decision.
   b. The situation being dealt with requires immediate decision.
   c. Team members have the ability to implement decisions made.
   d. The team members follow the procedural guide step by step.
10. A nursing team is providing care in an assisted living cottage house facility. What are the duties of the charge nurse with respect to implementing care for the 12 clients in the cottage? (Select all that apply.)
   a. Developing plans to meet the needs of all the clients.
   b. Developing plans to handle complex types of emergencies.
   c. Assigning staff based on the requirements of the clients and the abilities of the staff members.
   d. Assisting staff members to provide care for the clients.
   e. Preparing reports on nurses' duties, clients, and conferences.